INTERVIEWING CLIENTS ACROSS CULTURES

Interviewing Clients across Cultures

A Practitioner's Guide

LISA ARONSON FONTES

THE GUILFORD PRESS
New York   London

© 2008 The Guilford Press
A Division of Guilford Publications, Inc.
72 Spring Street, New York, NY 10012
www.guilford.com

Printed in the United States of America

This book is printed on acid-free paper.

Last digit is print number: 9 8 7 6 5

Library of Congress Cataloging-in-Publication Data

Fontes, Lisa Aronson.
  Interviewing clients across cultures : a practitioner's guide / Lisa Aronson Fontes.
    p. cm.
  Includes bibliographical references and index.
  ISBN 978-1-59385-710-3 (hardcover : alk. paper)
  ISBN 978-1-60623-405-1 (paperback : alk. paper)
  1. Interviewing. 2. Ethnopsychology. 3. Cross-cultural counseling. I. Title.
  BF637.I5F67 2008
  158'.39—dc22

                                                    2008002131

To be free is not merely to cast off one's chains, but to live in a way that respects and enhances the freedom of others.

—Nelson Mandela

About the Author

Lisa Aronson Fontes, PhD, is a Core Faculty Member in the PsyD Program in Clinical Psychology at Union Institute & University in Brattleboro, Vermont. She has dedicated almost two decades to making the social service, mental health, criminal justice, and medical systems more responsive to culturally diverse people. Dr. Fontes edited *Sexual Abuse in Nine North American Cultures: Treatment and Prevention* (Sage, 1995), authored *Child Abuse and Culture: Working with Diverse Families* (Guilford, 2005), and has written numerous journal articles and book chapters on cultural issues in child maltreatment and violence against women, cross-cultural research, and ethics. She has worked as a family, individual, and group psychotherapist, and has conducted research in Santiago, Chile, and with Puerto Ricans, African Americans, and European Americans in the United States. In 2007 Dr. Fontes was awarded a Fulbright Foundation Fellowship, which she completed in Buenos Aires, Argentina. Fluent in Spanish and Portuguese, she is a popular conference speaker and workshop facilitator.

Acknowledgments

Although I write best when sitting alone uninterrupted for long periods, this is a luxury I can rarely afford. I feel blessed to have a full and busy life, pulled away from my writing by coworkers, students, friends, and family, especially my magnificent children. I could never write without the help and support of a village of people who are geographically far and near. I feel grateful beyond words to have work that fascinates me more each day, to have the time to develop ideas, to have opportunities to share these ideas with others, and to have bright and outspoken colleagues who humble me as I see so clearly the limitations of my own knowledge. Although many people have influenced me over time, here I acknowledge those people who have contributed to this particular book.

I thank the anonymous reviewers for their thoughtful, blunt, and insightful comments, and my friends and colleagues who read and commented on specific sections of this manuscript, offered me examples, and/or shared their writing and ideas, including Karen Anderson, Jan Cambridge, Christi Collins, Kathy Conlon, Ilia Cornier, Niki Delson, Kathleen Faller, Bert Fernández, Elizabeth Fernández-O'Brien, Carlos Fontes, María Gallagher, Kim Gerould, Roberto Irizarry, Irv Levinson, José Lopez, Mohamud Mohamed, Bill Moore, Carol Plummer, Gretchen Rossman, Richard Seelig, Rita Sommers-Flannagan, Lisa Suzuki, Anne Velázquez, and Michael Williamson. A heartfelt *gracias* to Magdalena Gomez, *mi hermana*—write that novel!

I thank my African friends and colleagues who have taught me the meaning of resilience, especially Mohamud Mohamed, Nasir Arush, Yasmin Ahmed, Sorie Koroma, and their struggling brothers and sisters in Springfield, Massachusetts. Warmest wishes to Stella Ojera, in Gulu, Uganda, who does so much to help her community heal the wounds of war. A portion of my royalties from this book will go to her organization, the Acholi Community Empowerment Network.

Thanks to my colleagues Janine Roberts, Fred Piercy, and Rachel Hare-Mustin, whose guidance and faith in me continues to help me commit words to paper.

I bow in deep gratitude to my wonderful colleagues in the PsyD Program at Union Institute & University—Bill Lax, Richard Sears, and BeeGee Lynch—who have fulfilled my dreams by creating a workplace where our ideals and commitments can flourish. Special thanks to my coworker and buddy Magui O'Neill-Arana, who shares her brilliant ideas and friendship on a daily basis as well as her support, examples, and *arroz con gandules*.

I am grateful to Jane Keislar, Paul Gordon, Louise Farkas, Cassie Bosse, and my remarkable editor Jim Nageotte at The Guilford Press. I sing your praises.

I thank the Five College Women's Studies Research Center, whose one-semester associateship gave me an opportunity to learn from others and gather my thoughts in a feminist community of support, and the Fulbright Foundation, whose support enabled my son and me to taste what it means to be an immigrant in the great city of Buenos Aires. Thanks also to my bright and resourceful colleagues there: Ruth Teubal, Alicia Gandulia, and Irene Intebi.

Personal gratitude to Carlos, Carmina, Moisés, and Alda Fontes, who blessed my life for more than a quarter century and who showed me how to approach the strains of immigration with dignity; to Muriel Fox, my mother, who has been with me every step of the way, who has read the manuscript of this book multiple times, and to whom I grow closer every day; and to my brother, Eric Aronson, who inspires me with his deeply lived commitment to justice.

Warm hugs to Michael Williamson, who makes my life possible and happy through all we share together. The future beckons.

My most profound admiration and appreciation to my children: Ana Lua Aronson Fontes, who not only is the funniest person I know, but also inspires me with her huge heart, her smarts, her commitment to social justice, and the myriad ways she finds to help, lead, and teach others. Marlena Aronson Fontes, who wows me with her outspokenness and her way with words. I cannot wait to read *your* books! Gabriel Sol Aronson Fontes, who is the source of so much joy. Your diligent struggles in a new land and language motivated me to include a chapter on children. *Vencerás, m'ijo.*

This book was written in the sincere hope that I will live to see a world where inequality is obsolete and justice is the norm.

Contents

1 A Guide to Interviewing across Cultures

Have you ever been involved in an "interview from hell," where the interviewer and interviewee didn't understand each other, didn't feel comfortable with each other, and didn't exchange information efficiently or accurately? This can happen to any of us, even when both parties are the same gender, age, religion, and ethnic background. But it's even more likely to occur when there are cultural differences between the two parties. This book is designed to help prevent uncomfortable misunderstandings from sabotaging your interview and to teach you how to overcome the barriers created by cultural differences.

In your work you probably conduct interviews—at least sometimes, and maybe often—with people who are not "just like" you. They may differ in some obvious way such as race, age, or gender or in less immediately noticeable ways such as religion, ethnicity, sexual orientation, health status, educational background, or social class. Despite such differences, if you are well prepared and motivated, your cross-cultural interviews can achieve your goals.

This book has more to do with the *process* of cross-cultural interviewing than with its *content*. The content will vary according to the focus of the interview: physical or mental health, social welfare, criminal justice, education, or the law. Each of us pays attention to different factors, depending on what we need to learn from the interview.

Most interviews are designed to guide important decisions such as determining guilt, devising medical or mental health treatment plans, deciding custody or the disposition of social work cases, making hiring or college admissions decisions, or influencing someone's access to services. Many interviews are evaluative, designed to determine the level or kinds of care or services needed or the qualifications of the interviewee. Journalists and researchers conduct interviews to collect data and shape their ideas.

The purpose of interviews usually goes beyond just *gathering information*, although that is a crucial part of why we interview. In addition, we're also *building a relationship*. Most of the time, we're trying to do this *efficiently* in a context of too few resources—too little time, staff, facilities, and money. Often, we're expected to produce reports or make decisions quickly based on our interviews. Thus we don't have the luxury of fishing around carelessly. We need to be especially focused and well prepared for cross-cultural interviews.

Consider the following examples:

- A doctor or nurse interviews a child and his parents to figure out how to ease the child's suffering.
- A custody evaluator interviews divorcing parents and other family members to help develop a viable parenting plan.
- A social worker interviews a homeless family that needs a variety of services.
- A counselor conducts an intake session with a person who presents (voluntarily or in response to a court mandate) for treatment.
- A psychotherapist interviews a new client who has suicidal thoughts.
- A police officer interrogates a person suspected of having committed a crime.
- A forensic interviewer questions a possible victim of child abuse.
- A school psychologist or counselor queries a child and her family as part of an educational assessment.
- An attorney interviews potential clients about the feasibility of representing them.

In all these cases, the interview has to produce information that is accurate and relevant, which requires a productive working relationship. The process cannot take too much time, and it must use the limited resources at hand. Usually, the initial interview provides a platform that supports future additional interventions.

Interviews are driven by these three realities: our need to get information, our need to create a useful working relationship, and our need to make it happen in situations that may be far from optimal. Often the circumstances are politically charged. For instance, various groups may be seeking outcomes that conflict with each other.

Voltaire urges us to judge people by their questions rather than their answers. This notion highlights the inescapable fact that our questions and our style of questioning reflect who we are as people. We need to look in an imaginary mirror as we ask our questions. Do we express not only skillful professionalism but also respect and caring? Only if we succeed in conveying this impression will people answer our questions openly and provide the information we need.

The people we interview may be different from us in small and large ways. This difference may be so significant that we need to plan carefully to adjust our tactics, demeanor, approach, tone, language, office seating arrangements, body language, and so forth, to get the job done right.

The word "interview" itself comes from the joining of the prefix "inter," meaning between or among, with the word "view," meaning a seeing, looking, or inspection. That is, an interview is the intermingling of distinct ways of seeing; this is especially clear in a cross-cultural context. We must ask ourselves how our knowledge or lack of knowledge of people from a given culture affects the interview process.

A MULTICULTURAL FRAMEWORK

Most of us have been trained to conduct interviews using a universalist approach. That is, we learned to interview people in the same way regardless of their specific culture. This approach emphasizes the similarities among peoples and ignores their differences. At first, it might seem that we are treating people more fairly if we interview all of them in the same way. Unfortunately, this approach usually ends up shortchanging interviewees who come from minority cultural groups. That's because a one-size-fits-all approach is based on interview styles, formats, and questions that were modeled on the majority group. This book is filled with examples of why this does not work. The simplest example would be interviewing all people in the English language when some of them do not understand English. To use another straightforward example, if we habitually shake hands with interviewees before we speak with them, not realizing that this is offensive to certain religious groups, we would sabotage our effort to establish rapport with people from those groups.

Often, *culture specific* trainings can lead people to see difference among groups and lose touch with both universal issues and individualism. When all we see is cultural difference, we are apt to miss factors that mark people as individuals, such as personalities, dreams, age, gender, sexual orientation, and personal history. When we overemphasize culture to the exclusion of other factors, we risk treating some people as if they're exotic or stereotypical. We have an obligation to learn about the interviewee's culture. At the same time, we have an obligation to consider each person's *individuality* without being hampered by oversimplified stereotypes.

When we use a multicultural approach to interviewing, we see people both as individuals *and* as members of cultures. We see individuals within the context of their cultures, and know that this enhances our work. But we don't need to abandon all we have learned about interviewing. Like interviewees, we, too, are cultural beings. We bring our own habits, preferences, and worldviews into our interviews. This book also helps interviewers be mindful of the ways our own cultures shape our mindsets.

HOW INTERVIEWS DIFFER FROM OTHER KINDS OF CONVERSATIONS

An interview can be formal or informal, carefully planned, or relatively spontaneous. Although interviews often appear to differ little from other kinds of conversations, they do have important distinguishing characteristics. We need to keep these characteristics in mind when planning and conducting our work:

1. The conversation has a definite purpose. The interviewer has particular goals in mind. The interviewee may share the same goals or may be hoping for a completely different outcome.

2. The interviewer and interviewee have a defined relationship. This relationship usually involves some kind of hierarchy, and most often the interviewer is the more powerful participant. The interviewer determines which questions will be asked and when, and how the results will be presented. The stakes are ordinarily much higher for the interviewee than for the interviewer.

3. Information flows primarily in one direction—from the interviewee to the interviewer. Certainly many interviewers take advantage of the situation to inform the interviewee about matters such as services available or processes and procedures that might follow from the discussion. However, the primary purpose of the interview is to gather information from the interviewee. As one of my professors told me in graduate school, "If you're doing more talking than the interviewee, you may be conducting a lecture but you're not conducting an interview."

4. The interviewer plans and organizes the interaction, directing the conversation with specific goals in mind. True, the interviewee can exert a

certain amount of control by being more or less willing to discuss certain topics. But it's the interviewer who structures the process.

5. The interviewer follows guidelines concerning confidentiality, but interviewees are usually free to reveal to others as much as they want about what transpired. That is, while patients interviewed by a psychiatrist can tell anyone they want about what was said during the interview, the psychiatrist is restricted by ethical guidelines and legal mandates to limit severely what he or she communicates about the interview and to whom.

As professionals, we know that interviews are unlike other kinds of conversations; but this may not be readily apparent to someone who is not familiar with our particular kind of interview. For example:

> The Gomez family arrived at a municipal office to complete an application for housing. The parents thought they were requesting an apartment they were entitled to receive—they did not understand that they were also being evaluated for their suitability to live in the housing units and their eligibility for a government rent subsidy. As the administrator asked increasingly intimate questions, such as the sources of the family's income and whether anyone in the family had been convicted of crimes, Mr. Gomez grew concerned and angry. The line of questioning made him suspicious about the nature of the housing office and the intentions of the person behind the desk. He did not understand that this situation was an interview and that these questions were directed to *all* applicants and thus formed part of the usual process. Because of his lack of familiarity with the norms of the interview, he answered in a hostile manner and was not able to present himself in the best possible light.

ORIENTATION TO THIS BOOK

Various chapters in this book will help you avoid an interview situation like the one that frustrated Mr. Gomez and his interviewer. For instance, Chapter 2 discusses preparing for an interview, the information that needs to be gathered beforehand, who should be invited to participate, and other initial decisions. Chapter 3 discusses biases and boundary issues that may distort the interviewing relationship. Chapter 4 focuses on building the interview relationship: how to establish rapport and convey respect, concentrating on the early parts of an interview. With the proper preparation before an interview and the right orientation at the beginning, the Gomez family would have understood the nature of the interview more clearly, would have been more comfortable with the interviewing situation, and—because of the friendlier relationship—probably would have cooperated more fully with the interviewer. In short, the interview would have been more successful.

Chapter 5 continues with the theme of the relationship by focusing on nonverbal communication: how to avoid offending in the way you use your body in interviews and how to interpret the interviewee's nonverbal signals. Chapter 6 addresses interviewing people who have a different native language from the one used in the interview. It discusses some of the research on memory and feelings when people speak in their native language versus a language they acquired later, and ways interviewers can achieve the best possible results when speaking with someone whose native language is different. Chapter 7 discusses some of the challenges of using language interpreters in interviews, and ways to make the interpreted interviews successful. Chapter 8 is concerned with reasons why interviewees may be reluctant to discuss certain topic areas and ways to handle these challenges. Chapter 9 focuses on special issues in interviewing children and adolescents and supplements the topics related to youth that are scattered throughout the book. Chapter 10 gives tips on how to write and present unbiased reports. Chapter 11 discusses issues that are particularly relevant for people from specific professions. Chapter 12 discusses some of the most common misunderstandings that occur in cross-cultural interviews and ways to avoid these. The "Afterword" offers further encouragement and professional development suggestions for those working to become more culturally competent as interviewers.

Each chapter contains a discussion of the topic, including a variety of text boxes designed to provide in-depth information on a particular area. Many of these text boxes are highly practical and can be used to guide your interviewing practice. The chapters also contain a section "Questions to Think about and Discuss." If you hate this kind of section, please just skip over it. People who read this book individually may find that such a section helps them reconsider some of the complexities discussed in the chapter and apply the issues to their own work. My books are also often adopted in academic courses, and these questions may be used to spark discussions or writing assignments in the college or university context. Finally, agencies sometimes use my books to structure regular meetings on cultural competency, asking the staff to read one chapter a month, for instance, and then organizing the discussions around the chapter questions. Each chapter concludes with a list of related resources for further reading. These are mostly books, because books are often easiest for people to obtain through their libraries. Where books on the topic are not available, I have listed a chapter, article, or online resource.

This book overflows with examples. The names and identifying information have been changed, and in some cases these are composites designed to illustrate several principles at once. These examples have been drawn from my own clinical work, research, supervision, and trainings. Where the examples are not from my own work their source has, of course, been cited.

CULTURAL COMPETENCE IS AN ETHICAL ISSUE

Everyday interviewing decisions (even minor ones) concern ethical principles, and should be considered seriously. We need to be especially cautious when working with a person from a culture that is different from our own, where we are less apt to understand the full implications of what we say and do. The risk of accidentally stumbling into an ethical minefield is greater in cross-cultural encounters.

Interviewing decisions with ethical implications concern gifts, interpreters, assessment instruments, and our choice of words in writing or testifying about an interview. In my attempt to avoid jargon I don't always name the ethical principle being discussed in this book. These include respect for persons, deception, coercion, confidentiality, safety, privacy, justice, beneficence, and nonmalfeasance.

Most major professional organizations include the provision of culturally competent services in their list of ethical mandates. In that sense, this is a book on professional ethics, and ethical issues abound in every chapter.

CASE EXAMPLES: CROSS-CULTURAL INTERVIEWS THAT CRASHED

In this next section I provide somewhat extreme case examples of cross-cultural interviews that failed and refer you to chapters in this book that would be helpful to interviewers who face similar challenges.

Hassan: Educational Testing with a Hitch

Hassan, a 16-year-old Somali refugee whose official records say he is 14, became known as a bit of a troublemaker at his school in Columbus, Ohio. His family moved to Columbus 2 years ago after spending a dozen years in a refugee camp in Kenya. Because of his consistent low academic grades, Hassan was about to be held back in sixth grade, meaning he would be placed in a class with 12-year-olds. He was clearly well along in puberty and already towered above his classmates. He told his guidance counselor and his teacher that he simply would not stay back another year—that he would drop out entirely rather than be held back. At a loss as to how to help Hassan, the counselor referred him for a comprehensive learning assessment.

The school district did not have experience or a clear policy concerning testing students in a language other than English or Spanish. The district's one Somali tutor, Siyat, had secured permission for the assessment from Hassan's mother. The mother had never set foot in a school, could neither read nor write in any language, and could speak only a few words of English. She spent most of her time at home with her five children. Siyat was asked to serve as interpreter for tests to be administered in English. Siyat's English was itself rather basic, and he knew nothing about educational testing. During the assessment he chided Hassan for not being able to complete certain tasks, warned him that if he didn't start doing better he'd be stuck in a class with little children, and inadvertently provided incorrect instructions from time to time because he did not understand the tasks.

The tester had no idea what the interpreter, Siyat, was saying but felt she had no choice but to trust him. For her part, she was at a loss as to how to handle the unusual testing conditions. She didn't know what to do about the slower timing of the tests necessitated by the interpretation process. She was aware that certain vocabulary was beyond Hassan's grasp, such as the words "drizzle" and "nightmare" which appeared in a reading passage, but didn't know how to factor in his status as a novice in the English language. Hassan grew more and more frustrated. At one point the school guidance counselor walked into the testing room and began to speak with the school psychologist. Siyat was certain they were speaking about him. When they laughed and smiled while looking in his direction, he grew disgusted and stormed out.

This discouraging story illustrates numerous issues that are discussed in greater depth throughout this book. First, having inaccurate documents is common to many immigrants and refugees from less industrialized nations. (This is discussed in Chapter 2, "Preparing for the Interview".) Second, a youngster's history of trauma as a survivor of war and refugee camps can easily be missed by educational institutions that see him in his current context but fail to understand the implications of his early life. Hassan's difficult history and the precarious position in which he and his family still find themselves could contribute to a situation in which the child would appear in school to be a troublemaker or intellectually deficient, when neither of these judgments would be correct. (These are discussed in Chapter 9, "Interviewing Culturally Diverse Children and Adolescents.") Although Hassan's mother's permission was formally sought for the assessment, it is unlikely that she understood the full implications of the assessment or the options available to her. The testing situation itself was rife with problems, many of which are discussed in Chapter 7, on interpretation. And finally, Chapter 5 on nonverbal communication discusses ways to avoid the kind of misunderstandings that were created by the psychologist and counselor's misguided exchange of knowing looks.

Elena: Applying for a Job in Human Services

Elena Sanchez was excited about her upcoming interview for a new job in human services. She was optimistic that there would be a good fit between her interests and qualifications and the position she sought. She reviewed the agency website in advance, printed out an extra copy of her résumé, and checked out how she looked in her best suit one final time in the mirror, satisfied that she would make a good impression.

Sam Jones, the human resources officer, was looking forward to interviewing Elena, optimistic that he would then be able to pass on her materials to the committee that would conduct the final screening. His agency had been criticized for not being sufficiently diverse ethnically and for not having enough staff who could work comfortably with their Spanish-speaking clients, and so Sam was especially pleased when he came across Elena's résumé among the applications, as her name certainly sounded Hispanic.

When Sam greeted Elena, he suddenly felt confused. She looked White. She didn't seem to have an accent. He was distracted as he asked her questions about her work history, trying to figure out her ethnic background. He pointed out that her résumé said that she spoke Spanish and asked her where she learned it. "In high school and college. I spent my junior year in Mexico and I'm completely fluent. I use it every day," she replied. "Do you have any other relationship with Mexico?" he asked. "I visit at least once a year—I love Mexico!" she answered.

Sam was feeling frustrated by his inability to determine Elena's background. Finally he asked her, "And what's your ethnic background?" Elena looked at him, stupefied, knowing the question was illegal. "I would like you to consider me based on my qualifications, not my background," she replied. At that moment, Elena decided to withdraw her employment application and called an end to the interview. She knew she could be good at the job and she knew she could work well with the Spanish-speaking clients, but she had no intention of accepting a job where the decision to hire her hinged on her ethnicity—this was not an agency environment she would enjoy.

Sam wondered what had gone wrong and mused to himself that

he still couldn't tell "what" Elena was. Maybe she was a second- or third-generation Latina immigrant. Maybe she acquired her last name through marriage. Maybe she was the product of a mixed couple, Latino and something else. He never found out. The agency missed out on someone who would have been a valuable employee.

In this case example we see a well-meaning interviewer who has unwittingly alienated a potential employee. The section on taboo topics in Chapter 8 and common misunderstandings in Chapter 12 might have helped Sam avoid making the mistakes he did.

Clara: Distortion in a Mental Health Assessment

Clara, 25, grew up in a poor family in Rio de Janeiro, Brazil. She is now living in a college town in the midwestern United States where she moved with her husband, a college professor 20 years her senior, and two children, ages 3 and 5. She had dropped out of high school in Rio shortly before the day she met her husband—he approached the stand where she was selling juice in a park and immediately grew entranced with her. They had originally planned for her to take her GED (General Educational Development) test and attend college, but she became pregnant shortly after arriving in the United States and settled instead for taking a few classes in English as a Second Language. She said she spent her days caring for the house and children, cooking the elaborate meals her husband enjoyed, and surfing Brazilian websites on her home computer. Her husband had encouraged her to seek psychotherapy for her frequent tearful and angry outbursts.

In the therapy intake session Clara seemed irritable and emotional, occasionally sobbing loudly, sighing deeply, and clenching her fists. She described her intense worries about the future of her marriage. She feared that her husband would abandon her and cut off all contact with the children, leaving them in difficult economic straits and very much alone, as her own father had done to her mother. She was also afraid he might send her back to Brazil, where she said she would be ashamed to show her face, and where she believed her prospects for economic security were even slimmer than in the United States. Clara said she spoke to no one about her concerns other than God and her grandmother, who had died the year before. Clara told the therapist that she knelt before an altar each day, lit a candle, and prayed to her grandmother, the Virgin Mary, and several saints for protection.

The therapist, Jean, was a married Lutheran midwesterner in her 50s who had recently completed a graduate degree in counseling, having returned to school after her children left home for college. Jean had little personal or professional experience with people from backgrounds unlike her own but had a good heart and was committed to doing right by her clients. Jean asked Clara if her husband was "also Black." Clara didn't seem to understand the question and when Jean explained that she was asking about race, Clara replied that she herself was "not Black" but rather was "light brown." When Jean asked Clara for details about her relationship with her husband, including her satisfaction with their sex life, Clara stared at the floor and grew silent. After that question, Clara answered mostly in monosyllables and avoided eye contact.

Jean felt uncomfortable with Clara and attributed her discomfort to Clara's apparently disordered personality. Jean thought Clara was histrionic (overly dramatic) and overly dependent on her husband. She thought Clara's speaking with her dead grandmother was a sign of a possible psychosis and death wish. She thought Clara's fears about deportation and her "peculiar" responses to the questions about race and sex indicated paranoia or a thought disorder. Jean's overall impression was that Clara had one or more personality disorders and was inappropriate for psychotherapy. Jean thought Clara would be better served by a psychiatric consultation to determine which medications might reduce her depressive, anxious, and possibly psychotic symptoms. Jean shared her conclusions with Clara. Jean also encouraged Clara to join one of the local churches so she would feel less isolated. Clara walked out of the clinic and never returned. That night, when Clara's husband asked about her appointment, Clara replied that the lady was a pervert who thought she was crazy and wanted to give her drugs and convert her to religion. "Just like I expected," she said. In her report on the intake, Jean wrote that Clara was a "Black mother of two, with apparent histrionic and paranoid tendencies, who appears unable to establish a therapeutic alliance. I recommend a psychiatric evaluation for possible depression with psychotic features."

Jean misinterpreted Clara's nonverbal emotional expressions as indicative of a personality disorder. Rather, they may have simply been the way her culture expresses her feelings of dislocation, sadness, and worry about the future. (Cultural variations in emotional expression and nonverbal communication are discussed in Chapters 5 and 6, respectively.) Second, Jean asked Clara direct questions about her race and sexuality, without seeming to understand the sensitive nature of these questions and the different ways these issues are handled in different cultures. (Styles of questioning and how to handle taboos are discussed in Chapter 4, "Setting the Right Tone," and Chapter 8 on addressing reluctance, respectively.) Finally, Jean appeared to underestimate the power of her position as a mental health counselor and the complexity of referrals to a psychiatrist and to church. (These kinds of issues are discussed throughout the book.)

CONCLUDING OBSERVATIONS

These brief descriptions of interviews provide us with windows through which we can view various failures to connect well across cultures. The consequences of such failures depend on the purpose of the interview but may include interviewees not being able to develop their potential and facing serious unnecessary problems. The consequences of failed interviews for the interviewer include frustration, feelings of impotence, lost opportunity, and an inability to deliver services at the highest professional level. The societal costs are innumerable. They include depriving society of the full gifts of its members, possible consequent increases in crime, tensions across cultural groups, and general strife and alienation.

While this book is intended to offer practical suggestions and help you overcome technical difficulties in cross-cultural interviews, I hope it will also convey some of the spirit needed in cross-cultural contacts. We know that in some interviews we will be exposed to descriptions of emotional and physical pain, injustice, and horror—forms of suffering that were previously unfamiliar to us. We may sit with people who are in agonizing predicaments and whose emotions are raw. We may be facing our own prejudices and inherited discomforts. Sometimes we may tend to focus too much on the technical aspects of interviews so we can avoid the difficult feelings that would otherwise emerge in discussing sensitive topics (Gunaratnam, 2003a). We have to make certain that we are not so busy being "technically correct" that we lose touch with our own—and the interviewee's—humanity.

Questions to Think about and Discuss

1. What are the three major concerns in interviews, whatever their professional context?
2. Discuss differences between interviews and other kinds of conversations.
3. Describe a successful interview that you conducted with someone who differs from you. Describe the differences, how you handled them, and the reason you think the interview was successful.
4. Describe an interview you conducted with someone who differs from you that you think was less than successful. Describe the differences between you and the interviewee, how you handled them, and the reason you think the interview was not successful.

RECOMMENDED ADDITIONAL READING

Sue, S., & Sue, D. (2007). *Counseling the culturally diverse (5th edition)*. New York: Wiley.

Webb, N. B. (2001). *Culturally diverse parent–child and family relationships*. New York: Columbia University Press.

2 Preparing for the Interview

This chapter discusses preparing for and initiating an interview, deciding whom to include in an interview, and creating welcoming environments for interviewees from a variety of cultural groups. It also describes some of the other cultural issues that may affect the initiation of the interview and ways to handle these. Preparing well for an interview will reduce the number of unfortunate surprises and improve the quality and quantity of information obtained.

PRIOR INFORMATION

Depending on your context, if you have access to previous medical, social work, legal, or other records, it is usually helpful to review these documents before meeting the interviewee. At the same time, you should expect to be surprised by interviewees, and do *not* assume that the information contained in their file is correct. Other professionals may have been careless or prejudiced, had inadequate linguistic interpretation, been confused, or failed to establish the necessary rapport to obtain truthful information. In one particularly vivid study, half of a community sample of Puerto Rican children was rated as mentally ill when the assessments were not conducted in a culturally competent way (Bird et al., 1988). Imagine how these children's diagnoses could follow and haunt the children throughout their lives! All too often, one erroneous note in a file is perpetuated indefinitely as subsequent professionals elaborate on that initial incorrect impression.

I consider a case file with previous information as simply one source of data, which I confirm, disconfirm, or elaborate on during my subsequent conversations with the interviewee and collateral contacts. Following is an example of inaccurate information leading to an incorrect intervention:

> A family's social worker called a school and left a message asking the nurse to meet with a new Somali student, Abdulahi, to check for bruises from a bicycle accident sustained over the weekend. The boy didn't speak English yet, having recently moved to the United States. Abdulahi looked extremely nervous as he entered the nurse's office, shifting his weight from one leg to the other, sweating and trembling. The nurse examined his arms, hands, and face carefully and found no evidence of bruising. The boy seemed terrified when the nurse asked him to lift up his shirt and then examined his belly and back. The nurse then called the social worker and reported that Abdulahi seemed to be fine, although he appeared extremely anxious. Two weeks later the social worker discovered that it was Abdulahi's brother, Mohamed, who had fallen off the bicycle and who had, indeed, sustained injuries that should have been treated. They also learned that Abdulahi assumed he was being summoned out of the classroom by the teacher to receive a beating, as was common in schools in the refugee camps where he had grown up; and this impression was reinforced when he was asked to lift up his shirt. He did not understand the nurse's role in the school, nor the nature of the encounter. In this case an essential detail that was reported incorrectly—here the name of the target child—resulted in a failure to meet one child's needs and the frightening of another child.

Many of us have horror stories of incorrect information leading to clumsy errors of this kind. The best known of these anecdotes is the surgeon who ends up operating on the wrong leg. However, no profession is immune. I have seen police reports that left out important information from recorded interviews; family histories that confused incidents involving various parental figures; and school charts where recording errors resulted in the improper tracking of children. When documents are moved from one system to another there is even greater likelihood of error. For instance, many nations grade in a system of 1–20, where even the highest-performing students rarely score higher than 17, the great majority of students score around 13, and failure is common. If these scores are mistranslated into the U.S. system and a "13" is considered failure, clearly the foreign student will be mistakenly penalized.

Individuals' and families' prior records and reputations can influence us in ways we may not realize. All of us are subject to confirmatory bias, which is the tendency to notice things that confirm the ideas we already hold, and fail to notice things that disconfirm it (see Chapter 3 on biases and boundaries for a further discussion of biases). Because I am aware of this bias, I purposely try to identify aspects of the person I'm interviewing that *disconfirm* or contradict earlier notes in a file. I am not disrespecting the work of my colleagues. Rather, I realize that people grow and change, and I want to allow the interviewee to make a fresh impression. The prior records help orient me to some of the areas I may need to investigate, but I don't assume they provide a complete or accurate portrait of the person I will be interviewing.

WHAT ELSE DO WE NEED TO PREPARE?

The suggestions given in this section are not intended to be exhaustive. Rather, they call attention to those interview preparations that are most influenced by culture.

First, we should make sure we have on hand all the appropriate forms in the interviewee's own language. And, we should make sure we have a foreign language interpreter available, if necessary (see Chapter 7 on interpreting).

If we are using any special equipment for the interview, such as one-way mirrors, video cameras, or microphones, we should give some thought to how we will inform the interviewees about these items and obtain their permission to use them. Whatever their age, interviewees have a right to know that the interview is being recorded, and why. Some will refuse. If the interviewee is a minor, depending on the circumstances, the adult responsible for the child may have to give consent for the recording of the interview, but the child should still be informed about the recording and asked to assent to being recorded. Some interviewers avoid telling children that their interviews are being recorded or observed because of their concern that such information would intimidate them and inhibit them from speaking freely. I strongly believe that we have a moral and ethical obligation to tell children as much as we can about the process we are asking them to undergo (in a way that is developmentally appropriate). They have the right to refuse to participate. If they later discovered that their words or images had been recorded without their knowledge, they would feel misled and would be less likely to cooperate with future investigations or interventions (Fontes, 2004; King & Churchill, 2000).

Adults may also refuse to be video- or audiotaped because they worry about where the tapes might end up and who will have access to them, or because they have previously undergone upsetting recorded interrogations. Some people might have religious objections. For instance, the Amish, Pentecostals, and several other Christian groups have objected to videotaping and even the taking of still photographs because they believe it constitutes the taking of a "graven image," which is forbidden. Some traditional peoples believe that taking a photograph or being videotaped is akin to taking a person's soul. Some Muslim women refuse to have their image recorded without full or partial veiling of the head or face to preserve their modesty, because they do not show their faces to unrelated men. General privacy concerns may also make people hesitant to allow the video or audio recording of their interview. In most circumstances people have the legal right not to be recorded without their express permission. In any case, ethically, when a person prefers not to be recorded, this wish should be respected.

I once assisted in a focus group study that included Latinos with varying levels of acculturation (Fontes, Cruz, & Tabachnick, 2001). We found that the participants who came from low-income families in developing countries were less comfortable with the technological aspects of the interviewing process, such as the one-way mirrors and videotaping. They appeared to be more tense and guarded throughout the interview process. When people are less familiar with technology, we may need to spend extra time orienting them, taking them to meet the observers behind the one-way mirror, for instance, or giving them an opportunity to look into the viewfinder of the video camera. If we can make the technological aspects of the interview seem less foreign to interviewees, they may be better able to relax.

HANDLING INITIAL PAPERWORK

Some settings require that the interviewee fill out extensive forms prior to meeting with you. Others require that you ask the interviewee a series of questions to fill out initial paperwork when you meet together. Still others do not require extensive paperwork, or they rely on the interviewer to fill out the forms independently at the conclusion of the interview. Although filling out the paperwork may be required and "pro forma," even this procedure needs to be approached tactfully. In many Middle Eastern countries, a person's word or a handshake is considered more valuable and more honorable than a written signature on a document. Therefore, when we hand recent immigrants from some Middle Eastern countries a series of documents requiring that they affirm their intention to pay for sessions, for instance, or their understanding of the confidentiality rules, or their consent to treatment, and so on, it may be interpreted as doubting their word. The person may smile and hand the stack back to us, saying, "Of course, doctor, you have my word, this is fine." Alternatively, the person may sign the forms without reading them, believing that reading them would convey mistrust to the professional. Many American Indians are quite skeptical of written agreements, because of U.S. history of breaking treaties, and dismiss the paperwork as unimportant while looking carefully for *interpersonal* signs as to whether the individual interviewer can be trusted.

Even when interviewees would rather not handle paperwork, we may need to insist that the documents get filled out. It may help to admit gently that we recognize that the paperwork is a burden, but we need to complete it as part of our job. We should also be aware of the possibility that the person does not read, does not read English, does not read well enough to understand the form, has visual impairments, or has forgotten his or her reading glasses and therefore needs verbal help with the paperwork.

If the paperwork appears to cause conflict and stress, we should limit ourselves at the outset to those forms that are absolutely necessary and consider either postponing or forgoing altogether the less essential paperwork.

DECIDING WHOM TO INTERVIEW

When we work with culturally diverse families, we should make sure our vision of who the family is (and, possibly, who should be included in assessment and treatment) encompasses *all* relevant parties. Some families will want to include extended family members and godparents in all interactions with professionals. This can lead sometimes to unexpected predicaments. For example, sometimes members of the extended family, clergy, or a friend may offer to sit in on an interview "to help," when the actual intention is to monitor what is said. A battering husband may insist that his mother accompany his wife to her appointments to make sure she does not mention the violence. Or, a church elder may attend an interview ostensibly to serve as a cultural bridge or interpreter, when his true intention is to silence certain topics.

On the downside, it complicates an interview if you involve additional family members. It can be difficult to coordinate multiple conversations and conflicting viewpoints. Chaos may reign unless the interviewer takes on the role of orchestra conductor, amplifying and quieting different people's voices at various moments. This can be a delicate process. If people who are ranked highly in a family (such as a father) are shushed by someone who seems to be of a lower social status (such as a young female), this could greatly anger the father, and maybe the entire family. It would be important, then, to explain the "rules" of the interview before it begins, and to explain that one of the interviewer's jobs will be to ensure that every person gets a chance to speak, and that this might require asking individuals to be silent for a time. Even so, the interviewer should proceed patiently and tactfully.

I encourage you to welcome people into the interview who have been chosen by the family, but in some cases it's also preferable to hold separate individual conversations with family members. Try to understand the true dynamic of the various interpersonal relationships so you can be as well informed as to the possible risks of including different people. This is not always an easy or straightforward process and may require speaking with various family members individually, observing family interactions, and consulting with involved professionals.

On the plus side, welcoming additional people to the interview may calm and reassure the primary interviewees, may provide additional sources of information, and may extend the interviewer's influence in the family and community. Holding an interview with more than one person present offers us an opportunity to observe interactions among the interviewees, providing a more complete picture of family functioning.

Where different members of a family or couple possess differing levels of language fluency, it is easy to give more weight to statements from those who speak the interview language better. It is also easy to allow the more fluent speaker to "speak for" the person who is less fluent. We should be careful not to fall into this trap, and we should obtain the interpreting we need so we can accurately assess the situation. Often men in immigrant families have more formal schooling, more opportunities to learn the new language, and more comfort conversing with authorities. We must be sure we do not overlook the voices and needs of women in the family if this is the case.

SETTING FOR THE INTERVIEW

Some of us have a choice about where we conduct interviews, while others do not, depending on our professional roles and agency practices. Guidelines generally recommend that interviews be conducted in a neutral environment. However, they rarely explain what characteristics make an environment "neutral," and for whom. Most likely, no site is entirely neutral. Rather, the interviewees have positive and negative associations with whatever site we choose. A good interviewer has to be aware of how a particular setting may influence an interview and take into account the influence of the site when reaching conclusions about the interview.

One of my first psychotherapy jobs was as an emergency services clinician in a small city. During working hours we interviewed people in crisis in our mental health clinic offices. On the night shifts and on weekends we interviewed people at the hospital emergency room, in the police station, in their homes, or in the waiting room of the local psychiatric hospital—

depending on the person's location when the call came in, the outcome to their situation that we thought likely, and the degree of threat they presented. Each of these settings seemed to shape the interviewees' as well as my own perspectives. (This is an example of the actor–observer bias. That is, if I interview someone in the police station I may be more aware of the question of physical threat, whereas if I interview someone in a mental hospital I may become more aware of mental illness issues—and attribute these concerns to characteristics of the interviewee, rather than the setting.) I had to work hard to brush away the influence of the setting so I could evaluate the person in crisis as accurately as possible.

When we interview a person only one time and in one location, we obtain a snapshot of that person at that time and in that place. It is necessarily just one limited picture, and our ability to draw inferences about the person from just one contact is severely limited.

Those of us who have the possibility of interviewing "offsite" may be able to offer two or three choices to the interviewee, to find out where he or she would rather meet. For example, a social worker who needs to interview a child could offer to meet the child either in a private room at school or at the agency office. Police who need to take a victim's statement could offer to meet the victim in his or her home or at the station. People who frequently conduct interviews in the field are encouraged to develop a variety of interview sites in places that may be familiar to interviewees from different ethnic groups and income levels, including places of worship, schools, children's advocacy centers, and medical centers. Professionals who practice in areas that are racially, culturally, or economically segregated should be sure to establish a number of possible interview locations within each community. Clients will be uncomfortable if they're required to enter an unknown neighborhood to talk about a difficult subject.

If police are involved in the interview, in most situations they should be dressed in plain clothes. With rare exceptions, interviewees should be protected from seeing scenes that may be frightening and intimidating (e.g., seeing armed officers or people in handcuffs or shackles). Research has found that when interviewers are warm and friendly their interviews will be more likely to produce correct information, and interviewees will be more willing to correct the interviewer's mistakes if necessary (Davis & Bottoms, 2002).

Creating Welcoming Environments

While hanging an "ethnic" tapestry in the waiting room is not sufficient to make an ethnic minority client feel welcome, it is one small thing that you can do. We should help people from diverse groups to feel welcomed and at home as they walk into our agencies, and the decor can help set the tone. Books, magazines, artwork, signs, photographs, and posters in the rooms and hallways should reflect the variety of cultures served. People from minority ethnic and racial groups will frequently scan their environment for visible signs that the agency recognizes their existence and needs. For instance, are the signs printed in Spanish as well as English? Are a variety of holidays represented in the decorations, or only Christian holidays such as Christmas? Is there a copy of *Essence Magazine* next to the copy of the *Ladies Home Journal*? Are there foods in the cafeteria that will appeal to people from a variety of ethnic groups—for instance, rice as well as noodles? Are foods available for people who do not eat pork or shellfish for religious reasons, such as observant Muslims and Jews? Does the agency provide extended hours for those who cannot afford to take time off from work during the day? Are interpreters readily available? Can the client speak to the intake worker without fear of others overhearing? Is there a diaper changing table in the bathroom? Is there a private area where modest women can nurse? Is there a play area where families with children can wait comfortably for their appointment?

Flags and patriotic slogans and symbols adorn many waiting rooms and buildings in the United States, particularly since the September 11, 2001, terrorist attacks. Some interviewers may feel a desire to express their patriotic sentiments strongly. They may have trouble understanding how offputting these nationalistic symbols can be to some people from other countries, depending on their immigration experiences. This was driven home to me when I conducted a weeklong training for Spanish-speaking interviewers in a conference room with an enormous U.S. flag hanging on the wall. The participants from El Salvador and Nicaragua let me know that terrible things had been done in their country in the name of that flag. Upon my request, a staff member removed the flag for the next day's sessions. On the third morning, an administrator informed me that some U.S. employees were upset that the flag had been taken down and the administrator insisted on hanging it up again. Clearly, displaying flags is a heartfelt issue for many people.

Here is an example of a situation in which the display of a national flag alienated a family:

> A Lebanese family was contacted when their daughter's third-grade teacher was found to have sexually fondled another child in the class. The parents brought in their daughter for an interview at the local Children's Advocacy Center to determine if she, too, had been abused. The family was planning to cooperate until they entered the center and saw a big American flag hanging in the lobby and patriotic banners decorating the waiting room.

The parents suddenly felt uncomfortable. They met with the interviewer and told her, simply, that they had changed their minds and would not allow their daughter to be interviewed. (Fontes, 2005a, p. 202)

We will never know how many people decide not to seek our services, refuse our services, or decline to cooperate fully because they do not feel at ease in our agencies. My recommendation is that we err on the side of being as welcoming and inclusive to as many people as possible in our professional lives, and therefore patriotic and political symbols are not appropriate in most workplaces, particularly those that serve immigrant clients. We should do whatever we can do extend a warm welcome to all potential clients. (We can use patriotic symbols in our homes and personal vehicles if we wish—that is a different matter.)

I would hate to give the impression that people who object to flags and other nationalistic symbols are opposed to their new country. On the contrary, many immigrants to the United States and other countries are extremely grateful to live in their new land, while at the same feeling uncomfortable with nationalistic symbols. Some minority religious groups, including Jehovah's Witnesses, also reject the display of flags.

Appropriate Displays

What *should* you display in your office? Of course, it depends on your position and the norms of your profession. Some interviewers choose to hang their academic diplomas on their walls. Diplomas can convey expertness, authority, and professionalism that will be important to some clients, and particularly to those clients who may be less familiar with your profession. Some interviewers keep professional books and journals in their offices, to contribute further to their credibility. Whether or not you choose to display personal photographs of family members or other personal articles depends on your profession. Many people in law enforcement choose not to, because they don't want to put their family members at risk. Many people in mental health professions also choose not to display personal pictures because they believe it influences the client's perception of them. Interviewers in fields such as medicine, education, human services, and human resources may not feel constrained in the same way and may decide to display personal family pictures in order to humanize the environment. It is important to remember that each picture is a statement. It makes a statement if you display a picture of yourself with your family in scanty bathing suits on a luxurious-looking boat, in contrast to a simple family picture in a nondescript setting. Just make sure you think through what you're communicating with your decor.

In People's Homes

When interviewing people in their home, it is important to remind yourself that you *are* in their home. If you are arriving on a rainy, snowy, or muddy day, be sure to wipe off your feet carefully before stepping inside. If you see shoes lined up at the door and notice that the family walks around in stocking feet or slippers, ask if they would like you to take off your shoes, where possible. Avoid stepping into a home until you have been invited to do so. If you need to go in and have not yet been invited, ask, "May I step inside?" before doing so. Once inside the door, do not walk further into the home until invited to do so verbally or with a gesture that indicates, "Come on in." Or, if necessary, ask permission again to go further inside. In this way you are acknowledging that the person is in control of his or her own space. In most Spanish- and Portuguese-speaking countries, one says, *Con permiso* or *Com licença,* respectively (meaning, "With your permission"), before stepping into a home, even when invited to do so. The equivalent in English would be "May I?" or "Excuse me." These phrases acknowledge the residents' reign over their home, and that even an invited guest is imposing.

Once you are inside the home, if you are encouraged to sit, ask first, "Where would you like me to sit?" In some families a particular chair may belong to the father or an elder, and it would be an affront to sit in it. A colleague who brings animals to his therapeutic visits to nursing homes recently told me about bringing a rabbit to a home and sitting in a centrally located chair so the residents could approach him and pet the rabbit. One developmentally delayed man entered the room and began pounding his fist into his hand and stomping his feet as he grew increasingly agitated. One of the aides then politely told my colleague that the seat he had chosen informally "belongs to" the client who was becoming agitated. The bottom line—ask before sitting.

Once you have been invited into a home, many families will offer you something to eat or drink. They may ask if you'd like something, or they may simply set out a tray with cookies and tea, or set an extra place at the table if they are about to eat. In some cases it is against agency policy to accept food. Rigid agency guidelines of this kind can put you in a bind. You might find yourself needing to choose between following agency policy or bonding with a family by accepting a refreshment. How you resolve this dilemma will affect how you are received by the family. Culturally, some families will feel insulted if you do not accept some kind of token offering from them—a glass of water, a cup of tea, or a soda. A social worker recently told me that he has eaten his way to trust through every immigrant group in California. He smiled as he recounted how happy it made the families feel to share their food with him, and he described as an advantage his love of spicy food. A home visitor in Appalachia told me recently about how a family was so grateful for her visits that they presented her with several squirrels which they had skinned and cleaned especially for her, so she could bring them home and cook them up. She accepted them warmly (but declined to actually eat them). The meal table is often the center of family life; joining a family at their table will help you join them in their environment and give you an opportunity to observe their interactions in a more relaxed setting.

A recently retired police officer who spent years investigating sexual assault and statutory rape cases told me that she learned enough Spanish to be able to say when she came into a Spanish-speaking home and smelled food cooking, "That smells great! Is that rice and beans or chicken or something else?" She felt this demonstration of a little bit of cultural, linguistic, and culinary familiarity increased the likelihood that she would be trusted.

On the other hand, in many cultures it is considered impolite to accept food the first time it is offered. If you are planning to accept the food, then a safe position when offered food would be to say something like, "I don't want to put you to any trouble." Then if the person offers again, you can accept with "Just a little, thank you." If you do not want to accept the food then you can say, "I just ate but I would love a glass of water, thank you very much."

In traditional Asian homes, feel free to compliment someone on the home in general, as you would in any one else's house, for instance, "What a lovely home you have!" or "I love how the light comes in through your windows." However, if you offer compliments about a particular household object, the host may feel compelled to give it to you as a gift (Chan & Lee, 2004). I visited the home of a Japanese family friend, once and commented on a tiny pair of lacquered shoes. The hostess told me she had worn them as a child in Japan and insisted on giving them to me, to my great chagrin.

RESPECTING VALUES, NEGOTIATING MEANINGS, AND AVOIDING PROFESSIONAL ETHNOCENTRISM

When we step into the interviewer role we do not suddenly cease to be cultural beings. Rather, we bring along with us our own personal attitudes about what is normal, natural, and "the way things are and should be," even though many of these viewpoints may have cultural underpinnings. This attitude is called "ethnocentrism." Because schools and the media generally reflect majority values and norms, people who come from the domi-nant groups (in most Western countries this translates as White, main-stream Christian, born in the country where they live, middle class, and heterosexual) are particularly likely to see the way they act as "normal" and to see others who act in different ways as strange, abnormal, or in need of intervention. In Western countries the values of European groups have tended to be regarded as normal, whereas values of other groups have historically been considered "ethnic" and a deviation from normality (McGoldrick, Giordano, & García-Preto, 2005). Those who have power appear to have no culture, whereas those without power are seen as cul-tural beings, or "ethnic" (Volpp, 2005).

The dominant culture is so pervasive that it can be taken for granted as easily as the air we breathe. Therefore, it is especially incumbent upon members of the dominant culture (and all of us who have received training in that culture) to be self-reflective and respectful when working with peo-ple who may have a different set of values and beliefs. We must take care not to be judgmental about an interviewee's life decisions and predicaments that may seem strange to us simply because of our lack of familiarity with them. Consider the following examples where we see differences between the professional and the interviewee that are due to ethnic culture, religion, or social class:

- An African American mother holds her son firmly by both arms and says, "Now you are going to listen to the teacher and do what she says, you hear?" as she drops him off on the first day of kindergar-ten. The mother then kisses the boy on the forehead. The mother hangs the boy's jacket up on his hook and tells the teacher that he's a good child and won't cause any trouble. The White teacher frowns at the mother, upset by the mother's tone which the teacher feels is overly stern and harsh. The teacher fails to realize that direct but loving guidance with an emphasis on the importance of education is common in African American families (Boyd-Franklin, 2003).
- A police officer reports unsanitary conditions in the home of a Chi-nese family because poultry is hanging in several windows, dripping onto trays. This officer had never known the joys of Peking duck, which owes its crispness to one or more days of advance hanging to remove the grease.
- A visiting nurse describes the apartment of a Haitian family as "un-comfortably hot," and mentions that they continued to wear their summer clothes and flip-flops in the home, without realizing that this is the family's first winter in Boston. Although they own sweat-ers and warm clothes, they bundle themselves up only when they

leave their apartment. Indoors they keep their apartment temperature high enough so they can wear the clothes they have always worn at home in their native land.

- A social worker who is interviewing a family in their home may be put off by what appears to be extreme chaos, with a jumble of children from different families walking in and out, loud music playing, piles of laundry being folded on all available surfaces, and clothes everywhere. However, for the family "laundry day" is a day of celebration when the cousins drive over from the other side of town to do their laundry, share a meal, and allow the children to play together.

- A guardian *ad litem* negatively evaluates a mother's parenting, reporting as a sign of neglect that the mother "has always managed to work the night shift," rather than framing her efforts positively as a deliberate attempt to bring home enough income to keep her family sheltered (Azar, 2006).

The more we know about a family's background and their cultural traditions, the less likely we are to condemn practices simply because they are unfamiliar.

It is not always easy to differentiate, however, between practices that are unfamiliar but harmless and practices that are problematic or in need of intervention. For example, a social worker may observe a Malaysian wife deferring consistently to her husband and son in a family therapy session. Is this a culturally rooted practice that is oppressing the wife and mother and making conflict in the family, shutting down the mother's ability to live life in the way she chooses? Or, is this a culturally rooted practice that feels natural and unproblematic to the mother? Or, does this pattern reveal some form of pathology in this particular family, such as a husband and son who physically or emotionally abuse the mother? And how should the interviewer describe this dynamic in a report? It is no easy task. The interviewer who has information about Malaysian families in general as well as information about this family in particular will be better able to make these determinations.

When in doubt about whether a practice is culturally rooted, consult with someone who is more familiar with the culture, while protecting the interviewee's confidentiality. Also consult with members of the family separately, to determine how each is affected by the way they are living. If an interviewer has but brief contact with a family, the interviewer may be able to do no more than describe what is observed, without drawing conclusions.

I have to remind myself continually that a situation that seems problematic to me may not be problematic to the interviewee at all. For instance, I was raised to see teen pregnancy and youthful childbearing as undesirable and likely to produce negative outcomes, and statistically this association holds true for many problems in the United States. But of course youthful childbearing is not necessarily problematic for all families at all times. Koul (2002) describes growing up in the Kashmir region of India:

> The children are young, the parents are young, and the grandparents are young, and there is always a great grandparent or two somewhere in the house. There is a lot of coming and going, family life occupies our days and we love it. (p. 60)

While statistical information on problems and populations is interesting, we must evaluate each situation on its own merits.

It can be extremely challenging to interview a person who has radically different values from your own. The topics that create the most controversy in society can create similar conflict in the interview room, including sex roles, abortion, war, corporal punishment, religion, drugs, alcohol, money, and politics. It can be hard to put aside one's own values and fears, so the interview remains a forum for getting to know the interviewee, rather than converting it into a forum for expressing our own personal values. Some elements of the interviewee's values will be relevant to the topic of the interview and therefore merit exploration, whereas others are irrelevant and serve as a distraction.

Some cultural practices are downright harmful, however, and deserve to be a focus of professional attention. It is easier to see practices as "cultural" when they concern a practice that is from a cultural group that is different from one's own. Harmful cultural practices common to Western industrialized nations include allowing children to spend too many hours watching television and playing computer games, which reduces time for learning and contributes to obesity. Other harmful cultural practices in Western industrialized nations include pressuring young girls to be thin, which contributes to eating disorders. For people from these nations, these practices do not seem "cultural," they just seem like the way things are.

Interviewers may encounter a variety of dangerous cultural practices in their work which do merit exploration, depending on the interview's purpose. These practices include female genital cutting, which can contribute to pain, disease, and even death for women and girls, abusive disciplinary practices, child marriage, forced marriage, and certain forms of traditional medicine in the absence of proven medical care.

What criteria can an interviewer use to determine when a cultural practice is worth exploring?

Is information about the practice relevant to the interview's purpose?

Is a vulnerable person at risk for physical or psychological harm which requires reporting to authorities (e.g., a child, elder, or person with disabilities)?

Is a person at risk for harm (even if that person is not in a category which requires reporting to authorities)?

How likely is harm to ensue from the practice?

Is the practice illegal?

Is the practice a violation of a universal human rights principle?

How avoidable is the practice?

These issues are complicated indeed. I supervised a school counseling trainee who was completing her internship in a middle school with many Rastafarian families, which supported their children's use of marijuana. After much soul searching and consulting with the local district attorney, the school counseling department decided *not* to inquire of families about their use of marijuana, but rather they distributed literature about the potential harms of smoking in general and marijuana in particular and tried to help the young people themselves learn about the dangers of various substances, including alcohol and marijuana. The school advocated strongly for healthful habits, such as eating well, sleeping sufficiently, and avoiding mind-altering substances, particularly during the school week, when they could interfere with school performance. The counseling and health education departments presented this material in a culturally respectful way, without singling out members of a particular ethnic group. They knew the problem of intoxication during school hours was not limited to one group.

WHO IS COMING TO SEE ME?: BACKGROUND CULTURAL INFORMATION

Why should we assume that an individual's identity
is natural and fixed rather than chosen, constructed by
society, or in flux?
—MARTHA MINOW

We should gather information about the interviewee's cultural background before the first meeting, whenever possible. Helpful facts include the person's age, religion, household composition, country of origin, and—where relevant—date and circumstances of immigration and degree of English fluency. Racial information is not enough because culture is not defined by skin color. For instance, the culture of a Black person from the Dominican Republic is different from that of an African American person who grew up in New York City. A little background reading on the person's ethnic, cultural, and religious group can enhance our understanding before the first meeting. For Native Americans, inquire as to whether they are affiliated with a tribe and if they were raised on or off a reservation. Also ask if they adhere to cultural or tribal traditions and practices, and if they form part of a community with other members of their tribe where they are living now.

Try to determine the history of the interviewee's ethnic group in your particular area. When did this group begin to arrive? Where did they come from? Why did they move to your area? How were they first received? Did they suffer from any trauma before, during, or after they emigrated? In general, how are children from this community doing in the schools? Do they come from a particular ethnic group within a nation (e.g., Mayas in Guatemala or Mexico, Bantus in Somalia, Jews in Russia, Japanese or ethnic Hawaiians in Hawaii)?

General information about a group's culture can be obtained from the Internet, from reliable books and articles (many of which are cited at the end of this book), and from people who come from the same culture, as long as confidentiality is maintained. When I begin to work with people from a given group, I also try to immerse myself in the arts of that culture, including music, visual arts, movies, poetry, and fiction. These give me a sense of the "flavor" of that country or culture, as it is interpreted by an artist. Familiarity with a culture can help us guard against misunderstanding in all phases of the interview—such as choosing alienating or offensive survey instruments, greeting the interviewee improperly, or presenting the results in a harmful way. True, we cannot become a member of a cultural group that is not our own. However, when we make an effort toward greater cultural understanding we greatly strengthen the foundation for our cross-cultural interview and the subsequent report.

With some people, national origin may be less important to their identity than their ethnicity. That is, people of Hindu origin can be from India, Africa, or the Caribbean; Chinese people hail from China, Hong Kong, Taiwan, Singapore, the Philippines, and so on. This is complicated, however, because ethnic Chinese from Taiwan may be insulted if you call them "Chinese." Historical events have created in them a pride in their separate identity as Taiwanese. A person of Lebanese descent who has grown up in Trinidad may feel more Lebanese than Trinidadian, or not—we cannot know without asking. For some people, their religion is a crucial part of their identity, particularly in religiously divided nations where there is tension among groups, such as in Bosnia, Nigeria, India, the Sudan, and Ireland. As always, it is best to ask people how they identify themselves rather than choose the categories ourselves.

It can also be helpful to find out about people's generational status. Japanese Americans refer to the first generation of immigrants to the United States as *Issei*. The *Nisei* were the first generation to be born in the United States. *Sansei* are the third generation, and *Yonsei* and *Gosei* are the fourth and fifth generation, respectively (Shibusawa, 2005). While not all languages have special terms to describe generational status, most people from immigrant families are acutely aware of the differences among the generations. When working with immigrant families, try to determine who immigrated when and from where—this will help you understand some of the issues and stressors they may be facing. (In states in which there are laws prohibiting discrimination against people because of national origin, this line of questioning may not be appropriate in a job interview. It could even be illegal.)

ASSESSING CULTURE AND ACCULTURATION

If the person you are interviewing is from a minority cultural group, you will want to collect relevant information about their culture and acculturation: how much the person is integrated into the dominant culture in the area where you work, and how much he or she retains of the culture of origin. Figure 2.1 shows different acculturation positions and some of the elements that we can consider when we are trying to determine how acculturated a given person might be.

Additionally, depending on the purpose of the interview, you may want to collect information on the acculturation patterns of other members of the interviewee's family, and on possible conflicts resulting from differences in acculturation. You may be able to gather some of this information from other providers or from a file folder before the first contact.

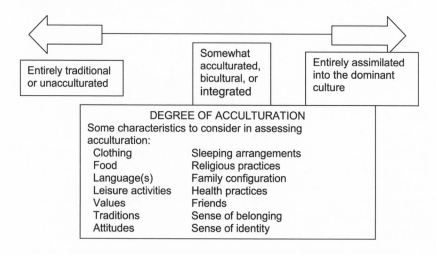

FIGURE 2.1. Acculturation spectrum.

Models exist for thorough assessments of culture, and in some cases a thorough assessment of this kind would be desirable. For instance, the Cultural Assessment Interview Protocol (Grieger, 2008), recommended for counseling situations, outlines a comprehensive assessment including the client's attitudes toward helping, cultural identity, level of acculturation, family structure and expectations, racial/cultural identity development, experience with bias, immigration issues, and existential/spiritual issues. This model also includes an assessment of the counselor/client dyad taking into account counselor characteristics and behaviors and the implications of cultural differences between the counselor and the client.

Inquiring about Culture and Acculturation

Be sure to ask these questions tactfully so they will not sound like an interrogation. Try to sprinkle them naturally in a conversation, rather than firing them off one after another. Of course, not all these questions will be relevant in all settings.

- Where were you born?
- Who do you consider family?
- What was the first language you learned to speak?
- Tell me about the other language(s) you speak.[1]
- What language or languages are spoken in your home? (It is important not to make assumptions here. Some people who identify as Native American will speak Navajo in the home with a grandparent, others will speak English, and still others will speak Spanish because some members of their family come from Mexico.)
- What is your religion? How observant are you in regard to practicing that religion?
- What activities do you enjoy when you are not working?
- How do you identify yourself culturally?
- What aspects of being _____ [use term for culture used by the interviewee] are most important to you?
- How would you describe your home and neighborhood?
- Who do you usually turn to for help when facing a problem?
- What are your goals for this interview today?

Additional questions for immigrant clients:

- Where did you live before you moved to this country?
- When did you first come to live in this country?
- In total, how many years have you lived in this country?
- What was the immigration process like?[2]
- How has the immigration process affected your family? (Probe for differences among family members, where relevant.)
- How are you (your family) adjusting to life in this country?

- Tell me about the ties you have with _____ (the country of origin).
- Are there any problems related to immigration or your status in this country that would be helpful for me to know about?

---

[1] It is important not to make assumptions. While most people from Ecuador speak Spanish, others speak Quechua; some people from Bolivia speak Aymara; and some people from Mexico speak Nahuatl, Maya, or a host of other indigenous languages, rather than Spanish. A person from Cape Verde may be more comfortable speaking French than Portuguese or Kriolou because he has lived most of his life in Senegal. Some immigrants who are more comfortable in other languages speak English at home because they have been told it will facilitate their children's adaptation to school, or because they are eager to blend in among their neighbors.

[2] The circumstances of immigration can be important because they influence how interviewees feel about their new country and authorities in it. For instance, interviewees who immigrated to attend graduate school are apt to have a high level of education and be integrated into official systems. On the other hand, interviewees who were smuggled across the border to work in sweatshops, factories, farms, or brothels may be suspicious of authorities, fearful of official systems, prone to flee, or in need of immediate protection. Questions about the circumstances of immigration could stimulate traumatic memories and should be asked with great care, depending on the purpose of the interview.

Answers to some of the questions in the text box will help you understand how comfortable the interviewee feels in the dominant culture, and therefore how much of an adjustment you need to make to the standard interviewing process.

People who are from ethnic minority groups but are not themselves immigrants also face decisions daily about how to integrate their minority culture with their lives in the majority culture. This may merit exploration, depending on the nature of your interview. For instance, many children and even great grandchildren of Cape Verdean immigrants structure their social lives around their Catholic churches and community centers that are dedicated solely to Cape Verdean members. Prayer services, community volunteering, socials, parties, and festivals will occupy a great deal of the members' time, enabling them to live abroad while nestled in Cape Verdean communities and maintaining the ability to speak Kriolou. Other Cape Verdeans are completely integrated into the dominant society, and while their neighbors might guess that they have foreign roots because of their last names, they blend easily into their ethnically mixed communities.

American Indians also run the gamut. Some live on reservations and foster the traditions of their ancestors, whereas others also live on reservations but live much like other, non-Indian Americans. Many live in cities or in rural areas far from reservations, where some maintain tribal traditions and friendships. Others connect to nontribal people and lifestyles and consider their roots little more than a historical artifact.

We can think of a spectrum, with people who are completely separate from the dominant culture and unassimilated on one side, people who are completely assimilated on the other side, and people who are somewhat acculturated in the middle. While this spectrum is useful, it is also too simplistic, as we discuss below.

A basic model suggests that people handle the challenges of acculturation in five general ways (Sue & Sue, 2002):

1. *Traditionalism*: People maintain, practice, and value the traditions of their culture of origin. This approach is common among people who immigrate in their later years:

> Antonio, for instance, emigrated from Greece in his 50s to join a son and his family in the United States. He became discouraged and gave up on learning English after years of frustrating attempts. He lost interest in his new country, acquired a satellite dish, and began watching Greek television and listening to Greek radio stations. He spoke constantly of retiring to Greece and saved his money and vacation days all year so he could visit his homeland as much as possible. He delighted in Greek food and holidays, and although he recognized the advantages of some aspects of his new country, he thought of himself as entirely separate from them. His position could be described as traditionalist.

2. *Transitional period*: During a transitional period, people participate in their original culture and their new one but don't feel at home in either, and find themselves questioning both. In an emotional sense, they are "neither here nor there." For example:

> Abbar, a Muslim teenager from Pakistan, is irritated by all the fuss around Christmas in his new country, with a Secret Santa program in his classroom, and Christmas decorations and carols surrounding him constantly for more than a month. When people wish him "Merry Christmas," which they seem to do everywhere he turns, he wishes them the same, and he feels the good cheer implied in the statement. At the same time, he feels as if the words are hollow and quite separate from him, and he is slightly depressed to feel so invisible in his new country. But when his father's three brothers and all their wives and children crowd into his small apartment for three days to celebrate the Muslim holy day of Eid al-Adha, the Feast of Sacrifice, which occurs around the same time of year as Christmas, Abbar feels that it's a backward tradition. He is embarrassed when his family roasts a goat in the parking lot of their apartment complex in front of all the neighbors. He hates having his cousins squeeze into his room to sleep at night. On one hand he enjoys the traditions of his home culture, and on the other hand he is uncomfortable with the way they set him apart.

3. *Marginality:* Some people are unsuccessful in meeting the demands of the old and the new culture and become alienated from both. Some of these people will not be able to hold jobs, may become homeless, and may abuse substances or become involved in criminal activity. Many of the immigrants who become marginal have trauma histories that have not been treated or resolved, and these interfere with their functioning. For example:

Soledad was born in 1983 to a peasant family in El Salvador that was fleeing political violence. She remembers fetching water one day as a young child and seeing a family friend shot dead in front of her. She says she kept walking so as not to attract attention, but she feels that his spirit follows her. She says she has experienced *nervios* ever since, having bad dreams, waking in a panic, and jumping at loud noises. Soledad's shack collapsed in the earthquake of 2001, and she and her husband and daughter were rendered homeless. She says her husband at that time began drinking alcohol more heavily and beating her more severely. Afraid for her life, she left her daughter with her mother and snuck across the U.S. border, making her way to her sister's home in a small town in Michigan. She began working in the local grape farm and jelly processing plant, and experienced what she described as the calmest period of her life for a few months. However, she was terribly worried about her daughter. When her sister's husband began pressing her for sexual favors, she moved in with a Mexican man at work. Although he was a legal resident of the United States, they could not find a way to legalize her immigration status. She was haunted by thoughts and images of her daughter, of the shooting she had witnessed in her childhood, of the beatings she endured in her first marriage, and of her multiple losses in the earthquake. She became paranoid and angry toward the man she lived with and disruptive at work. After she was fired, she hitched a ride to Chicago, where she is now homeless. Soledad was rendered unable to function successfully because of her trauma history, and the ways in which immigration law and poverty forced the dissolution of her family. She could not function either as a full member of U.S. society or as a full member of society either in El Salvador or in immigrant communities in the United States.

4. *Assimilation:* People who are assimilating assume the customs and practices of their new culture and reject and devalue their heritage. Immigrant parents with this orientation often fail to teach their children their first language and may view their first language and the traditions of their country of origin as backward and unappealing. For example:

When he was a child, Vito's Italian mother and Puerto Rican father thought he should learn only English and become as American as possible as soon as possible. Although they spoke a mixture of Italian and Spanish to each other in private, with their children and in front of others the two spoke English only. As soon as they could afford it they moved into a neighborhood with few immigrant families. As an adult now, Vito regrets having grown up so assimilated, but says he has little "heart connection" to the culture of either of his parents.

5. *Biculturalism*: Bicultural people create a sense of identity drawing on elements of their original and new cultures. They may speak both languages, celebrate two sets of holidays, and eat the foods of their new culture and their original homeland, or they may create new traditions that include a melding of both. For example:

Mira grew up in an India family in Milwaukee. Her parents spoke to her in Hindi at home, served Indian food, had her take classes in traditional Indian dance, and celebrated Indian holidays. As a college student now, she happily serves Indian dishes to her friends and hosts Indian students who are spending a semester on her campus during their first days, as they get used to their new environment. Her friends are from a variety of ethnic backgrounds and she appreciates American music and fashion. She feels fortunate to benefit from the richness of the U.S. and Indian cultures.

Many bicultural people have a *blended* identity, having forged a unique identity by blending elements of each culture, like Mira above, but staying relatively consistent as an individual in each context. Other bilingual people use a bicultural strategy called *alternation* (LaFromboise, Coleman, & Gerton, 1993). In this model, a person is considered able to know, understand, and behave like a member of two different cultures and alter his or her behavior to fit the relevant context. In practice, this often means acting one way at home (or with members of the home culture) and another way when in school, work, or in other public contexts.

These ways of approaching acculturation are not fixed. People may adopt different approaches at various stages in their lives. Often, during a period of crisis, people return to the ways of their childhood or ancestors:

Susana, a Navajo woman, grew up on the reservation and moved to Los Angeles in her late teens where she met and married a Jewish man. They raised their children as Americans without much regard for either of the parents' backgrounds. After 30 years of marriage Susana's husband died. Grieving deeply, she moved back to the reservation; and two of her grown daughters followed her there, where they now work as social workers and are raising their own children steeped in Navajo ways.

As this example illustrates, people's relationship to their cultures is dynamic, changing, and multidirectional. Families do not simply become more acculturated or assimilated over time. Indeed, many young Jews have chosen to be more religiously observant than their parents. Similarly, many young African Americans have taken on African names and celebrate Kwanzaa and other African-rooted traditions, in this way expressing greater separation from the dominant culture and more connection to their African roots than their parents' generation.

Within a given family, we commonly find people who acculturate at different paces or in different ways from each other. This has been called *dissonant acculturation*, where linguistic and other acculturation gaps develop within families that exacerbate intergenerational conflicts and misunderstanding and may cause a role reversal in which more acculturated children caretake their less acculturated parents (Portes & Rumbaut, 2001). For example:

> After just 2 years in Boston, 9-year-old Carolina spoke more English and was more at home in U.S. culture than her Salvadoran mother. Carolina soon began to answer the phone, read the mail, and negotiate with the landlord on behalf of her family, which gave her undue power within the family and created conflicts.

Differing levels of acculturation do not necessarily create conflicts in families. Many people are remarkably resilient and successful at handling acculturation issues as individuals, and families:

> The Lee family runs a Korean restaurant. Their employees are mostly Korean, their suppliers are mostly Korean, and their customers are both Korean and from other cultures. The parents attend a Korean church and largely take a traditionalist approach to acculturation. The older son, Kwan, who works as a waiter in the family restaurant most evenings after high school, proudly announces to all the non-Korean customers that he cannot give recommendations on the food because he doesn't like Korean food, and he wishes his parents ran an Italian restaurant. He avoids waiting on Korean customers, although he speaks Korean. He asks his friends to call him Chuck instead of Kwan. He holds an assertively assimilationist position. His older sister, Yung Hee, has been away for 2 years at college. During her time away she

has come to appreciate her Korean roots at the same time as she has become more fluent in English and more comfortable and secure as part of an "American" youth culture. She has become bicultural.

The Lee family juggles cultural complexity with aplomb. The parents instill in their children a pride in their Korean culture, and yet they seem to accept that their children will become more acculturated than they are themselves. Kwan appears to be rejecting aspects of his ethnic culture, at least in public, but this does not worry his parents too much. They understand that concerns about being "different" are common to adolescents. They expect he will come to embrace aspects of his Korean self as he matures, just like his sister.

CONCLUDING OBSERVATIONS

Decisions that were made before the interview has even begun can have a tremendous impact on the interview itself. These decisions include requesting and reviewing prior records, deciding who will be present during an interview, and deciding where the interview will take place. We should remember that people who are less familiar with our work setting will be at a distinct disadvantage when meeting with us. It would be important to convey as clearly as possible the intentions of the interview and whether the relationship will be ongoing in some way or just a one-time contact. Even if we have discussed some of these issues previously on the telephone, they are worth reiterating in person. People who don't speak English fluently or who are hard of hearing may have a particularly difficult time absorbing information gleaned on the phone.

The interviewer's goals may match or differ from the goals of the interviewee, the interviewee's family, the interviewee's cultural group, and the referral source. Often interviews begin with crossed signals. Mental health clinicians think they are doing an intake for psychological help while the interviewee wants to buttress an asylum claim. A police officer thinks he is being friendly as a form of community outreach, but the people he addresses on the sidewalk think they are being hassled and considered suspects. An educator asks parents to come into school as a routine part of getting to know the pupils' families, whereas the parents believe they are about to be informed of their child's misbehavior. These misunderstandings occur all the time, and can be partially averted through carefully preparing the interviewees.

We should inform interviewees of the likely and possible outcomes of the interview. One psychologist was called by a Puerto Rican mother 5 days after a 20-minute intake interview at a mental health clinic, complaining that her child hadn't changed yet. The mother thought the interview would be like a simple medical appointment—one visit and the cure would be imminent (M. O'Neill, personal communication, June 2007).

As we interact with people, whether in their homes, in our offices, or in some other place, we must be careful not to reject or judge harshly certain of their customs simply because they are unfamiliar to us. Learning about a person's cultural group, family, and individual history will help us understand them. Questions about their degree of acculturation and how they live their culture or cultures on a daily basis will help us know how to adjust our interviews. As in so much of life, doing our homework before an interview so we arrive fully prepared will help us do a better job and conduct a more productive, valid, and pleasant interview.

Questions to Think about and Discuss

1. What are some of the ways prior records can help orient you before an interview?
2. What are some of the potential hazards of relying on prior records for information?
3. Remember an occasion when you interviewed more than one person at a time. What were some of the advantages and disadvantages of conducting the interview this way?
4. Discuss the advantages and disadvantages of interviewing a person in his or her home as compared to conducting an interview in your office.
5. Think of a person from a particular cultural background. Consider the way that person's degree of acculturation or acculturation style might affect the interview process in your setting.

RECOMMENDED ADDITIONAL READING

Lynch, E. W., & Hanson, M. J. (Eds.). (2004). *Developing cross-cultural competence: A guide for working with children and their families* (3rd ed.). Baltimore: Brookes.

Portes, A., & Rumbaut, R. G. (2001). *Legacies: The story of the immigrant second generation*. Los Angeles: University of California Press.

Sommers-Flanagan, J., & Sommers-Flanagan, R. (2003). *Clinical interviewing* (3rd ed.). New York: Wiley.

3 Biases and Boundary Issues

This chapter focuses on biases and boundary issues that can affect the interviewing process. Biases distort what we see, how we act, the weight we give to particular behaviors or statements, and how we write about the interviews. Some biases are basic processes within our own psyches. They affect our colleagues, our interviewees, and ourselves.

Appropriate boundaries can be difficult to determine in many human encounters, particularly where they involve people from distinct cultural groups. Boundary violations can be a cause or a result of various biases in interviews.

BIASES

Several kinds of bias can create distortions in our interviews (Miller, 1984). These include *motivational bias*, in which the interviewer or the interviewee is motivated to provide a particular kind of outcome to please a person or group. As an example of motivational bias on the part of an interviewer, a police officer might want to find incriminating evidence against a suspect because of pressure from a commanding officer to "get the guy." Or, consider an entitlement officer who has been told her office needs to cut its caseload by 20%, and thus she is eager to find evidence in interviews that the interviewee does not need certain services. Examples of motivational bias *for interviewees* include eagerly searching the interviewer's face for indications of "the best answer" in order to make a favorable impression. These problems of motivational bias are described frequently throughout this book as we discuss ways to check our own motivations and those of the interviewee to make sure they are as free from coercion and distortion as possible.

Motivational biases sometimes have a cultural element. Sometimes staff members of an organization are told they need to increase or decrease the number of people from a particular group who obtain a service or who are subject to a penalty. This might influence interviewers to code interviewees incorrectly, assigning them to the wrong cultural group, or it might influence them to skew the outcome of an interview in subtle ways. Interviewees may also be subject to cultural motivational biases. For instance, they might be motivated to perform better (or worse) when interviewed by a person from a particular ethnic group.

Notational bias can also lead us to distorted impressions. This refers to the instruments we use for measuring and our terms, categories, forms, and so on. We discuss this subject at greater length in Chapter 10 on writing reports.

A third class of biases is referred to as *cognitive biases*. These are thinking errors caused by the simplified information processing strategies that people use; these affect our ability to engage in thinking processes such as remembering and estimating. *Observational biases* are a subcategory of cognitive biases that limit and distort our ability to observe properly.

UNBIASED OBSERVING

I once complained to an art teacher about not being able to draw. She said that it was all a question of *seeing*; if I could learn to see accurately I would be able to draw. I think the relationship between seeing and drawing is parallel to the relationship between observing in interviews and writing notes. That is, if we can be truly present for the person in front of us in an interview and observe that person without distortion, we will be far more likely to write about that person without bias. Unfortunately, several psychological processes together increase the likelihood of discriminatory biases in our observations when we interview people from social groups that differ from our own.

The first stage of memory is encoding, where we perceive things sufficiently to commit them to memory. We may notice details through any of our senses. This stage may be tinged with serious bias when we interview people from differing backgrounds. What we notice and fail to notice as we conduct our interview and take notes will influence our final report.

Observational and Cognitive Biases That Can Affect Interviewing, Taking Notes, and Writing Reports

- *Confirmatory bias* is the tendency to notice what we expect to see, while ignoring or discounting the rest. This tendency is one reason that stereotypes persist—we are apt to notice aspects of individuals that confirm our stereotypes about members of that group.
- *Fundamental attribution error* is the tendency to view others' actions as stemming from their personalities or other enduring characteristics, while underestimating the influence of *the situation*. This can be problematic when, for instance, we write a report based on one interview with a person without checking with other documents, additional interviews, or other sources of information. If the interviewee felt particularly sad, angry, weary, physically ill, sleepy, or suspicious in that one interview for some reason, or was so paralyzed with anxiety that he or she did not perform well, we might have a tendency to assume this is an enduring characteristic, rather than a transitory result of the particular situation.
- *Halo effect* is the tendency to allow one aspect of a person's appearance or personality to "spill over" and influence our global evaluation of that person. For instance, good-looking people are often seen as more outgoing and kinder than people who are considered less attractive. This also works with more negative characteristics, so that people who are considered less attractive are assumed to have other negative characteristics. It is easy to see how this tendency might distort an interview report. If, for instance, an interviewee's clothes give off a food aroma that's disagreeable to the interviewer, or if the interviewee wears clothes that the interviewer considers in poor taste, or if the person uses language awkwardly, the interviewer might tend to rate that person more negatively on a variety of other unrelated characteristics. Interviewers might be similarly biased by an interviewee's skin color, accent, or other external, superficial characteristics: These might bias our perceptions of the entire interview, and influence the interviewer's ratings of more important characteristics (such as trustworthiness, honesty, and intelligence).
- *In-group bias* is giving preferential treatment to others whom a person perceives as being from his or her own group. As interviewers, we could show in-group bias without even being aware of it. In any given day I could—unintentionally—focus more on people who are similar to me in age, sex, race, social class, political orientation, religion, or other characteristics. I might just feel more comfortable with these people who are similar to me and therefore feel more disposed to helping them.
- *Self-fulfilling prophecy* is the tendency to engage in behaviors that elicit results that will confirm our own beliefs. This can work in a negative or a positive way. For instance, a physician might approach an Italian or Latina woman brusquely if he has

an expectation that this patient will speak excessively about unrelated matters, engaging in what a physician described to me once as "the mama mia syndrome" (Fontes, 2005a, p. 8). In response to the doctor's interruptions and curt approach, this patient might feel a need to convey as much detail as possible: She senses the doctor will not take all factors into account unless she insists on describing them all to him in detail. In a more positive vein, an interviewer who approaches an interview situation optimistically may unconsciously create the conditions that lead to a successful interview.

It is easy to see how these cognitive biases could skew the results of an interview. The cognitive biases described here are natural, human, and—at the same time—problematic and may result in unfair outcomes. However, there are ways we can correct for cognitive biases. Increased self-knowledge will help us see our own specific areas of ignorance and teach us where we need to stretch ourselves to eliminate our prejudices. Increased self-knowledge makes it easier to reach out to people from different groups and watch ourselves to make sure we are behaving fairly.

Additionally, we can fortify ourselves against confirmation bias by checking in with ourselves honestly before an interview. "What am I expecting this person to be like? What will I be looking out for?" Once we've engaged in this first step, then we need to make sure we notice *and record in our notes* any aspects of the person, or statements the person makes, that *defy* our stereotypes. I am not suggesting that you purposely distort what you see and record. Rather, we all need to be aware of potential bias in our observations and to take great care to be unbiased in recording what we hear and observe.

True emotional empathy and intellectual understanding will help us correct for the fundamental attribution error. We will be able to see the constraints that may be inhibiting the interviewee's capacity to perform "up to speed" (for instance, language difficulties or nervousness about the interview) and we will be sure to inquire about possible problems. We will be humble enough to assume that one interview alone will not reveal to us how an interviewee "really is," and we will seek additional information from other sources, where appropriate.

Immigrants, survivors of terrorism and natural disasters, and other people who have undergone recent tumultuous changes in their lives may be particularly likely to suffer the negative consequences of confirmation bias and the fundamental attribution error. We must be wary of assuming that dysfunctional behavior is due to "who they are" rather than a reaction to extraordinary circumstances in their lives. It can be helpful to ask interviewees about how things used to be "before"—before the move, before the attack, before the disaster, before they were living in a homeless shelter.

If, indeed, their functioning deteriorated suddenly with the change, this is well worth noting. It suggests that with improved circumstances and support, they are likely to be able to return to their level of functioning that existed before the traumatic event.

For example, immigration is a "highly disorganizing experience" (Maiter & George, 2003, p. 426). Studies show that immigration can disrupt parent–child relations, intensify intergenerational conflict, and increase high-risk behavior among adolescents. (Immigration can also be a highly positive experience, and certainly not all people who move from one country to another suffer unhappy dislocations.) Therefore, it is important when we interview a family of relatively recent immigrants, to take into account that this family is functioning in a particular way at this particular time in their history. Their current behavior may be an aberration rather than a reflection of their potential.

We can avoid negative self-fulfilling prophecies by replacing them with positive ones. We should assume from the start that all our interviews will be successful, and that we'll be able to achieve the necessary rapport.

SPECIAL CONNECTIONS AND BOUNDARY ISSUES

The separation between the interviewer and the interviewee may seem artificial to people from cultures that emphasize collectivism rather than individuality, which can create challenges around maintaining professional boundaries. "From an African American perspective, the helper and the helpee are not separated from one another but are bound together both emotionally and spiritually" (Sue & Sue, 2002, p. 65). People who share this perspective, which I believe includes people from a variety of cultural groups, may not understand or accept the notion that the interviewer is trying to be "objective" or "scientific" and doesn't have a personal interest in the outcome of the interview. The interviewee may openly ask you for advice about what kinds of answers would achieve their desired results, or the interviewee may look for subtle signs from you as to which answer is "best" or which answer will assure a favorable outcome.

In many developing countries and in much of Eastern Europe, official systems run on the basis of connections. That is, you get what you need based on whom you know, whom your family knows, your membership in a particular political party, and in some cases, whom you bribe. Interviewees who are immigrants may feel despairing because they don't have the kinds of connections or social status that they believe would earn them the best treatment in their new countries. They may believe they are doomed to "fail" the interview without links to powerful officials. Conversely, an interviewee may believe that a caring interviewer can intervene personally and make everything turn out all right (in Portuguese this would be called giving a *jeitinho*, or a helping hand). Or interviewees may feel that their social status entitles them to avoid an interview or obtain the best possible outcome. In a police interview, for example, a man may point out that he was also a police officer in his country of origin and assume this will give him special privileges.

It is important for us to be aware of how cultural issues interact with our professional boundaries, even when working with interviewees from the same ethnic culture as our own. I am not advocating for an overly rigid set of boundaries. On the contrary, I think it is important to maintain flexibility. For instance, depending on the circumstances, an interviewer might decide to read or translate a letter for an interviewee who needs assistance, or make a helpful telephone call, or be flexible about the starting time of meetings. At the same time, bending rules or overstepping one's role can lead to problems for both the interviewer and the interviewee. You might want to ask yourself the following questions when you find yourself loosening your professional boundaries:

- Is this really in the interviewee's best interest?
- Why am I being less firm in setting boundaries with this person than with others?
- What are the possible ramifications of my looser boundaries for me, the client, the client's family, and other members of the community?
- Am I committing an ethical violation by loosening this boundary, or am I simply and defensibly going out of my way to be helpful to a person who needs extra assistance?
- Am I tempted to keep my actions secret from my supervisor or colleagues?

Thinking about the foregoing questions may help you make decisions regarding boundaries. When in doubt, consult colleagues and supervisors.

ETHNIC MATCHING

Organizations sometimes believe they can resolve cultural dilemmas simply by matching clients and professionals (or interviewers and interviewees) for race or ethnicity. While I am a strong supporter of ethnically diverse workplaces for a variety of reasons, several problems are created by matching for ethnicity or race too automatically. First of all, if we choose the people to conduct interviews based on interviewees' race or ethnicity, we are denying the importance of other aspects of interviewees and essentially say-ing that their race or ethnicity is the only or most important aspect of who they are. Also, matching for ethnicity usually means that clients or inter-viewees from minority groups will have fewer options about whom they work with. That is, people from the majority group may be matched with someone who has a special understanding of their issues or advanced train-ing in how to work with their issues, whereas people from minority groups who are matched on the basis of race or ethnicity alone will not be given as wide a range of choices, or perhaps no choice at all. Also, matching for eth-nicity does not by itself ensure the quality of connection or communication; and it can distract from other aspects of the interview, such as power imbal-ances and other pressures (Gunaratnam, 2003a).

Some writers have advocated for matching professionals to clients ac-cording to their race or ethnicity, suggesting that a professional from the same ethnic background will be able to understand the interviewee better, will automatically have better rapport with people from the same group, and will have greater interest in the well-being of people from their own community. In short, matching is seen as a way to reduce the interpersonal distance between two people, which is assumed to lead to more accurate in-terviews and services (Gunaratnam, 2003a). Other experts have questioned such assumptions. For instance, De Souza (1996) writes that ethnic match-ing in mental health care is "reductionistic and simplistic" (p. 8). She sug-gests that matching people on the basis of their race or color reduces indi-viduals to their cultural characteristics, and might lead us to "forget the human aspect which is integral to our work" (De Souza, 1996, p. 8). Oth-ers have pointed out that people may not be so happy to see someone from their own ethnic group in a professional role. They may doubt the qualifi-cations or status of a member of a minority group, may fear gossip, may feel the person is too acculturated or too removed from their ethnic roots to be helpful, or may be concerned about the professional's political or per-sonal connections within a small community.

Research into racial or ethnic matching has found mixed results (e.g., Sue, Fujino, Hu, Takeuchi, & Zane, 1991). In some studies the practitio-ner's competence and personal qualities were found to be more important than racial or ethnic similarity. In other instances, racial or ethnic similarity appear to be important in interviews (Dunkerly & Dalenberg, 1999). In yet others, children were found to be more likely to disclose child sexual abuse to an interviewer of a different race (Springman & Wherry, 2006). Clearly, these issues are complex and much remains to be discovered about the ad-vantages and disadvantages of ethnic matching in interviews with people of various ages and backgrounds, and in different settings.

When racial or ethnic matching is seen as the only or the most important way to achieve cultural competence, sometimes organizations become less vigilant in taking a host of other steps that would advance cultural competence. Advocating for the end to discrimination may come to be seen as the exclusive province of the few staff members from minority groups who have been hired, as if these matters are no longer the responsibility of others. Having an ethnically diverse work force is an important step for an organization to achieve cultural competence, but it is not the only answer.

Even if matching for certain similarities were desirable, it can be hard to know which aspect of identity is most important for any particular interviewee. Gender, age, education, social class, personality, skin color, degree of acculturation, sexual orientation, lifestyle, politics, religion, values, regional or generational differences, sense of humor, and language ability can also affect rapport. All of these are axes of difference, and it can be hard to predetermine which is most important for any given interviewee discussing any particular topic at a given point in time.

In some cases, two people from the same ethnic group or nation may come from different clans or religions, and these differences may make a working relationship next to impossible. For instance, in my area an agency recently hired a social worker from the Sudan to help with Sudanese refugees. The refugees uniformly refused to work with her because she came from a region and group that had caused the refugees' original displacement in their native country. They could not trust this social worker. They still saw her as part of the enemy, and they preferred working with U.S. professionals with the help of an interpreter rather than working with this Sudanese social worker who spoke their language but came from a rival ethnic group.

WORKING WITH SOMEONE FROM THE "SAME" CULTURE

Some professionals find it especially challenging to maintain adequate boundaries with interviewees from their own ethnic group, whether that group belongs to the majority or to a minority culture. We may especially want them to get the job they are seeking or to benefit from the services that are available. We may be tempted to deny, minimize, or overlook problems because we find it too hard to admit publicly that people who are "like me" have these problems. We may want to protect these "similar" individuals from getting caught up in the child welfare, criminal justice, mental health, or other official systems. We may also hesitate to admit to our colleagues that these people—who may feel like extended family—have done wrong. We may find ourselves empathizing so strongly with the difficult situation in which these interviewees find themselves that we overlook problems that require intervention. Or we may be tempted to accept what interviewees say at face value without doubt, in a way we wouldn't do for members of another group.

Conversely, some professionals who have overcome poverty, racism, and other obstacles themselves dismiss as a "sob story" the explanations of families from a similar background. An attitude of "I made it, why can't you?" may surface.

It can be difficult, at times, to obtain complete information from people who are like us. An ethnically similar interviewee might say, "You know how it is," and decline to elaborate, assuming that a racial, cultural, religious, or sexual orientation similarity gives us automatic insight into their plight and obviates the need for elaboration. This can also show up conversely, where professionals believe they know all about an interviewee's situation because of their shared background and therefore are not open to learning about the person's specific situation.

Sometimes interviewees ask for special treatment, based on commonalities. A father from Puerto Rico may say to a social worker who is also Puerto Rican, "'Mano (brother), give me a break here. We boricuas have to stick together." Similarly, a White upper-middle-class mother might use her self-assurance and sense of entitlement to try to convey to a White social worker that she, unlike some of those parents, can address a problem by herself or with the help of a private therapist or physician, and she is not the kind of mother who needs authorities poking into her business.

Some interviewers describe difficulty speaking about sexual or other sensitive issues with members of their own group because it is like insulting one's own family to bring up certain topics or use forbidden words. (I have also heard people assert the opposite: that it is easier for them to discuss sensitive topics with members of their own group.)

In many situations, of course, it can be an advantage to come from the same ethnic, racial, cultural, or other identity group as the interviewee. Richie (1996) describes her identity as a Black woman giving her an easier time establishing rapport with incarcerated battered Black women. A Jewish attorney described reaching out to a Jewish judge by saying he wanted to make a "Rachmonas plea," referring to a humble, beseeching plea for mercy discussed in the Bible. He was relying on their shared common cultural knowledge as a way of establishing a special link. A Mexican police officer described what he called an infallible technique for getting confessions from Central American and Mexican sex offenders. He says they cry and confess when he tells them, "God knows what you did." He takes advantage of his knowledge of the offenders' culture and religion to make them tell the truth. These are all examples of cultural commonalities facilitating communication.

SELF-DISCLOSURE

How much interviewers self-disclose varies with their personal style and the circumstances of the interview. Sometimes self-disclosure makes the interviewer appear more human. For instance, a physical therapist might say to a patient, "I broke my wrist too last year. I know how much it can hurt." This is apt to be noncontroversial and nonproblematic. However, it would be a different matter for a mental health clinician to say to a client, "I also suffer from paranoid delusions." In the mental health context, this would be seen as a distraction from the client's concerns, and would reduce the professional's credibility. American Indian clients expect professionals to identify where they are from (Sutton & Broken Nose, 2005).

It can be difficult to know what a particular self-disclosure will mean for an interviewee at any particular time. As distinct from certain kinds of ongoing relationships, self-disclosures in an interview could be an annoying diversion, unless they are of the most superficial type, such as, "I agree! I can't wait until the winter's over."

A study of physicians' self-disclosure revealed that contrary to what they intended, when doctors spoke about themselves it inhibited rather than facilitated a discussion of the patients' concerns (Kolata, 2007). Most of the time when the doctor injected personal information, the conversation never returned to the problem under discussion before the interruption. There is no reason to think physicians are unique here. Before we volunteer information about ourselves, it is important to think about whether the self-revelation is apt to serve the interviewee.

Wearing Religious Symbols

The appropriate boundary between our "professional" and our "private" selves is discussed in a variety of ways throughout this book. Traditionally trained psychotherapists typically avoid self-disclosure of all types and therefore try to wear clothes and decorate their offices in ways that reveal little about themselves in the interest of neutrality. In business, medical, and other settings, the norms may be less clear.

How much should we carry our own religious (or political or other) convictions into our work lives? Clearly, the answer to these questions varies with the setting. Counselors who work in pastoral care centers would be expected to use their religious values in their sessions, and even in some cases to wear garb that identifies their position in the institution. In secular work settings, however, most of us should avoid wearing our religious (or political) affiliations on our sleeves. I support people's right to wear a cross, a star of David, a hand of Fatima, a figo, or any other religious or ethnic symbol that they choose and that they believe protects them, or pleases them, in any setting they choose. However, I do not believe these should be *displayed* in settings in which we are trying to be welcoming to diverse groups of people. I would hope that—as much as possible—people would choose to tuck these items out of sight (e.g., wear their symbol on a necklace long enough to slip under their shirt). For me, this is not a matter of hiding one's own identity so much as it is a commitment to demonstrating in every way possible that we are open to all come before us—even if they differ from us.

Of course, some religions *require* the use of items that are necessarily visible to all, such as a *hijab* (headscarf) for a Muslim woman, a *kipa* (skullcap) for a Jewish man, or a *pagri* (turban) for a Sikh. But these items are required by these faiths for religious observance and cannot be concealed, which is different from a voluntary expression of religious affiliation that could easily be kept out of sight. Even for people from the same religion as the person conducting the interview, the open display of a religious item can be disconcerting. I have known Catholics who felt inhibited speaking with interviewers who openly wore crosses because they feared the interviewer would be judging them from an orthodox Catholic perspective, which they themselves had abandoned.

I realize not everyone will agree with my position on this, and I believe there is room for reasonable, thoughtful people to disagree. However, I would especially like to encourage people who are from dominant groups (White, Christian, native born, etc.) to give careful thought to the way in which their use of symbols that reflect their position in this dominant group (e.g., the National flag or a crucifix) may intimidate people from less dominant groups. Here is an example:

> In the town where I live we recently interviewed a number of candidates for elementary school principal. One candidate wore her crucifix outside her shirt in both her public interviews. This caused consternation among the Jewish, Muslim, and atheist families. Finally, with great trepidation, a parent asked this candidate whether she was aware of the religious diversity in the community and whether she would be able to support all our children. Her answer was satisfactory and she was hired, but many of us were disturbed that she continued to wear her cross outside her shirt at subsequent public events. We could not understand why she felt that her desire to display her cross was more important than the need to appear open to all groups. It remains to be seen whether she is as open to diversity as her words indicated, in contradiction to her persistent public displaying of her cross. Many of us hope she will tuck her cross into her shirt so children from all faiths can immediately feel that she is on their side and that they belong

in the school—that neither the school nor its principal prefers children of certain faiths over others. Additionally, when religious minority children see Christian symbols in public places, it serves as a reminder to them that they are in a minority.

Avoiding symbols that might be interpreted as indicating a preference for one group of people over another is a way of welcoming all and insulting no one.

BRIBES AND GIFTS

An interviewee who understands that bribes are illegal in your country might still try to discern if there is some favor he can do, some gift he can offer, some form of *baksheesh* he can provide as a token of appreciation in exchange for favorable treatment. While outright bribes are illegal throughout the world, some form of gifts or money to curry favors is standard operating procedure in many places. (For an example close to home, we need look no further than the common practice of pharmaceutical companies giving physicians meals, holidays, and other gifts.) If you are offered a gift or money from someone who comes from a country where such behavior is expected or even mandatory, you may respond with a number of possible reactions. Avoid becoming angry or defensive and view this as a teaching moment. While thanking the interviewee for this offer, explain that it would be unethical for you to accept the gift. Make sure the interviewee understands that the gift is not necessary and may not be acceptable in your country or in your agency. If you have agency guidelines around what to do in this kind of situation, of course, they should be followed.

On the other hand, in some cultures people routinely give small gifts to professionals to express their gratitude without the expectation of any form of reciprocation. For instance, many teachers in North America are surprised when parents of their Japanese, Korean, and Thai students present them with small, carefully wrapped gifts at the end of the school year. While these items typically have little monetary value, they are a culturally expected expression of gratitude. The parents would most likely be offended if such tokens were refused, and the gifts are not intended to garner special treatment for their children.

The Korean concept of *unhae* refers to this reciprocity: "favors that are graciously given and willingly returned" (Chan & Lee, 2004, p. 282). When a professional grants assistance to people who need it, those who benefited are seen as incurring a debt. Because the professional is unlikely to need a favor from them, interviewees or their family may express gratitude through giving gifts or inviting the professional to dinner. The refusal to accept such offers may be viewed as a rejection and cause the person who made the offer to lose face. You should think carefully about ways to be tactful and sensitive if you find yourself in such a position.

In many cultures, particular protocols govern the giving and receiving of gifts. For example, Koreans believe you should not open the gift in front of the giver. Japanese believe gifts should be given and received with both hands and with a slight bow.

It can be difficult to distinguish a gift of affection and gratitude from a gift offered to increase goodwill or even an out-and-out bribe. In general, if your agency has no policy against accepting gifts, if the gift is of minimal monetary value, if you can be certain that your behavior with this person will not change because you received the gift, if you do not feel a need to hide the gift from your colleagues or supervisors, and if you are certain the gift was not given with an expectation of special treatment, then it is probably alright to accept it. When in doubt, check with your colleagues and supervisors.

Sometimes, as professionals, we are tempted to give gifts to the clients with whom we work. I have known police officers and social workers who have bought groceries and even helped pay rent for families in need, counselors who have given stuffed animals and other toys to children, psychotherapists who have given books to clients, and so on. Most of our professional organizations offer guidance in this matter, and many of our agencies explicitly forbid us from giving gifts.

There are many kinds of gifts, and they mean different things. A basket of small toys, toothbrushes, or books from which children can select a gift on their way out of an interview or medical exam would not seem to generate much controversy—these items are offered to all children equally, and clearly there is no expectation of reciprocity.

We must ask ourselves about the meaning of giving different kinds of gifts. An attorney who traveled to Japan to take a deposition in a corporate case purposely bought a bottle of wine on the plane to offer to the man he was deposing. He had been told that such a gift—clearly purchased without great care or consideration—would be seen as an insult to the person who received it—and this was part of the attorney's plan to unsettle the deponent.

Before giving a gift to a child, we should ask the parents' permission. For some parents who cannot afford many toys, an adult from outside the family who offers a large gift to a child may be seen as trying to usurp the child's affection, or as making the parent lose face. I have known professionals who escorted impoverished child clients to a toy store to "buy any one thing you want." Of course, the child was delighted but the parents were dismayed, because they did not see themselves as ever being able to offer the same. Some toys—such as Barbies in short skirts, or weapons—may be seen as inappropriate and may be rejected by particular families.

Agencies sometimes facilitate the giving of gifts during the holidays to low-income children by implementing a program where families can request a particular toy for each child, which agency staff then purchase. The agency gives the toys to the parents along with wrapping paper, so the parents can wrap and give the gifts themselves. In this way, agency staff experience the pleasure of giving gifts to children they care about, the parents are enabled to offer gifts to their children that they might otherwise not be able to afford, and the family is able to retain its self-respect, avoiding the humiliation that can accompany open charity given from one hand to another. It may be less satisfying for the giver to present a gift anonymously in this way, but ideally the knowledge that it may be better received like this will compensate.

What Might a Gift Mean in the Context of an Interview?

- An offer of recognition or appreciation for the receiver's help or cooperation.
- A "no strings attached" effort to give the receiver something he or she needs.
- An effort to entice the receiver into a relationship of "debt," where the receiver ends up owing something to the giver.
- An effort to humiliate the receiver.
- A way to pressure the receiver into keeping silent, betraying others, giving a particular response, or engaging in other kinds of questionable behaviors.
- An offer with the expectation of sexual favors in return.

MAINTAINING BOUNDARIES IN CRISIS SITUATIONS

In her fascinating article on ethical issues in crisis interventions, Sommers-Flanagan (2007) describes the way crises and disasters raise the emotional intensity of interventions for all involved, and often occur under less scrutiny than interventions in noncrisis situations. Let's examine the possible cross-cultural implications for interviewers in crisis and humanitarian situations.

When in crisis, interviewees may possess lowered psychological defenses, and therefore they behave in unusual ways or reveal information that they would otherwise keep to themselves. While this may fit the interviewer's purposes, we must remember that this person will then have to live with the memory of what was revealed, and perhaps with any material consequences that might result such as ostracism from the community, threats of physical violence, and shame. We should treat the information with appropriate care and confidentiality.

When conducting interviews and interventions in crisis situations, the interviewers often face many of the same stressors as the interviewees and therefore may not be using their best judgment. Although the interviewers are likely to have an easier way out of the crisis context, they are still smelling the same smells and seeing the same sights as the interviewees. It is easy to feel intensely toward the people one is interviewing in a crisis context, mistakenly seeing the person as "all-good," a perfect victim, or as "all-bad," in some way deserving of his or her plight and unworthy of our help. This practice of splitting interviewees into these two distinct and nonoverlapping groups is even more likely to occur if we don't understand the cultures of the people we are interviewing. We may mistake an interviewee's gesture, such as falling upon us crying, as a sexual or romantic overture when it is simply an expression of despair and a desire to reach out to whoever offers support. Sommers-Flanagan admonishes us to resist fantasies that we are rescuers or superheros. I would add cautions about imagining ourselves personally repairing an interviewee's damaged ability to trust, or even taking over the role of spouse, lover, or parent of someone in desperate need. These situations are rife with potential for unethical behavior (e.g., exploitation).

By the same token, we may view an interviewee's gruff response or hostility as a sign that the person is bad, or angry with us specifically, when the person is simply despairing and angry at the world, or suspicious that we represent the same kind of authority that contributed to his or her misery in the first place. We may be insulted and disgusted by an interviewee's apparent lack of gratitude, particularly if we are intervening as an unpaid volunteer. Sometimes people in crisis may appear to us as greedy, when they disparage (or sometimes destroy!) what we have provided for them and demand more or better, or compare what we have provided for them unfavorably with what someone else provided for another person. Sometimes a person in crisis may behave callously or even cruelly to others who are less able to defend themselves, perhaps to the women or children in the family. We must be sure that we do not respond to an interviewee in crisis angrily or punitively or out of a personal need to inflict retribution or suffering. In short, we must not give in to aggressive impulses that may be stimulated by the crisis situation.

The ethical guidelines of our professions or the guidelines conveyed to us by our supervisors or agencies may seem irrelevant in the powerful con-

texts in which we find ourselves. In contexts of crisis and conflict, interviewers and interrogators sometimes forget or ignore essential documents
such as the Geneva Convention. They also sometimes forget their own humanity. Ethical breeches in crisis situations are as egregious as in other circumstances. We need to check in with colleagues, supervisors, and our own
conscience in order to maintain the ethical standards that interviews require of us, even in crisis situations.

CONCLUDING OBSERVATIONS

We want our interviews to be fair and just. How we achieve this is not
straightforward, however. We ourselves are subject to biases, as are our collateral contacts and the interviewees themselves. Stakeholders who have an
interest in the outcome of the interview are unlikely to give us purely objective, unbiased information; thus so we need to take this into account as we
incorporate information from other sources.

Similarly, the appropriate boundaries for the relationship with an interviewee may not always be easy to ascertain. As with all ethical issues, it
is vital to reason clearly by consulting with supervisors, colleagues, and ethical guidelines. When faced with an ethical dilemma, such as the temptation
to violate a professional boundary, it is important to have the integrity to
"do the right thing" even when it may be distasteful, disappointing, or in
some way risky to us. And it is important to document both our thinking
process and the actions taken when considering situations in which ethics
or boundaries are not clear.

These ethical issues of biases and boundaries are especially tricky when
working cross-culturally. We must be vigilant and cautious when these issues arise.

Questions to Think about and Discuss

1. Review the cognitive biases discussed in this chapter: confirmatory bias,
   fundamental attribution error, halo effect, in-group bias, and self-fulfilling prophecies. Discuss a situation in your own personal or professional
   life where you've seen one of these biases emerge.
2. What would you do if an interviewee offered you a gift of a homemade
   cake, for instance, and why? Suppose an interviewee offered you a silver
   key chain?
3. Imagine the following scenario: Steve is a member of your profession
   and is conducting his last interview of the day. The interviewee, who has
   a low income and no easy transportation, asks for a ride home. Steve has

a car. Should Steve give this interviewee a ride home? Why or why not? Which factors should be considered? Does it matter if the interviewee is a young woman or an older man?

RECOMMENDED ADDITIONAL READING

Dana, R. H. (2005). *Multicultural assessment: Principles, applications, and examples.* Mahwah, NJ: Erlbaum.

Sommers-Flanagan, R., & Sommers-Flanagan, J. (2006). *Becoming an ethical helping professional: Cultural and philosophical foundations.* New York: Wiley.

Sue, D. W. (2003). *Overcoming our racism: The journey to liberation.* New York: Jossey-Bass.

Yoshino, K. (2006). *Covering: The hidden assault on our civil rights.* New York: Random House.

4 Setting the Right Tone

*Building Rapport
and Conveying Respect*

Subtleties in the interviewer's tone, attitude, and word choice can make the interviewee feel ashamed, victimized, accused, bullied, humiliated, encouraged, empowered, exonerated, confirmed, or supported. In this chapter I explore ways to make sure the interviewing process results in connection rather than alienation. This will not only make the interview more pleasant but will also increase the amount of accurate information you obtain. Some of our approaches have to change when working across cultures.

Generally, we should minimize any possible aura of invasion or intrusion by paying special attention to our voice, phrasing, and a host of other elements that are discussed in this chapter and Chapter 5 on nonverbal communication. As much as possible, we should allow the respondents to recount and evaluate their experiences in their own way and at their own pace. Our inquiry must affirm the worth and value of the people we're interviewing.

DEMEANOR

The set of nonverbal behaviors that communicates your interest in the interviewee has been termed "attending behaviors" and is discussed in Chapter 5. Certainly, you help establish a relationship with an interviewee through attending behaviors such as making appropriate eye contact, nodding, and leaning forward. But if these actions are imposed too mechanically from the outside without inner feelings, they will be insufficient. Here, I am encouraging you to do more than simply demonstrate certain actions to look "as if" you care. I am encouraging you, rather, to try your best to open your heart and your humanity to the interviewees in front of you so you actually *do* care about their well-being. Whether the interviewee is someone who draws you in or repulses you, the quantity and quality of the information you garner will be improved if you can connect on a level of true feeling.

We continue to build rapport throughout an interview as new topics are raised and the relationship deepens. Many people become cold and distant when they step into their professional roles. I encourage you, instead, to appear warm, relaxed, supportive, and nonjudgmental, particularly in cross-cultural interviews where the interviewee may need substantial reassurance. You will want to communicate that you care, you are interested in what the interviewee has to say, and you can be trusted. You should show the interviewee a personal and specific caring for him or her as an individual, not merely a generalized empathy. This can be achieved by starting meetings with time to socialize, remembering details about interviewees' specific situations, and truly listening to their concerns.

The personal relationship is key to interviewing with people from most cultures. In Korean the concept *jeong* expresses a "combination of empathy, sympathy, compassion, emotional attachment, and tenderness, in varying degrees, according to the social context" (Kim & Ryu, 2005, p. 353). A Korean will be observing an interviewer for signs of *jeong*, which may be demonstrated by showing concern for another person's comfort and by revealing your own humanity. We have no word that is the exact equivalent of *jeong* in English. Regardless, interviewees sense this quality and respond well when it is present.

As an interviewer, you have your own agenda. The interview may be routine for you, or unusually important for some reason. However, try to keep in mind that the interview is apt to be vastly more central to the interviewee's life than to yours. Many interviews portend life-changing repercussions for interviewees, and this can make them frightened, defensive, nervous, angry, or overly compliant. We must take extra care to put interviewees at ease, to increase the likelihood that they will speak with us openly.

GIVING FULL ATTENTION AND TAKING NOTES

How rare it is for people to listen to each other with full attention! So often when we speak to each other in our personal and professional lives, we are doing other tasks at the same time, whether driving, washing dishes, listening to music, checking e-mail, or thinking about our plans for that evening. The formal interview presents the requirement, and opportunity, to pay full attention to the interviewee, to tune into this person with our full being. When we give them our full attention, people are more likely to speak with us openly. (The exception being interviews with young children, who sometimes prefer if we draw with a crayon or in some other way help them feel less "on the spot.")

As much as possible, we should avoid interruptions during interviews. Answering a phone or even checking a cellular phone to see who called, eating your lunch, filing your nails, opening a package of gum, or drinking cold or hot beverages without offering them to the interviewee—all of these interruptions may be considered rude to people from a variety of cultures.

You'll probably want to avoid having a desk between yourself and interviewees, unless you deliberately want to intimidate and distance yourself from them. If you are taking notes, you may wish to sit across the corner of a table. This arrangement allows you to rest your notes on the table, and permits easy eye contact as well as the option of looking away comfortably. Sitting at a table corner is less confrontational than sitting or standing across from interviewees and facing them directly.

If you take notes during your interview you should explain what you are writing and why. You can say, "What you are telling me today is really important. I am writing it down so I won't forget any of it and so I'll remember it all correctly." Especially for people who don't read or write well themselves, the act of taking notes may seem strange and offputting. Interviewees will sometimes want to glance at our notes, even if they cannot read English or decipher our handwriting, just to feel that they have some control. I recommend that we write our notes in such a way that if the person we're interviewing does ask to read them, we can feel comfortable handing over the notes during or after the interview. This degree of transparency requires making sure our notes are written respectfully and accurately. Don't forget that, even in situations in which we are reluctant to hand over our notes, the interviewee could probably, ultimately, have access to them through an attorney.

CONVEYING RESPECT

Experiences with discrimination lead many immigrants and people from ethnic, racial, or religious minority groups to be acutely sensitive to possible demonstrations of disrespect. For example:

There were a small number of Latinos in the elementary school attended by Roberto's son, Carlos. When Roberto arrived at school to pick up Carlos one day, the principal approached him and said, "Oh, you must be Yasmin's father. What a delightful little girl she is!" Roberto politely corrected the principal, but inside he was fuming. He told me later, "That's the problem with sending my son to a school where almost all the kids are White. The staff sees me with brown skin and they assume I must be the father of all the brown-skinned children there. The principal can't even tell the difference between one Latino and another. Yasmin's father is Puerto Rican, I'm Mexican—but to her we're all the same." While some might suggest that Roberto is being overly sensitive here and is responding too harshly to an innocent case of mistaken identity, others will identify with Roberto's sense that some people from the majority culture cannot distinguish among persons from a minority culture, and don't bother to learn who they truly are.

When this kind of experience is repeated over time it can produce a strong response, like an ill-fitting shoe eventually leading to a blister. (People from the majority group infrequently experience situations like this as well, where all "White people" or all blonde and blue-eyed people are assumed to have the same opportunities, attitudes and personalities, which is certainly not the case.) After multiple experiences of being overlooked or discriminated against, some people from minority groups alternate between feeling weary, angry, determined, defensive, and bemused. They bring these feelings with them to subsequent encounters, including our interviews.

People who blend into the majority group and have not experienced discrimination themselves may underestimate how constant, far-reaching, and distressing this discrimination can be. One Puerto Rican psychotherapist described the multiple burdens of her Latino clients in this way:

> The client is responding to a system which is totally unfair, responding to a really unfair and apathetic system in the school—that because he's in bilingual classes, he's stupid. Or because he speaks two languages but he doesn't speak English so well, he's stupid. And so you have to understand that . . . this, too, prevents him from getting ahead. The concept of hope [is difficult], when you have a whole oppressive system on top of you. (cited in Fontes, 1992, p. 68)

Becoming involved with certain agencies is often embarrassing and even humiliating for clients. By doing our utmost to convey respect, we can thwart these feelings of shame and help clients maintain and recover their dignity.

How do we know if we are behaving in a way that is respectful? We pay careful attention to what we say and how we present ourselves, and then we try to figure out how the interviewees hear us. To be able to try on the interviewees' shoes, we need to accept the idea of a mismatch between the way we want to be seen and heard and the image we are actually conveying. We must examine our demeanor when we pose questions, explain procedures, look inside cabinets, search cars, examine injuries, review transcripts, and fill out forms—and we should explore how these activities may feel from the interviewees' perspective. As we catch ourselves conveying any trace of disrespect, we must have the courage to try something new. In our professional roles we may still need to do things that interviewees would rather we did not do, but a respectful manner will make these actions easier to accept.

We should also check in regularly with the people we're interviewing, asking versions of, "How am I doing?" "How is it going?" "Are you okay?"

In most cultures, directions will be better received if they are preceded by a nicety such as "Please," or "Would you please," or "Be kind enough to." Direct orders such as "follow me" or "fill out this form" may be seen as rude and disrespectful. In general, we should go out of our ways to be courteous. In the United States, it is common to reply, "What?" when someone calls our name. For Arabic speakers, this sounds quite rude. In Arabic one replies to the calling of one's name with "Na'ahm" which conveys respect. If we are extra careful to respond politely to someone calling us by name, we might reply with, "Yes, Ms. Johnson?" rather than, "What?"

One Puerto Rican client I interviewed suggested that professionals aim to communicate the following:

> "I'm not here to judge you. I am not God. I am just a human being, just like you are. Whatever you've gone through, I'm here to help. And I'll let you know if I can help and I'll let you know if I can't help, but we'll try. And if we both work at it, we're going to get some place. . . . We have to both be together and be honest with each other, not try to pull one over on the other."

COUNTERACTING SHAME

While minority group characteristics are a source of pride at some moments, they can be a source of shame at others. "Rejection of who we are is a pressure we feel in all encounters," writes a Pakistani psychotherapist about the experience of "immigrant women of color" in Canada (Javed, 1995, p. 18). Shame is thought to have two components, the feeling of lack of *self*-worth and the feeling of lack of worth *in others' eyes* (social worth).

Members of ethnic and religious minority groups typically feel empowered by their identities in some contexts and delighted to be from cultures that are distinct from the mainstream. However, most members of minority groups have also experienced moments when they were shamed by others for not conforming to the dominant ideal. An African American student told me about the first racial incident she could remember, when a White kindergartener refused to hold her hand because it was brown. At the age of 6, my daughter was approached by another 6-year-old and told, "I don't want to hurt your feelings, but if you don't start believing in Jesus Christ you're going to go to hell." These instances get tucked away into a well of shame inside members of oppressed groups. Additional shaming experiences, like being followed by security guards in the supermarket or getting harassed or teased by classmates or coworkers, can bring this shame to the surface.

Numerous writers from ethnic minority cultures have described feelings of shame related to the negative connotations attached to their skin color, hair texture, eye shape, social status, accent, or name. In her novel about a Korean adoptee's search for her birth mother, for instance, Lee (2005) described endless taunting by Minnesota schoolmates including children pulling their eyes to the side and saying, "Chinese, Japanese, Dirty Knees," "Ching-Chong Chinaman," and other insults (p. 18). The protagonist wanted so much to blend in with her Minnesota classmates, she was shocked at times to see herself in a mirror and rediscover that she did not have blonde wavy hair.

In another example, let us consider all the layers of shame that might be experienced by a low-income Mexican American man:

> Diego has family members who are undocumented, and he lives in fear that their status might be discovered. He knows that his skin color, his accent, and his country of origin make him a target for members of certain groups. His dark hair and his short stature mark him as different from others. He works as a painter; and his clothes and hands often reveal his trade, which embarrasses him—he takes pride in dressing up neatly whenever he can. He finished high school in Mexico but was never able to resume schooling in the United States, so he feels ashamed when he returns to Mexico and meets with his former classmates who now have professional jobs. He wants to make sure his children attend college, and so he sends them to a parochial school,

and he knows they are ashamed to reveal his profession to their class-mates.

When antiforeigner sentiment intensifies, as it does from time to time, Diego is called names on the street and he's even had people spit at him. If he is involved with social service agencies, the police, or even medical professionals related to certain problems, he may feel shame around these issues as well. We need to understand and work through many layers of shame before we can expect Diego to reveal himself openly to us in an interview.

To counteract shame, we must welcome all facets of Diego's self into our interview. Through our demeanor we tell Diego that he is welcome. We let him know that we value his bilingualism, and that we do not think he is stupid if he misuses an English word. We inter-act with him so as to counteract his shame, and in no way do contrib-ute to it.

VOICE QUALITY, TONE, SPEED, AND VOLUME

In people who are right-handed, the left hemisphere of the brain hears words while the right side hears the melody of the words (Givens, 2005). Therefore, when we speak we are literally speaking to two different aspects of the listener's brain—one that processes our word meanings and the other that processes our voice quality and nonverbal signals. A pleasantly pitched and modulated voice communicates kindliness to one side of the inter-viewee's brain while our words communicate it to the other.

Around the world, people tend to use higher-pitched voices and speak in a sweet, sing-song manner with children when they are not angry. This language, "motherese," is considered friendly and would be appropriate with a young child. A sweet voice with a varying tone suggests that the in-terviewer does not have aggressive intentions. However, interviewers should be careful not to speak in this way to teens and adults—it could be consid-ered condescending.

Interviewers who speak in a dry, steady monotone may be perceived as unfriendly, cold, and intimidating:

> Devoid of inflection, a monotonal voice sounds unenthusiastic and bored.
> A loud voice sounds domineering and pushy. A tense voice sounds frus-trated, angry and rude. . . . Use the light voice to sound like you care.
> (Givens, 2005, pp. 85–86)

How you use your voice goes a long way to convey caring in a professional relationship. In most circumstances, you will want to use a gentle but firm voice. However, if the interviewee is extremely anxious you may choose to use a soothing voice; if the interviewee looks volatile you may choose to emphasize stability and calm by speaking in a steady way.

Listen to video- or audiotapes of your interviews from time to time and pay attention to what you really sound like during the process. Did the interviewee have to strain to hear because you were speaking so quietly? Were you speaking so loudly that you seemed to frighten or intimidate the interviewee? Was it hard to make out your words because you were mumbling, held your hand in front of your face, or were chewing gum? Was your voice kind and sympathetic? Did it convey support? If the person hesitated to talk, did you respond patiently to encourage more responsiveness, or were you impatient, threatening, pushy or dismissive? If the person was not a native speaker of English, should you have used an interpreter (see Chapter 7, "The Interpreted Interview"). If the person seemed to struggle with English words, did you use simple language but avoid sounding condescending?

A supportive tone of voice will encourage the interviewee to reveal sensitive information and cooperate with official systems. A critical or impatient tone can make an interviewee shut down emotionally and close the door to further intervention. (I may be especially sensitive to these issues, not only because of my exposure to people who are not native speakers of English but also because I have family members who are hard of hearing. Acquiring good speaking habits will improve our professional work with people who are hard of hearing, too.)

When we don't understand a language, it is common to think that it is spoken more quickly than our own language, as in the frequently heard comment in the United States, "Those people speak [Spanish] so quickly!" However, research shows that speed and slowness vary little according to the language. They are determined more by the emotions of the moment and the requirements of the situation (Roach, 1998).

Languages that are more guttural (such as Arabic, German, Dutch, and some East Asian tongues) can sound "harsh" or "unpleasant" to the unaccustomed ear (Giles & Niedzielski, 1998). Some languages such as Chinese and Vietnamese are tonal; the meaning of the word varies with its pitch. Speakers of guttural and tonal languages are often misperceived by English speakers to be angry because of the way they use their voices. Similarly, male speakers of Arabic and some African languages often sound as if they are yelling angrily because they tend to speak loudly. This may be true whether they are speaking in their first language or in English, as many people import the intonation and volume of their first language into the other languages they learn. An interviewer who is not accustomed to these language habits may find herself responding to an Arabic-speaking person as if he is angry, out of control, or aggressive, when that may not be the case. Ethiopians, East Indians, Filipinos, Bangladeshis, Pakistanis, and many American Indians are apt to speak softly and interpret as rude a person who uses a loud voice or who issues a loud direct command.

Italians, Greeks, Israelis, Puerto Ricans, Dominicans, Cubans, Brazilians, Poles, Jews, Arabs, and African Americans often engage in loud, animated, and passionate conversations. They may appear to outsiders to be volatile, antagonistic, or threatening when they are simply engaged in lively conversation. We should consider body language and the context and content of a conversation before making inferences as to a person's intent based on his or her speaking tone, volume, or expressiveness. To people from cultures that are accustomed to high levels of emotionalism, the "level-headedness" of the majority culture in the United States, Canada, England, and Northern Europe may be misinterpreted as a lack of interest or involvement.

Ethnic differences in the use of the voice can lead to misunderstandings in professional situations:

A White psychotherapist from a rather prim New England family told me recently about her early work with an African American family. She said she was constantly asking them to calm down and lower their voices. During the third session, the mother finally turned to her and said, "This is how we talk. Do you *mind*?" The therapist said she realized that she had been reading too much into the loud and passionate speech and, having perceived it as a threat, felt it as her duty to "contain" the family. She learned to become tuned in to her own responses and to suppress the ethnocentric ones. She has been working successfully with the family in the year since then. She says they continue to speak loudly in session, even when they are happy and enjoying each other, and will turn to her sometimes playfully and say, "Are we too loud for you today, Miss?"

Tone of voice and volume may also vary by gender. Women in France use a much higher pitch than women in the United States or Canada. This is not due to a difference in vocal chords but, rather, a product of social training. Among West Indians and Japanese, women in particular are expected to use a soft, nonassertive tone of voice. This can be tricky for women who are in a position of authority and feel a need to assert their influence but who do not wish to appear hostile. Women's deference to men is built into Japanese language, in that Japanese women use the same forms of speech with men as children use with adults.

PACE AND TIME

As much as possible, the interviewee should be allowed to set the pace; and we should listen for the interviewee's speaking rhythm. Often people need more time to answer questions than we might expect. People who are not native speakers of English but who are being interviewed in English may take longer than usual to respond as they search for the right words. This is likely to be true even if they have been speaking English for years, especially if they use their first language more often than English (Heredia & Brown, 2004) (see Chapter 8 on reluctance for a more complete discussion of pauses, hesitations, and silence in interviews).

For some people, the quality of an interaction is partly determined by the amount of time spent together. "The more time something takes, the better it always is," writes Koul (2002, p. 69), about beliefs in the Kashmir. Southern Europeans and Latin Americans who are less acculturated may spend quite a while in an interview telling stories and elaborating at length. They are apt to be angered by professionals who show impatience. One Puerto Rican woman who had been in psychotherapy with two different clinicians described sessions in this way:

> I felt so uncomfortable in that place, it's not funny, because she was working with papers and looking at the watch, the clock, doing some other things while I'm talking. "Go ahead! Keep on! Keep on talking!" And it made me feel like I had to constantly say something so I don't stay quiet, and her doing all the stuff instead of giving me her undivided attention. . . . Another time I had a man and it seemed like he was more interested in the time of when to end. . . . He kept looking at his watch . . . And boy, I would bawl my eyes out. . . . "Time's up!" . . . you have to give the person time. You can't rush things in. . . . I felt like I was rushed. They wanted to know the problem right away and try to figure out what to do next. (cited in Fontes, 1992, pp. 52–53)

I know it is difficult to avoid rushing or appearing rushed if you are constrained by large caseloads, deadlines, productivity quotas, busy schedules, or the pressures of managed care. Taking your time at the beginning of an interview to establish the relationship may help build the sense of trust that will make a bit of rushing later on seem less problematic. To accommodate the more relaxed sense of time of people from all cultures other than Northern Europe, the United States, and Canada, many professionals schedule longer sessions with their immigrant clients, particularly early in the course of their work together.

Sometimes you will find yourself needing to limit the speech of a particularly voluble interviewee. Among the many tactful ways to do this, I hope you can find one that fits your style. Possibilities include:

- "Because we don't have a lot of time today, I'm going to have to focus our conversation a bit."
- "I can see this is important to you. Maybe we can speak more about that later."
- "Does that fit in with what we were talking about, or is this a different direction?"
- "Let me return to . . . "
- "I want to make sure we at least touch on all the important topics today. Please forgive me if I ask you to fast forward to . . . "
- "I see we only have 15 minutes left, and I . . . "

Some conflicts over time can be avoided if you clarify explicitly the time constraints at the beginning of the interview. For example, "We'll have 45 minutes to talk today, but we can schedule another appointment if we need to," or "This process usually takes about 2 hours. Does that work for you?" You can also set up the expectations by saying something like, "I am going to be asking you a lot of questions today, and sometimes I might have to interrupt you so I can be sure to cover all the areas we need to cover. I hope I won't hurt your feelings if I do that." It is important to remember, however, that people from many cultures talk in more of a roundabout way than the linear kinds of conversations usually heard in Western industrialized countries. It would be a shame to interrupt what appears to be a digression if—in fact—the interviewee was making his or her best effort to answer the question posed.

Developing a trusting relationship with an interviewee from a culture different from your own may take more time and effort than usual. It may first require talking about family, or about practical issues and concerns that are not related specifically to the explicit content of the interview.

JOINING WITH ALL MEMBERS OF THE FAMILY

In most families, it will be helpful to honor the hierarchy by first greeting the older members of the family (parents or perhaps even grandparents) and then asking them to introduce the children (see the section on greetings in Chapter 5 on nonverbal communication). Often, it is helpful to acknowledge the father first.[1]

As you observe your clients in the waiting room and as you build rapport at the beginning of an interview, you will be assessing the interviewees' baseline demeanor—the gestures, postures, and ways of speaking that you observe while they are relatively relaxed. This baseline demeanor is helpful so you can note any significant changes that occur once the more stressful part of the interview begins. People who are restless or tense by temperament may fidget constantly. If these are constant habits, they should not be mistaken for indicators of deception or stress.

WHAT'S IN A NAME?: ADDRESSING PEOPLE APPROPRIATELY

Generally, when speaking with adults, we should address them by their last names, as Mr. or Ms. X, rather than assuming the familiarity of using first names. Particularly when working with older people who are from an oppressed group, such as African Americans, the familiarity of the first name might seem like an insult. For generations in the United States, White people addressed Black people by their first names while expecting to be addressed as "Sir," "Ma'am," or "Miss" in return. Therefore, adult African Americans are apt to feel insulted when professionals use first names with them without prior permission. And, finally, many women feel insulted when male professionals call them by their first names while introducing themselves by their last name—the women find this demeaning.

As egalitarian as we may try to be, the interviewer is the one who holds the power in the encounter. This reminds me of when I saw my new dentist for the first time. He is a relatively young man who—without asking my permission—started calling me by my first name. He shook my hand and said, "Hi Lisa, I'm Dr. Carver." This imbalance in forms of address felt demeaning and I was already intimidated enough just by being there! He held the potential to inflict pain on me, so I did not argue with his presentation,

---

[1]In some cultural groups, such as among the Amish, female professionals will be considered disrespectful if they address adult male family members directly. Men will typically attend important family meetings with their wives and children but if the professional is female, they may "watch over" the session, rather than participate actively. Conversely, among the Amish it would be considered inappropriate for a male professional to address a woman without her husband present. In this topic, as in so many others, true familiarity with the culture enables us to figure out the appropriate way to proceed.

although I thought, "We can be Dr. Carver and Dr. Fontes, or Lisa and Sam." The people we work with may feel the same way. We can ask to be addressed by our first names, if we so choose, but we should not assume this familiarity with adult clients unless they indicate that they, too, would like to be addressed by their first name. Even some young adults would rather not be addressed by their first name until they have given permission for this. Eighteen-year-old Cindy told me: "When the doctor called me by my first name the first time I met him, I thought he was being less respectful toward me because I'm young. I didn't like that but what could I do? He's the doctor."

We need to find out what specific names the clients want us to use. Many Spanish, Portuguese, Italian, and Southern United States names are double names, such as María Teresa, José Antonio, or Mary Sue. My eldest daughter's name is Ana Lua, and she introduces herself this way. When an adult replies with "Hi Ann" or "Annie" she feels cut off from this person— who didn't really bother to listen to her name or try to get it right.

Of course, many people are called by their nickname—but others despise the shortened versions of their names. Don't call William "Bill" unless you're sure he wants this. Make sure you address people in their preferred way, saying the name a few times if necessary until you can pronounce it correctly. Spanish, Portuguese, Polish, and other Slavic languages allow for a wide variety of nicknames derived from the original names, each with a different flavor. For example, in Portuguese Roberto can become Robertinho (little Roberto), Robertão (big Roberto), Beto, Robi, and so on. If you hear a nickname being used by a family member, check in with the person before you also use that name, lest you inadvertently call the person by an inappropriate moniker.

Chinese, Bangladeshi, and some other Asian names begin with the surname and end with what is called the "first name" in the West. So someone whose name is written Lo En Chen should be addressed as Mrs. Lo—not necessarily what you'd expect. Recording names improperly can lead to myriad problems in tracking people's identities and helping them obtain the benefits to which they're entitled. Do your best to ascertain through questions and documents the correct order of the person's name and the correct spelling.

In Russian and other Slavic cultures, names may have different endings depending on whether the person is male or female. However, some Slavic families have adopted the naming traditions of their new countries and have dropped the gendered endings on their names. It can be hard for people who are less familiar with the culture to keep all this straight. It's important to be aware of these possibilities and try our best.

Somalis and some other Muslim Africans usually name their children 3 days after birth. Somalis usually have three names: a given name followed by the father's given name and then the grandfather's. However, after immigrating most have adopted the English-speaking tradition of using their given name as their first name, the father's name as their middle name, and their grandfather's name as their last name. Somalis have one limited pool for all three names, so the same name could serve as a first, middle, or last name (Mohamed Ali Hassan or Hassan Mohamed Ali or Ali Hassan Mohamed or Ali Hassan Ali, etc.). With so few names to choose from, in any Somali community you will encounter numerous people with the same names. This can be a logistical challenge for organizations that are trying to distinguish among the Somalis with whom they work. Somali women do not change their name at marriage. Somalis who were conceived out of wedlock may have only one name because they have not been given a father's surname. A child without a recognized father is considered a disgrace, so the question of names becomes a sensitive one. Somali women whose children are a product of rape may assign their children a last name and claim to be widows to protect their own and their children's standing in the community. In an exception to the rule stated earlier about calling people by their last name plus an honorific, Somalis are apt to prefer being called by their first name—their given name—which they think of as their own name, as their last name is likely to be their grandfather's name and in their culture serves to identify "their roots" rather than themselves. As with everyone else, when in doubt, ask Somalis how they would like to be addressed.

PROFESSIONAL TITLES

In countries as diverse as Nigeria and Ecuador, it's especially important to greet someone (and particularly a man) by his professional title. So, for instance, if James Oyenike is a teacher he probably prefers to be greeted as "Professor Oyenike" rather than "Mr. Oyenike" or "James." And if Margarita Dávila has her bachelor's degree, she might prefer to be greeted as *licenciada Dávila* rather than Margarita. Titles in other countries may include some that are less common in the United States, such as attorney, chief, professor, officer, engineer, teacher, and nurse. In some parts of the world, to show respect and deference one might even exaggerate the other's title in greeting. So, for instance, although Pedro Neto has not yet finished his doctorate, his university students in Portugal are apt to call him *Doutor Profesor* Neto. It is better to err in the direction of assuming people have a higher status than they do, rather than the reverse. That is, assume that the Filipina woman one meets in the hospital is a physician rather than an aide.

Of course, you can always ask someone politely, "What is your position here?" if you are uncertain.

This inflation or exaggeration of titles can be awkward for professionals who are unaccustomed to this. For instance, a dental hygienist, a nurse, a physical therapist, a psychology intern, and a clinical social worker might all be regularly called "Dr. ____" by their patients and clients from Latin America, even though they have explained more than once that they are not doctors. Correct the person upon the first use, and at any other time when you feel he or she may be truly attributing to you more expertise than you have. In other situations, accept the honorific gracefully, as a sign of respect for your knowledge and status. Remember, too, sometimes people may call you "Doctor" or "professor" or "officer" because they don't remember your name!

In the Philippines, formal titles persist even after more personalized and informal relationships have been established (Santos & Chan, 2004, p. 328). That is, a physician will be called Dr. Ramos and a nurse will be called Nurse Ramírez even after they have become friendly with another person, in contrast to the United States where people move rapidly toward a first-name basis.

SAVING AND LOSING FACE

The twin concepts of "saving" and "losing" face may be difficult to grasp for people who are not familiar with East Asian cultures. These ideas have been exoticized as an exaggerated form of pride, or an excuse to become quick to anger. In Korean, the central concept is called *chae-myun*, and it "protects the dignity, honor, and self respect of the individual and family" (Kim & Ryu, 2005, p. 356). To protect the interviewer's *chae-myun*, a Korean will refrain from challenging or directly questioning the professional. Reciprocally, interviewers must attempt to avoid making the interviewee lose face by avoiding nonverbal behavior or challenging, confronting, or commenting in a way that could be interpreted as criticism or lack of respect. This will be especially true when interviewing Korean men, and it is not always easy to achieve. Tact is key.

In Western industrialized nations, being direct and assertive is considered a virtue. In Asia, behaving in this way may be seen as threatening group cohesion and as evidence of a lack of control and even bad character. Conversely:

> What appears as passivity or critical lack of assertiveness from an American viewpoint carries with it in many East Asian contexts a whole palette of

> highly positive associations, including intelligence, flexibility, managing
> face, cooperativeness, caring, and maturity. (Kim & Markus, 2002, p. 440)

Concerns about losing face will make some Asian interviewees initially hesitate to reveal information about problem areas. Chan and Lee (2004) recommend a circular approach in which the professional establishes mutual trust and respect and attends to small details that demonstrate genuine concern for the individual or family's well-being. This humanized relationship provides the setting in which a traditional Asian interviewee may be more comfortable discussing sensitive material (see Chapter 8 on overcoming reluctance).

Once a person's "face" has been breached, it can be difficult or impossible to recover within that relationship. On one unfortunate occasion I caused a neighbor to lose face in way that permanently damaged our relationship:

> My family and I lived in university housing along with many other young families from around the world. New neighbors from China moved into the next apartment. I went over to their door and welcomed them with a plate of cookies, noticing that they had just moved from the mainland and did not speak much English. The next day, they appeared at my door with a platter with a big steak on it. Being from a culture that emphasizes direct communication and frankness, I thanked them profusely for the steak but told them that my family did not eat meat. That was a big mistake! I had rejected their food—essentially communicating that their food was not good enough for me. They never spoke to me or my family again—I had caused them to lose face.

Traditional Asian interviewees may hesitate to choose an alternative or may postpone making a decision because of their anxiety about committing a social blunder that could result in their "losing face." When given options, a traditional Asian interviewee may seek the option that the professional seems to value most, looking for external clues as to the "right" course of action rather than turning inward to determine which path feels best (Chan & Lee, 2004).

Interviewers from societies where questions of shame and saving face are central may need to be vigilant about a possible tendency to "overprotect" interviewees by not inquiring about sensitive topics. As always, the desire to be tactful and respectful needs to be balanced with the value of certain information for the interview referral question.

Simply being involved in many of the systems where interviews are conducted causes interviewees to lose face. For example, interviews by police, social workers, physicians, and other health workers are often about topics that are shameful or might cause an interviewee to lose face. Even a job interview could be a challenge to the face of a Chinese man if—for instance—he was a physician in his home country and is seeking a job as a janitor in his new land. Certain kinds of questions increase the shame of some Asian interviewees and might cause them to lose face, such as questions about sexuality, certain diseases, finances, literacy, and so on (see Chapter 8 on addressing reluctance). The response to losing face can be anger, shame, resistance, or even suicide in extreme cases.

In a vivid article on a Korean woman's experience processing a rape in psychotherapy, Chan (1999) describes the shame the client, Kaya, felt revealing her experiences to the therapist, who was a Chinese American woman. She also describes the importance of addressing issues of shame and "face."

> I asked Kaya whether she felt as though she had lost face with me through relaying her experiences. She said she did not know since she was not sure that I could fully understand what losing face meant to her. I assured her that I understood the concept well, having been trained by my own family to act as honorably as possible and to avoid losing face and embarrassing the family at all costs. Kaya expressed relief that my cultural experiences enabled me to understand how much she feared losing face, as well as her reason for not revealing the incident to anyone else. When I told Kaya that my image of her had not been diminished in any way by her [rape] experience . . . she was somewhat taken aback. It was at these times that I understood my role as a therapist for Kaya and other Asian Americans to be a type of bridge between cultures. (p. 82)

Around a wide variety of topics, there is great potential for feelings of shame to enter, inhibit, and distort an interview. How we handle the shame issues may determine the success of the interview.

QUESTIONS ALSO SET THE TONE

It is not every question that deserves an answer.
            —PUBLILIUS SYRUS

Most interviews begin with asking questions; yet we rarely consider the overwhelming impact of the questions themselves. Whatever our intentions, questions are not neutral. Questions convey values and exert influence. Questions establish the professional relationship. They determine the scope of the discussion: what topics will be included or excluded. Questions establish power relations. They determine the exact nature of "the problem" and how you and the interviewee will refer to it. Questions embody intentions, and they arise from certain assumptions (Tomm, 1988).

Clearly, the questions we ask throughout an interview will depend, in large part, on the purpose and context of the interview and the age of the interviewee. The initial questions may range from those that appear to require a simple answer (e.g., "How old are you?") to slightly more complicated ones, (e.g., "How are you feeling today?") to ones that may require the interviewee to make some complex decisions before responding (e.g., "How would you describe yourself?").

Questions are a particular way to obtain information in an interview but certainly are not the only method. Posing questions is a directive mode of communicating because questions tell the interviewee what to talk about at that moment. When you ask a question, you are taking control of the conversation (Sommers-Flanagan & Sommers-Flanagan, 2003). In some circumstances, this may be desirable. For instance, sometimes you'll need detailed information about a particular issue at a given time, or sometimes you'll want to limit the ramblings of a particularly verbose interviewee. Questions are a way of focusing an interview, or a portion of an interview.

Questions can also be comforting to a person in crisis. I worked on a psychiatric crisis team early in my career. My supervisor suggested that asking very detailed questions about a person's symptoms, thoughts, behaviors, and feelings would be reassuring—just as it can be reassuring when a physician asks detailed questions during a medical consultation. It conveys that the professional will be able to determine what is wrong and provide some relief. Asking detailed questions and listening carefully to the answers also conveys to the interviewee that you are paying close attention.

Questions are sometimes problematic in interviews, however, because when one question is posed after another, they can make interviewees feel as if they are being interrogated. Questions also place the interviewee in the passive position of being the provider of information that will then be collected and acted upon by the interviewer. This passivity may be advantageous in certain circumstances such as the emergency assessment discussed previously, where a person in crisis needs to know that he or she will be kept safe. However, inducing passivity in an interviewee can be highly undesirable in other situations. For instance, if you are conducting psychiatric or educational assessments and you begin the process with many focused questions, interviewees are apt to appear quite passive and may not be able to demonstrate their full capacity for initiative, curiosity, and resourcefulness. Or, if you begin a psychotherapeutic relationship with a client with many questions, you may be inducing an attitude in your clients of, "Okay, Dr., *you* tell me what to do, then."

One psychology professor I know challenged his interns to conduct entire intake interviews without a single question. The students became fluent in other, less formal ways of gathering information, such as, "So your doctor suggested that you come see me," instead of "Why did your doctor suggest that you come see me" and "I notice you're looking somewhat sad as you discuss your children" rather than "How do you feel about your children?" These are sometimes called *implied* or *indirect* questions, and they can seem less pushy and interrogatory than direct questions.

Sometimes we are tempted to deviate from our usual interview process because of a hunch or an instinct that tells us to pursue a new topic. We must be careful here, because asking questions impulsively may lead us into areas that are unethical or—to put it plainly—simply none of our business.

Types of Questions[2]

Question type	Example	Goal	Cultural comments
Indirect or implied	1. Some children feel nervous when they meet with me. 2. You said you witnessed a mugging.	Helps person relax, normalizes feelings, encourages discussion of the situation.	If people seem to need more direction, follow up with, "Please tell me about. . . . "
Grand tour	1. Tell me about coming to the United States. 2. What do I need to know about you?	Opens up a broad area of discussion, encourages interviewee's own words and concepts.	Grand tour questions can teach a great deal about the interviewee's perspective and priorities.
Hypothetical	1. Imagine that your problem is solved . . . 2. If you had a magic wand . . .	Invites interviewee to imagine a particular outcome or to express desired outcome.	Can be tricky for people who don't speak English well or for people with developmental delays.
Questions about change	1. How did his death change you? 2. Is that different from the way you responded in the past?	Provides information about prior functioning. Reminds interviewee that things were different at one time and that change is part of life.	People who do not speak English well may have difficulty with the verb tenses.

Presupposing questions	1. In what ways do you feel at home in school? 2. How has drinking alcohol impacted you? 3. How will this new job change you?	Avoids negation. May be seen as leading in forensic contexts.	It is important not to engage in ethnic or social class presuppositions (e.g., to assume that everyone celebrates Christmas or has his or her own bedroom).
Categorizing questions	1. What kinds of friends do you have? 2. What kinds of things do you do on the weekend?	Shows how the interviewee sorts out his or her world into categories.	How people sort their world can reveal fascinating cultural information.
Compare and contrast	1. What's different about living here compared to X? 2. In what ways are your sons different from each other?	Elicits comparisons.	Can be helpful for establishing differences in cultural norms. People may hesitate to say negative things about your culture or country if they're afraid they'll hurt your feelings.
Illustrative examples	1. Describe a time when . . . 2. Give me an example of that . . .	Invites interviewee to discuss specific and concrete occurrences.	Requesting details in this way can help you understand people's lives better.
Illustrative extremes	1. What was most difficult about . . . ? 2. Describe the best . . . 3. Tell me about the worst incident.	Uncovers the limits or range of certain behaviors or situations.	If you ask about negative extremes, be prepared for information that may upset you and the interviewee.
Present	1. How are we doing? 2. What are you feeling right now?	Elicits information about the interview process. Shows interest in the person's current state.	Important to assess the interview process as it proceeds so you can make adjustments.
Future	1. What would you like to happen next? 2. What will this look like a year from now? 3. How will you feel about this in 10 years?	Assesses person's future orientation and plans. Emphasizes possibility of change. Helps client put events into perspective.	Helps you understand the implications of an event for a person. Allows person to define next steps and alerts you to possible outcomes.

Controversial	1. I'm going to ask you a difficult question . . . 2. Some people might say . . .	Opens up difficult areas and can provoke a strong response.	Use caution with these questions if you're not familiar with the culture. These could be offensive.

[2] Thanks to Gretchen Rossman for sharing her insights on interviewing.

If we are seen as prying unnecessarily or overly curious, we may damage our working alliance with an interviewee. For instance, we might be tempted to inquire about a person mentioned by an interviewee because we think we may know him or her, or we may tempted to ask more questions about sexuality than we need to ask because we find it exciting, or we may want to ask about a cultural practice because we're curious, although it has no bearing on the interview. We must be sure we are asking questions to accomplish our professional goals and with concern for the interviewee—not to satisfy our own interest.

Sometimes interviewees think we are asking questions for our own prurient reasons when, in fact, there is a rationale. Prefacing our questions with, "Now I'm going to ask you about X because . . . " may help interviewees understand our motives.

Questions should be seen as one technique among many for soliciting information. In most interview situations, questions will be among your very best and most essential tools. In this next section we look at ways to begin interviews that maximize the free exchange of information.

Narrative Training

Forensic interviewing specialists recommend that we engage in what they call "narrative training" from the beginning of an interview. This means using open-ended questions from the outset to train the respondent to provide narrative responses, rather than responding with just one word or very short answers. In typical interviews the first questions often elicit short-answers. They may be yes or no questions, such as, "Are you John Smith?"; short answer questions, such as, "How long have you been living in Orangetown?"; or option-posing questions, such as, "Would you say you feel very happy, happy, or not at all happy"? By opening the interview with these kinds of questions we are in effect training interviewees to provide us with short answers; and they may have trouble switching to longer narratives later when we say, for example, "Tell me everything that happened on Thursday night," or "How would you say you're doing in school?"

With narrative training you are encouraged to take advantage of the early part of an interview to help the interviewee get accustomed to giving longer narratives. For instance, you can say, "Please tell me about your family," or "What brings you here today?" rather than asking more close-ended questions. Research demonstrates the effectiveness of this approach with children and teens (Orbach & Lamb, 2000). By beginning with open-ended questions that elicit a longer narrative, you are alerting the interviewee to the preferred pattern of responding for the interview.

Eliciting Free Narratives

Perhaps the most extensive research on interviewing has been conducted in the forensic context of interviewing children about possible sexual abuse. These interviews yield testimony that is often vital to court cases, and therefore numerous aspects of how to obtain the most accurate details have been studied. This research offers lessons that I believe are relevant to other contexts and to interviewing adults as well. Unfortunately, little of this forensic interviewing research has focused on cultural issues.

The literature on forensic interviewing of children suggests that if you are hoping to elicit the interviewee's version of events, to hear the interviewee talk about a sexual assault, for instance, you will probably want to begin by asking "general" or "invitational" questions that elicit a "free narrative." When you ask a broad, open-ended question in this way, the information is likely to come from the interviewee's own mind and experience—it has not been suggested by the interviewer (Saywitz, Goodman, & Lyon, 2002). An example of a general question is, "Is there something I can help you with?" or "Do you know why you are here today?" An invitational question is just slightly more specific, in that it assumes that there may be an event or experience. An example of an invitational question is, "I heard something may have happened to you. Please tell me everything you remember about it." In a medical interview context, a general question would be, "Tell me about your health." An invitational question would be, "What brings you here today?"

Proponents of narrative interviewing suggest that the perspective of interviewees is best revealed when they are allowed to use their own spontaneous language to discuss their situations (Bauer, 1996). To do this, we will want to pull ourselves out of the interview as much as possible by asking questions in such a way that interviewees will begin to speak out in their own words—creating a "free narrative." That is, we allow the interviewee to speak with as little prompting as possible. Asking broader questions and allowing time for a long answer enables interviewees to speak without having their thoughts interrupted or sidetracked by us. Later, when the general outline has been gathered, we will probably need to fill in the blanks with more focused questions. (Open-ended questions may not be effective with young children, with people who have developmental disabilities, or with people who are too intimidated to speak freely. See Chapter 8 on overcoming reluctance for more information on these topics.)

Encouraging a free narrative may be especially important when working with people who are not accustomed to speaking freely and openly for long periods of time. In many cultures people do less speaking, in general, than in Western industrialized nations, and particularly in the United States. Also, in most cultures people in subordinate positions, such as women, children, and people with a low income or social status, do less speaking when meeting with people of a more dominant status. If your interview is contradicting these norms, it is important to set up clear expectations from the get-go. However, we should also be careful not to push people into speaking in a way that is uncomfortable for them. If our efforts at eliciting a free narrative fail, we can switch to more focused and direct questions.

CONCLUDING OBSERVATIONS

We set the foundation for a successful interview at the beginning, by making clear the process and goals of the interview. The more information you can provide about the context of the communication, the better it will be for the interviewee. In simple terms, tell the interviewees about the role and position of the interviewer and how the information will be used. Tell them as much as you can about the procedures governing the conversation, such as the time frame and expectations. Let them know if this is a one-time interview or the beginning of a long-standing relationship. Allow them to ask you questions.

We build rapport with interviewees by addressing them appropriately, conveying respect, speaking with them in a welcoming tone of voice, and choosing our questions carefully. Of course, a respectful atmosphere is not limited to the first few minutes of an interview or the first session, if there will be more. Rather, respect must be sustained over time through listening compassionately, keeping your word (don't promise what you cannot deliver), and allowing interviewees to establish the pace of the interview as much as possible. Show that you are listening to and remember what the person said, by returning to topics discussed earlier, where this is appropriate. Demonstrate appreciation of the person's language and cultural traditions, where you can, and try to engage in appropriate nonverbal behavior (discussed in the next chapter). Once the groundwork for a productive interview relationship has been established, the next steps will be easier to construct.

Questions to Think about and Discuss

1. You are about to interview a Pakistani father, mother, and two children in your office. Describe three things you will to do to convey respect.
2. Why is it important to convey respect in interviews? How does it help you achieve your goals as an interviewer?
3. From the paperwork you have been given, you are not sure which is the first, last, or middle name of the person you are about to interview. How will you know how to address him or her? What might you say?
4. What are some steps you can take early in an interview to encourage an interviewee to speak freely?

RECOMMENDED ADDITIONAL READING

For this topic, reading about the specific cultures whose members you are going to work with may prove especially helpful. The following books provide information about people from a variety of specific cultures (divided by chapter):

Boyd-Franklin, N. (2003). *Black families in therapy* (2nd ed.). New York: Guilford Press.

Falicov, C. J. (1998). *Latino families in therapy.* New York: Guilford Press.

Lee, E. (1997). *Working with Asian Americans: A guide for clinicians.* New York: Guilford Press.

5 Beyond Words
Nonverbal Communication in Interviews

Juan looks up in the waiting room when his name is called. The interviewer, Linda, introduces herself, smiles, and motions for Juan to follow her. Chances are that before they have even entered the interview room they have sized each other up. They have evaluated each other's body language, appearance, manner of speaking, and way of relating. They have noticed and unconsciously processed each others' "aroma cues" if any are readily apparent; these are scents including the odors of the body, food, alcohol, cigarettes, perfume, and aftershave. Juan and Linda may have formed some kind of opinion about whether the other is kind or unfriendly, passive or assertive, or masculine or feminine. Based on their initial impression, they may have reached some tentative conclusion about whether the interview will be a pleasure or a chore, and whether it is likely to have a favorable outcome.

As a result of various biases discussed in Chapter 3, a subtle nonverbal cue that makes us like or dislike a person, and makes the person like or dislike us, can be amplified over the course of an interview and serve as a filter to future information. Ultimately, a minor detail that may not even have reached a conscious level of awareness can influence the course of the interview and the subsequent report far more than it should. If we can become aware of these nonverbal signals—both those we transmit and those we receive—we are far less likely to allow them to influence us unduly.

When the interviewer and interviewee come from different cultures, these cues may be misinterpreted in both directions, sometimes making it difficult to exchange information accurately, and often preventing the creation of a solid working relationship. Learning how to convey accurate and appropriate nonverbal communication may be best absorbed by living on a daily basis with people from the culture in question; through intensive observation of habits and protocols in a variety of situations. Of course, when we work with multicultural populations, such immersion in each culture is likely to be impossible.

This chapter will help you understand nonverbal communication in the interview setting with people from a variety of cultural groups. It will improve your ability to convey what you want through nonverbal channels such as gestures, posture, and touch. It will also help you understand others' nonverbal signals. And, finally, by bringing this realm into greater awareness, it will help you avoid misinterpreting nonverbal signals or sending out offensive communications of your own.

THE NONVERBAL WORLD

Linguists and anthropologists refer to the realm of communication beyond language as "the nonverbal world." This has been described as the "hidden place off the written transcript, where meaning lies not in vocabulary but in unspoken signals and cues" (Givens, 2006). We cannot stop communicating nonverbally while we're in the presence of another person. We are constantly conveying signals through our posture, hand gestures, and facial expression, whether we are still or moving, speaking or remaining silent. Even when we think we are "just listening," we are talking through our bodies, and interviewees watch us as we listen, trying to gauge our response. They are trying to find out how much attention we are paying, whether we like them, whether we believe them, if we are horrified or amused by what they are telling us, if we find them interesting and appealing, and so on.

Nonverbal communication has four primary functions: expressing emotion, conveying interpersonal attitudes such as like/dislike or dominance/submission, presenting one's personality to others, and supplementing speech for the purpose of managing turn taking, attention, shifts in topic, and so on. Nonverbal communication is also important in rituals such as greeting, leave taking, and ending conversations (Knapp & Hall, 2005).

Desmond Morris (1994), an early and important investigator of nonverbal communication, wrote: "It is spoken language that divides the world and body language that unites it" (p. 47). Even if we do not share the same spoken language as another person, we often can gauge their feelings from their nonverbal communication. Unfortunately, however, we sometimes "read" the nonverbal cues inaccurately.

Much nonverbal language is universally understood across cultures, and some of it we even share with primates. In a fascinating example of a gesture employed by chimpanzees and used in many human societies today, chimpanzees greet each other by stretching out a limp hand and offering the back of it to be kissed. A friendly chimp will press its mouth softly against the knuckles of its greeter (Morris, 1994). Verbal language, in contrast, distinguishes us from most other animals, and a spoken language can be understood only by people who are familiar with it.

Some nonverbal communication is learned, such as saluting a commanding officer; some is innate and resembles the behaviors of other primates, such as sneering in contempt. Most nonverbal behavior is a mixed product of both nature and culture. These mixed behaviors include crying, laughing, smiling, and sighing, among others. These originate as innate actions, but their timing, intensity, and use are shaped by culture. I became acutely aware of this disparity recently when a friend adopted several children from Ethiopia and invited an Ethiopian man over to the house to speak with the newly adopted children about life in the United States. He explained in Amharic, the children's language, that in the United States sneezing loud is considered impolite and Americans make an effort to sneeze quietly and discretely, in contrast to Ethiopia where a robust, hardy sneeze is acceptable. It had never before occurred to me that the way I sneezed was shaped by my culture! But then I realized that I sneeze differently depending on whether I am alone, with family, or in a formal situation. Even sneezing—which feels so innate and involuntary—communicates something about the sneezer to those who witness it. Another example is burping. Although burping also feels involuntary, anyone who has ever watched 10-year-olds having a burping contest can attest to the way burps are also shaped by the social context.

Sometimes when we are uncomfortable in a conversation but are not sure why, it is due to culturally based differences in nonverbal communication. It is important to avoid interpreting these crossed signals in a way that stigmatizes or disadvantages the people with whom we are working. Conversely, we must avoid conveying offputting or insulting messages through our nonverbal behavior that might damage an interview, often without our awareness.

This chapter will help you communicate nonverbally more effectively with culturally diverse interviewees, both as a sender and receiver of messages.

GESTURES

Humans make at least 3,000 different gestures with their hands and fingers alone, not including the specific sign language signals employed in languages by people who are deaf (Morris, 1994). Linguists, anthropologists, and others who have studied nonverbal language have found that although humans as a species engage in hundreds of thousands of different gestures and movements, each of us as an individual has a surprisingly small gesture and movement vocabulary, which we repeat regularly. That is, each one of us smiles, sits down, wipes our noses, and puts on our shoes in almost the same way every time (Morris, 1994).

Gesturing helps us do more than communicate; it can help us think. This may explain why people often gesture even when speaking on the telephone, when their gestures cannot be seen. Gesturing while speaking has been found to assist people in remembering and thinking through problems. In a small study of children and adults, participants performed 20% better on a memory test when allowed to gesture with their hands while explaining a math problem. The subjects who were required to keep their hands still did not perform as well (Goldin-Meadow, 2003). The author of the study suggested that gesturing makes it easier for us to think because it enlists spatial and other nonverbal areas of the brain.

Many people who grow up speaking one language use the gestures from that language even when they are speaking their second language. This can be confusing for an interviewer who is unfamiliar with nonverbal communication in the original culture. For instance, an interviewer might ask a Salvadoran teenager a question, to which the teenager responds with a shrug of the shoulders. The uninformed interviewer may assume that this gesture means, "I don't know," whereas for many Latinos it means, "I don't care," or "I don't want to talk about it," which is a very different message. Gang members frequently use gestures to communicate with each other in codes that others don't understand. Next we examine common gestures that are sometimes misinterpreted and ways to avoid these crossed signals.

Pointing and Beckoning

In court, an attorney may ask a Chinese witness to point to the assailant and expect the witness to point with her index finger. Among people from many Asian countries, including India, China, Indonesia, and the Philippines, it is impolite to point with a finger; and the witness is apt to point with her chin and lips instead, or with an open hand. Afghanis and many Native Americans also consider it impolite to point to a person with the finger (Lipson & Askaryar, 2005; Axtell, 1998; Shusta, Levine, Wong, & Harris, 2005).

We need to be especially careful about pointing. Frequently, native speakers of English point a finger at their conversation partners to drive home a message or to indicate whom they are addressing. I sat in on an interview recently where every time the interviewer wanted to address a different member of a Somali family, she would look down at her clipboard to check the name, turn to face the person, and then point her finger at the person and say, for instance, "You, Ahmed, did you . . . ?" Unfortunately, her pointing was resented by the family and considered disrespectful. Portuguese men also sometimes point a finger at the person they are addressing, which feels rather aggressive to me, and I have to remind myself that it is not an aggressive gesture in Portuguese culture.

Nigerians censor children by pointing or waving a finger at them but consider such gestures insulting when used with adults (Ogbu, 2005). People from some Arab cultures, on the other hand, may point and shake a finger at others for emphasis; this gesture might seem offensive to people from other cultures, even though it is not intended to be insulting (Meleis, 2005). In cross-cultural encounters in general, it is probably wise to avoid sticking out a finger at someone to emphasize a point. And when we need to indicate a particular individual, it may be better to signal in his or her direction with a full hand rather than pointing with a single finger.

What gesture can you use to call someone over from the waiting room into your office, let's say? Curling the index finger to beckon someone as many people do in the United States can be an extremely insulting gesture. This is true not only in China but also in Australia, Malaysia, Indonesia, and some countries in Eastern Europe. If you wish to motion someone to come over, in most countries it is best to hold the hand out, palm downward, and pull the fingers in briskly as if you were scratching.

Risky Gestures

Some gestures that are common and conventional in the United States are considered rude by people from other countries. For example, the "A-OK" sign created by making a circle of the thumb and index finger with the other fingers outstretched is considered obscene in Brazil and Russia, means "zero" in France, and indicates "money" in Japan. In Arab countries, shaking this "OK" sign at someone can be interpreted as giving the person the evil eye. The thumbs-up sign means "up yours" to people from many African nations, Australians, Iranians, Bangladeshis, and others. In Germany and Japan, an upright thumb signals the number "1." The thumb extended to the side is the symbol for hitchhiking in the United States.

In the United States, many people, and especially men, offhandedly slap one fist into their other open palm or slap an open palm onto a fist, as an idle gesture with no particular meaning. This gesture is considered obscene in France, Italy, Chile, and other countries (Axtell, 1998). Raising a single closed fist in the air is considered obscene in many countries, including much of the Arab world and Pakistan (Axtell, 1998). Crossing the middle and index finger, which is a gesture of good luck in the United States, is a sexually obscene gesture in some countries in Asia, as is making a "V" for victory with the index and middle finger (Chan & Lee, 2004). Holding up a hand and twisting it as if screwing in a lightbulb indicates "so-so" or "sort-of" in many cultures. Among Arabs it means, "What are you saying?"

When in doubt, it is probably wise to avoid using a lot of gestures in our conversations with people from other cultures, and to explain things as simply and clearly as we can with words instead. This feels counter-intuitive, as we tend to rely on gestures when speaking with someone who is just learning English. However, avoiding gestures that may be misinterpreted is probably the safest policy.

Variations in nonverbal communication are endless and fascinating. Of course, interviewers cannot possibly learn all gestures for all cultures. But we should try to learn the most important gestures used by the major ethnic groups in our area—even if we work through interpreters—so we can better follow the emotional tone of a conversation and avoid discomfort and misunderstandings.

Inquiring about Gestures

Sometimes interviewees give us a signal through their body language that we have touched a nerve or hit upon an important topic. For instance, even if people don't tell us verbally what's going on they might show a sudden change of facial expression, squirm in their chair, cross and uncross their legs, or change the angling of their torso. These movements may indicate an unspoken mood, feeling, or opinion that merits further exploration. And sometimes people use a nonverbal gesture—such as a wink or a hand signal whose meaning we don't comprehend. We can use verbal questions to inquire about these gestures. For instance, we could say, "I noticed that you frowned when I asked about your cousin. Why is that?" Or, in response to an unfamiliar gesture, "I'm not sure what you mean when you use your hand that way. Can you give words to that for me, please?"

We give off frequent nonverbal signals without even being aware of it. When we ask some people about gestures, especially children, they may not even be sure what we're referring to, so these verbal questions about gestures may or may not be helpful.

GREETING AND LEAVE TAKING

Customs around greeting and leave taking across cultures could fill a chapter by themselves. In much of the world the process of greeting a person or a group of people is of greater importance and takes a longer time than in the United States and Canada. Often people ask about each other's well-being and the well-being of their families every time they meet, even if only a day has passed since their last encounter. In much of Latin America and southern Europe, men stand when a woman walks into the room as a way of demonstrating respect. In these same countries, friends greet each other warmly with an embrace or air-kiss when they see each other, even if they have seen each other just a few hours earlier. These greetings may seem highly ritualized to the unaccustomed.

Telephone greetings may be ritualized in a similar way. Among traditional Portuguese, for instance, people who know each other's family usually say, "How are you? How is your family?" every time they meet or speak on the phone, before launching into the business at hand. The reply is usually brief, either "fine, fine," or maybe a succinct report on a specific family member. The inquiry serves to demonstrate caring more than genuinely probing for information. In contrast, greetings in the United States and Canada often feel rushed, cold, and unfriendly to people from other countries.

Once two people have connected, whether professionally or socially, in many cultures their greeting becomes correspondingly much warmer. For example, for Sudanese children, playing soccer together one day may count as a tight bond and Sudanese boys will be insulted or think it's a sign of prejudice or hostility when an American who was their teammate the day before just waves "hello" very casually when they meet again (Potter, 2002). Similarly, a family from Sudan or certain other African countries who casually encounters in the supermarket a professional they have met once before may be insulted if that professional merely nods and continues with her shopping, rather than offering an effusive warm greeting. This harkens back to the personal nature of professional encounters discussed at other times in this book. If they have taken a liking to the professional and find that person helpful, people from many countries, such as Mexico, allow that person into their friendship circle and see that person as a sort of friend, rather than simply a competent person who is doing his or her job.

In general, try to greet people in order of seniority or status, which means that usually we should begin with the father or grandfather, if he is present. When first meeting people, feel free to smile briefly and nod. Handing people your business card can help them learn your name. Even if they cannot read, the card will still provide them with a way to contact you.

Whether, when, and how people shake hands varies by culture. In the United States men tend to shake hands more than women, and the preferred handshake is usually firm but brief. In many parts of Africa, however, the handshake is prolonged but the contact is light. An American woman who shakes the hand of a Somali, Sudanese, or Kenyan man, for instance, and then finds that he continues holding her hand for a long time may suspect that he is flirting with her, when this may not be his intention at all. If the American breaks off the handshake prematurely, the African may feel that she is behaving in an unfriendly manner. Japanese and Koreans tend to shake hands with a light grip and with their eyes averted.

In many countries older children and especially boys are expected to shake hands to greet adults. I have walked into the home of a Somali family and been surprised when the father, mother, and even children as young as 3 shook my hand on my way in and out the door.

In parts of Europe (France, Spain, Portugal, Italy, Russia, etc.) and parts of Latin America, the Middle East, and Africa, even people who do not know each other kiss each other on the cheek one or more times when meeting for the first time or seeing each other again. This might be true even of coworkers who spent the day together in the office and then see each other at night in a social situation. And they may kiss each other again when saying "good-bye," even if the encounter was a brief one. In some countries this is a true kiss on the cheek; in others it is more of a touching of the cheeks with an "air kiss." In Argentina people greet each other almost constantly with air kisses, just one kiss on the cheek between women, between women and men, between men who know each other well, and from adults to children of either sex. I have seen kisses exchanged in this way in Argentina even among people with relatively distant and formal relationships, such as the secretary of a school with a new student and his mother, among mothers as they greet each other when picking up children at school, and among new work acquaintances. In other countries, two or even three kisses is the custom. Kissing is less apt to be used in a strictly professional encounter. On the other hand, in many countries the decision as to who kisses whom, when, and how is more tightly scripted than might meet the eye of a casual observer. For instance, in many places women may kiss women in this way but not men. Or, people may shake hands the first time they meet and do "air kisses" upon subsequent meetings. Over time, when families from many countries come to trust professionals, they may greet them with a kiss on the cheek and/or a hug, essentially welcoming them into their circle of affection. Whenever possible, this affection should be received in the spirit of innocent appreciation in which it was given. When in doubt, take your cues from the people with whom you are working.

Some professionals maintain a policy of "no kissing and no hugging under any circumstances." They may believe that this policy protects them from accusations of sexual harassment and also that it sets up secure boundaries with people whose boundaries have been violated by sexual abuse or other assaults. Some professionals who make home visits try to avoid hugging in greetings in an effort to emphasize that, although the visit occurs in the home, it is a professional relationship and not a friendship. If you or your agency have a policy of no kissing or hugging and you are concerned that your interviewees will feel hurt by what they see as your physical aloofness, try to devise another manner of greeting that is warm and personal. For instance, some professionals will give children with whom they work a "high five" when they greet them and say, "I'm so glad to see you!"

Like greetings, leave taking in many cultures is similarly prolonged and important. A Chilean saying articulates this difference, *Los gringos se van sin despedirse y los chilenos se despiden sin irse* [Americans leave without saying "good-bye," and Chileans say "good-bye" without leaving]. This refrain highlights the tendency in the United States to leave a party or meeting without saying a personal good-bye to everyone present, in contrast to a Chilean tendency to become so involved in individual "good-byes" that the person leaving ends up staying much longer than expected.

Again, true familiarity with the culture can help us know how to proceed. When a social or work occasion with Latin Americans or Africans is ending, I usually offer each person a handshake or a kiss on the cheek, depending on the circumstances, as a sign of respect and affection. Some Muslim and Orthodox Jewish men would prefer a gesture of farewell from me that does not involve touching, such as a smile and a nod.

SHOWING ATTENTIVENESS

As mentioned in Chapter 4, the set of things we do and say to demonstrate that we are paying attention and following a conversation is called "attending behaviors." In all cultures, sitting forward in your chair is a way of demonstrating that you are paying close attention. Leaning back in your chair is apt to be perceived more negatively, as a sign of disinterest or lack of connection. Through your nonverbal communication you can convey that you are paying attention and understanding the interviewee's position, even if you don't agree with everything the interviewee says.

Avoid communicating impatience by shifting in your seat, rolling your eyes, cracking your knuckles, sighing, ruffling through your papers, tapping a pencil or pen or foot, swinging your foot, playing with a paperclip or other object, clicking your pen, or picking at your nails. In many cultures yawning, scratching, stretching, or grooming one's hair are considered rude personal behaviors that should not be displayed in public (comparable to picking one's nose or teeth or scratching one's bottom in the United States). People from many cultures consider chewing gum to be a crude and despicable habit.

Avoid allowing your paperwork to serve as a barrier between you and the interviewee. Rather, especially at the beginning of the interview and preferably at various points as the interview progresses, put down your clipboard, file, or chart and make sure you are connecting directly with the interviewee. Some interviewers become skilled at maintaining the person-to-person contact with the interviewee at the same time taking notes without glancing down. At all times the interviewee should feel that he or she as a human being is more important than the paperwork.

Koreans describe the ability to size each other up wordlessly as *nun-chi*, or measuring with the eyes (Lee, 2005; Kim & Ryu, 2005). They believe *nun-chi* allows them to read environmental cues to choose an appropriate course of action. Unless they are thoroughly acculturated, Koreans may feel anxious in social situations with people from other cultures because of their inability to read the social cues and therefore choose the best course of action. When meeting with a Korean person, you may notice that the person is paying careful attention to you, perhaps even while disguising this in a polite distance. The person may be looking eagerly for signs of what to do next.

POSTURE

Your posture—how you hold your back, shoulders, head, neck, and legs while sitting or standing—can convey a great deal about your authority, how much you like a person, how relaxed you are, and whether you pose a threat. One of the ways people define the group to which they belong is through their posture, as can be seen when watching a group of teenage girls who often share the same distinctive way of standing with one hip thrust forward and their head tilted to the side. What does your posture say about you, as you stand or sit during an interview? Around the world, squaring your shoulders, lifting your face and chin, and visibly standing tall are postures that indicate authority—which can be the preferable stance in some interviews. In other interviews, such as with young children, you might choose instead to emphasize warmth rather than authority, lowering yourself down to the child's level by sitting in a small chair or on the floor, leaning in toward the child rather than sitting back stiffly, and holding your arms and body in the most relaxed way possible.

Sitting back with both hands clamped behind your head can be seen as a display of dominance—that you do not need to demonstrate eagerness or attention because you are in full control of the encounter. In many cultures this would be seen as an overly familiar posture for an official interview. Whereas high-status communicators generally telegraph their dominance by maintaining a relaxed posture in the United States and Canada, in Japan they assume stiff, erect postures with feet firmly planted on the floor (Burgoon et al., 1989, p. 194).

Holding one's hands on the hips, which is also described as the "arms akimbo" posture, universally indicates authority, territoriality, or holding one's position (Givens, 2006). An interviewee who assumes this position may be indicating an unwillingness to cooperate, "Keep away from me" or "Step back." Some African American girls and women use a highly stylized one or two-handed version of this pose to indicate real or feigned contempt or disgust (Givens, 2006). We should be aware that if we stand arms akimbo we may distance and intimidate an interviewee.

Male interviewers may need to be particularly careful with their body posture, especially with women and children from cultures different from their own. Movements and postures that have no sexual connotation in one country can be interpreted as flirtatious or sexually inappropriate in other countries. For instance, men should avoid sitting with their legs spread wide open, which may be seen as putting their genitals on display, even though they are fully dressed. Men in many countries (and women in most) are raised to keep their legs together when sitting. Additionally, large men should be mindful of how they use their size, positioning themselves in as nonthreatening a posture as possible. Male law enforcement officers have often been trained to use their size to intimidate suspects. This would be inappropriate in situations with a frightened victim or a witness who needs reassurance rather than intimidation.

Feet are considered unclean in many cultures. If you accidentally bump or poke someone or something with your foot, apologize. Avoid placing feet on furniture. If you are conducting a physical exam, examine the feet last with rubber gloves if possible, and discard the gloves and wash hands before touching the patient again. This is particularly true with Roma (gypsy) patients (Sutherland, 2005).

In Singapore, Thailand, and Muslim countries of the Middle East, showing the bottoms of the feet either accidentally or on purpose while sitting down is considered a rude gesture meaning "you are beneath my feet." The bottom of the shoe is considered the filthiest part of the body. When meeting with people from the Middle East and Asia, interviewers should avoid pointing the soles of their feet at anyone, and instead sit with their soles on the ground.

GAIT

The manner in which we walk conveys a great deal about our mood, gender, culture, health, and age; yet it is so ingrained that we rarely think about it. Studies have found that people can identify another person's gender and sometimes nationality or ethnicity by the way he or she walks. One medical study comparing Chinese and Caucasian women in England found that the Caucasian women typically walked more quickly and exerted more force on their heels, contributing to their higher rates of arthritis (Chen, O'Connor, & Radin, 2003). Sometimes a person's gait is partially shaped by his or her culture's choice of footwear and clothing, as when women in industrialized countries wear spiky high-heeled shoes that contribute to a short stride and cautious step. Tibetan traditional clothing, *chupas*, which is essentially a long tight skirt, requires wearers to walk in a slow manner that is thought to develop calm dignity and to conserve energy (Tibetan Culture Preservation in Canada, website accessed September 20, 2006, from *www.geocities. com/tcpc2001ca/*).

Young African American men sometimes walk with a definite rhythm and swagger, "the cool pose." People unfamiliar with this posture and gait often misinterpret it as a sign of delinquency or defiance. Goleman (April 21, 1992) writes, "While the cool pose is often misread by teachers, principals and police officers as an attitude of defiance, psychologists who have studied it say it is a way for Black youths to maintain a sense of integrity and suppress rage at being blocked from usual routes to esteem and success" (cited in Shusta et al., 2005, p. 172). We need to be careful about the ways we interpret our interviewee's gait, and we need to give some thought to the way we ourselves walk when doing our work. There may be times when we want to swagger boldly, and other times when we choose to walk with a certain calm discretion, depending on what we want to communicate.

COMMUNICATING WITH THE EYES

Eye contact arouses strong emotions. Whether these feelings are of connection or threat depends on the circumstances. White middle-class Anglo-Americans often expect people to look them in the eye when holding a conversation. However, people in many cultures have been taught that it is disrespectful to look others in the eye, particularly if those others are in a position of authority or of a higher status. If an interviewer stares into someone's eyes and seeks out contact, the interviewee may believe that he or she is about to be punished or reprimanded. There may be some differences among Black and White people in the United States in regard to eye contact as well, with African American listeners tending to look away as people speak and White listeners tending more often to gaze into the speaker's eyes (Grossman, 1995). In general, in Native American cultures it is customary to avert one's eyes when speaking with elders and only occasionally to make direct eye contact. O'Dwyer (2001) suggests that "the Irish are likely to see constant eye contact as overly intrusive, penetrating, and ultimately disrespectful" (p. 210). He suggests that a more casual and distanced approach will be perceived as less threatening.

In Japan, listeners are taught to focus on a speaker's neck in order to avoid eye contact (Burgoon, Buller, & Woodall, 1995). In Korea and Japan, prolonged direct eye contact is considered impolite and even intimidating. One way to show concentration and attentiveness is to close the eyes in contemplation and nod the head slightly, up and down.

Interviewers should approach interviewees in a friendly, natural way but not actively seek out or avoid eye contact. Look at the interviewee comfortably but try not to stare fixedly at the person. By occasionally lowering your eyes or looking away you will give the person a chance to observe you, too.

The presence or absence of eye contact should not be used to judge truthfulness, attentiveness, or engagement. In many cultures children are especially unwilling to meet adults' eyes for more than a fleeting moment and people hesitate to make eye contact with people of the other sex, lest this be misconstrued as romantic or sexual interest. A Pakistani university admissions officer described sitting on a committee that was evaluating a Pakistani woman applicant who made eye contact with the female interviewers on the committee but not the males, even when responding to a question asked by one of the men. The committee was ready to deny admissions to this candidate based on this habit alone. The Pakistani admissions officer stepped in, explained that this was a cultural practice and was not likely to interfere with the candidate's ability to succeed in the university. She was granted admission (anonymous personal communication, 2005).

Winking can mean many things, even within a single nation, including sexual or romantic interest or complicity in a secret. In Chile, a wink often means "yes." Winking at a woman from India is considered demeaning. Among Vietnamese, winking is considered indecent, especially when directed at people of the other sex. In general, interviewers should avoid winking because it is an ambiguous communication that might easily be misinterpreted.

In many cultures, people use their eyes to check in with their loved ones or with people in a position of authority before they will respond to a question; this is called eye checking. Thus, for instance, if while interviewing a couple you ask a wife something, she may fleetingly glance at her husband before she responds, seeking his permission to speak or hoping he will guide the conversation. He may communicate his assent or dissent through moving his head slightly or narrowing his eyes. A child might also eye-check a parent or teacher before responding to a question. This eye checking does not indicate that the person is engaged in a deception. Rather, it is an indication of a cultural pattern of authority, and of the group orientation of many cultures that puts the group or family's needs ahead of those of one individual.

A "knowing glance" is when two people communicate a shared negative opinion of a person by looking at each other and making the same facial expression, such as narrowing or rolling their eyes, raising their eyebrows, or pursing their lips (Givens, 2006). Sometimes when two people in a dominant position, such as two interviewers, look at each other and exchange knowing glances, they may be perceived by the subordinate person as mocking or criticizing, even if this is not their intention. (An example of this was provided in the case of Hassan in Chapter 1.)

EXPRESSING EMOTIONS

Attending to the synchrony between what interviewees says verbally and their nonverbal communication has been recommended as a way of detecting truthfulness, mental state, and mental illness (Sattler, 1998). In some cultures, however, such as among the Japanese and British, people learn from childhood to suppress words and expressions that reveal their psychic state. Many Native Americans also show little emotional expression and may speak little—particularly with outsiders.

We should also note the "appropriate" nonverbal display to accompany a given emotion varies by culture. For example, in the United States most people hold their head down and look mournful when they are embarrassed or ashamed. In Japan, on the other hand, people may smile and laugh when they are experiencing shame and regret. It is not that the Japanese think the incident is funny but, rather, that laughing is a cultural way of expressing regret. Similarly, people in English-speaking industrialized nations generally look down, speak quietly, and frown when delivering bad news. In Japan, it is considered good manners to smile when conveying any kind of bad news (Wierzbicka, 1994). This might obviously leave an incorrect impression with someone who is not familiar with Japanese culture.

Cultures vary in how much people move their eyebrows, eyes, lips, heads, arms, and hands while they converse. Interviewers need to be careful about how they view a person who is either more or less expressive than they expect. Someone who is physically expressive may *seem* angry or theatrical, and someone who is more rigid may *seem* uncooperative, uncomfortable, or depressed. However, they may just be acting in the way they have learned in their culture.

Cultures with Confucian roots such as Japanese, Chinese, and Korean tend to value "walking the middle road," avoiding extremes of all kinds, including displays of emotion. They tend to express their emotions and opinions and even their desire to speak through subtle and indirect cues that people from other cultures may miss (Uba, 1994). People from these backgrounds tend to show little facial expression, moving their eyebrows, lips, and faces only slightly when they speak. With their relatively still faces, they may appear to have "flat affect" or to be uncooperative or lying to Westerners who are unused to these norms around emotional expressiveness (Axtell, 1998). For instance, a Chinese woman may recount a traumatic event without much expression on her face or in her voice. This does *not* mean that she is not feeling emotionally distressed—she is just declining to show it. Chan and Lee (2004) describe it this way:

> In general, the value placed on control of emotional expression contributes to a demeanor among selected Asian groups that is often interpreted by Eurocentric individuals as "flat," "stoic," "enigmatic," or even "inscrutable. . . . Koreans, for example, in keeping with the national character of the "Land of the Morning Calm," may present with a demeanor referred to as *myu-po-jung* (lack of facial expression). Casual smiling and direct eye contact when greeting or interacting with strangers is considered inappropriate. (p. 273)

In general, Jews, Latinos, and African Americans provide a contrasting picture. Veronica Abney, an African American psychoanalyst and social worker, describes being called down periodically to the emergency room of the Los Angeles hospital where she worked to help the White and Asian medical professionals speak with Black mothers whom they said were "hysterical" (personal communication, 1998). She describes encountering mothers who were, naturally, upset because their children were in the emergency room, and who expressed their distress with stronger displays of emotion than the emergency room personnel were accustomed to (e.g., weeping, breathing deeply, sighing, rubbing their faces, and calling out to

God). Pathologizing this behavior by labeling it "hysterical" is inaccurate and not helpful. Rather, Abney recommends that we empathize with the mothers' distress, offer them realistic reassurances, and help them contact family members, clergy, or friends for support.

In many cultures, people are emotionally expressive with family members and people they know and trust, and are apt to be more subdued among people they know less well. The longer people have lived in their new country and the more assimilated they are into mainstream culture, the more their emotional displays are apt to conform to the norms of the region where they live.

Many cultures tolerate women displaying a wider range of feelings than men. I remember watching my Jewish Polish immigrant grandfather weep openly when I was a child and feeling that in some way such behavior was "unseemly" for a man. His behavior can be contrasted with that of stereotypical men in the United States who have often been taught that "boys don't cry." U.S. boys are often "toughened up" through physically rough sports and corporal punishment, and they learn to restrain tears in these situations. Men who openly display a wider range of emotions such as sadness, disappointment, tenderness, and vulnerability may be suspected of being less masculine. Anyone who remembers back to the U.S. presidential election of 1972 will recall how tears in the eyes of vice presidential candidate Edwin Muskie cost him the Democratic nomination. There is some indication that these norms may be changing, as recently some male sports figures have wept openly in defeat or victory. Also, a number of male politicians in the United States have openly cried in public situations in recent years, winning admiration for their sensitivity.

Expressing emotions in front of others, including family members, is a source of shame for traditional Korean men. According to Im (2005), Koreans commonly believe that "men should cry only three times in their lives: when they are born, when their parents die, and when their country perishes" (p. 321).

Judges, asylum officers, police, and others often try to judge truthfulness by attending to a person's facial expressions. In addition to the cultural influences in degree of expressiveness like those mentioned previously, particular historical events can cause people to show a lower degree of expressiveness. For instance, people who have lived under the Khmer Rouge or in other extremely repressive political circumstances have often learned to betray as little as possible through their facial expressions. People who have been interrogated or tortured, and even people who live in situations of domestic violence, have often learned to keep their feelings "to themselves" to survive. Okawa (2008) describes a Bosnian refugee as saying she is "beyond tears."

EXPRESSING PAIN AND DISTRESS

People from many cultures have learned to be stoic and are unlikely to show how much something hurts through a pained expression. This can make it difficult for health and mental health care providers to use facial expressions to gauge the severity of a worry, illness, or pain. When an older Portuguese friend was suffering from kidney stones, for instance, I could read how much pain she was in by the sweat on her brow and the way she held her breath. When a doctor asked if she was in pain she simply said "Yes," without elaborating. She has told me with great pride how she did not cry out during two prolonged and complicated labors. This cultural stoicism can lead some patients to have their pain undertreated by health care providers. Chinese, Vietnamese, and Pacific Islanders are also apt to be stoic regarding pain, believing that the expression of pain is a sign of weakness (Lipson & Dibble, 2005). In Korean, *pal-ja* describes unchanging destiny, which a person must suffer without complaint (Kim & Ryu, 2005), as with Catholics who may believe suffering is their cross to bear.

The same kind of stoicism is likely to be true for the expression of "negative" feelings or psychological pain for people from some countries. When asked how she feels emotionally, for instance, a Portuguese woman is apt to answer "fine" and will elaborate only if a professional asks for more specifics, such as "Ms. Alves, last time we met, you said you felt sad. Show me with your hands how sad you feel. Do you have just a little sadness [show hands close to each other] or a lot [show hands far apart]?" It is easier for some people to discuss their physical and emotional pain when they are afforded an opportunity to externalize their feelings in this way—to discuss them as something outside themselves. However, the convention of asking people to quantify their pain or feelings on a numerical scale, for instance, "On a scale of 1 to 10, how would you rate your anxiety?" is apt to be difficult for people who have fewer years of formal schooling and may be unfamiliar with numerical rating systems. Instead, interviewers should ask them to show with their hands, or to explain verbally if they feel "not worried, a little worried, or very worried." Some people use a scale with pictures, such as the Wong–Baker FACES pain rating scale (Hockenberry, Wilson, & Winkelstein, 2005) and ask people to point to a face that shows how they are feeling (see Figure 5.1).

Puerto Ricans and Dominicans tend not to be stoic but rather are often loud and outspoken in their expression of physical pain, clutching or rubbing the affected area and calling or moaning "*Ay!*" or "*Ay bendito!*" (Juarbe, 2005). These expressions of pain should not be censored, belittled, or seen as exaggerations. They are real; they may just be more intensely ex-

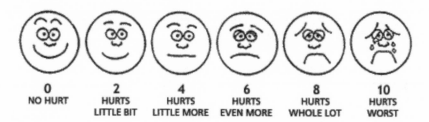

FIGURE 5.1. Wong-Baker FACES Pain Rating Scale. Point to each face using the words to describe the pain intensity. Ask the patient to choose the face that best describes his or her own pain and record the appropriate number. From Hockenberry, M. J., Wilson, D., & Winkelstein, M. L. *Wong's Essentials of Pediatric Nursing*, Ed. 7, St. Louis, 2005, p. 1259. Used with permission. Copyright, Mosby.

pressed by Puerto Ricans than by some others. Some Puerto Rican women have even been called "histrionic" because of their level of expressiveness. We must be cautious before we apply a label that indicates a personality disorder to a person who is behaving in a culturally congruent way.

Jews are often depicted as especially willing to discuss their emotional pain and life's difficulties (*kvetch*ing in Yiddish) (Wex, 2005). Woody Allen's character in his early movies portrays this trait comically. How one views kvetching depends in part on one's familiarity and comfort with the practice. To people unused to this interpersonal style, it may be unappealing and look as if Jews are "wearing their problems on their sleeve." However, for many Jews, discussing their problems is a way of bonding with another person. I complain a little to you, you complain a little to me, and in this way we have shared intimacies and cemented our relationship. To Jews, people who are less emotionally expressive may seem to be cold, impersonal, and withholding. (Jewish comedians tell numerous jokes about the lack of expressiveness among U.S. "WASPs.")

In many countries of the Middle East, patting the chest over the heart with the palm of the right hand means "I need help." "The action mimes a fast heartbeat, implying that the gesturer is in a state of panic" (Morris, 1994, p. 148). Arabs from the Middle East who are upset may put their hands to their face and cry out a phrase such as "God help us! God help us!" if there has been an emergency or shocking news. They also often reiterate statements for emphasis, or repeatedly use expressions such as "I swear by God." To someone who is unaccustomed to such habits, it can look as if the person is exaggerating for dramatic effect.

The take-home message of this discussion of emotional expression is that we must be careful not to apply our own cultural ideas about "the right way" to show what one is feeling to people of other backgrounds. Rather, we should take note of a variety of nonverbal indicators (facial expression, body movements, tone of voice) and also inquire verbally, to form as complete a picture as possible.

TOUCH

Touching behavior has been categorized into five different levels of intimacy: (1) functional–professional; (2) social–polite; (3) friendship–warmth; (4) love–intimacy; and (5) sexual arousal (Heslin, 1974). However, a touch that is considered social in one culture may be seen as intimate in another. In this section we examine different ways of touching and some rules around touch that might affect the interview process. As always, if you are seeking information about particular people from particular cultures, it is a good idea to read about that culture specifically, spend time among people from that culture, ask people from that culture about acceptable touching, and observe the particular individual or family you are working with, to find out their own specific norms. Even within a given culture people vary in how much they like to touch and be touched.

Typically in some cultures, such as among African Americans, when people are fond of each other they habitually engage in a lot of physical contact, such as touching a person's arm, hugging, and backslapping, and—for girls—touching each other's hair. With people they don't know or trust, however, they may seek the safety of less contact and relatively greater physical distance. White ethnic groups in the United States differ in how much they tend to touch each other.

Hoffman (1989) describes the different cultural norms around touching eloquently in her memoir of growing up as a Polish Jewish émigré in the United States:

> My mother says I'm becoming "English." This hurts me, because I know she means I'm becoming cold. I'm no colder than I've ever been, but I'm learning to be less demonstrative. . . . I learn my new reserve from people who take a step back when we talk, because I'm standing too close, crowding them. Cultural distances are different, I later learn in a sociology class, but I know it already. I learn restraint from Penny, who looks offended when I shake her by the arm in excitement, as if my gesture had been one of aggression instead of friendliness. I learn it from a girl who pulls away when I hook my arm through hers as we walk down the street—this movement of friendly intimacy is an embarrassment to her. (pp. 146–147)

When Hoffman describes "cold" she means unfeeling, and in her Jewish Polish context how deeply one feels and even one's state as a feeling person is partially communicated through touch and gestures. "In Polish culture, behavior that shows feeling is seen as the norm, not as a departure from the norm" (Wierzbicka, 1994, p. 158). Poles (and Slavic people in general) frequently kiss, hug, embrace, touch, and shower in verbal endearments the people they care about, because when one feels positively toward the person one is communicating with, one is expected to show it (Wierzbicka, 1994).

Touch is used more frequently and widely across many cultures than it is in the dominant culture in the United States and Canada. Puerto Ricans typically touch the upper body of the people with whom they are speaking, touching, grabbing, or tapping their hands, arms, or shoulders as part of the wide array of gestures that they use regularly in conversation. This may feel uncomfortable to people who are unused to this kind of physical intimacy, but its absence may make some Puerto Ricans feel as if the person with whom they are speaking is cold or unfriendly. Puerto Ricans who have lived for a long time on the mainland are apt to be bicultural in their touching—interacting more physically when among Latinos and less so with people from other groups.

Certain kinds of touch can be problematic. For example, in Canada and the United States, adults frequently pat children on the head as a sign of affection. But this is a demeaning gesture for some Chinese, Filipinos, South Asians, Indonesians, Central Americans, and African Americans; rubbing the head is seen as a caress befitting animals, not people. The top of the head is considered a sacred spot and off limits for casual touch by some Native Americans, Hawaiians, and the Khmer. Among the Hmong of Southeast Asia, one should not tickle a baby's feet or the baby will grow up to be a thief (Arax, 1996, cited in Chan & Lee, 2004).

Many professionals touch the people with whom they are working on the arm or shoulder as a gesture of support. Whereas in much of Latin America such a touch would be considered comforting, in much of Asia and the Middle East it could be considered patronizing and insulting.

In many countries in the Middle East and Africa it is considered impolite to greet or touch someone with the left hand or to pass money or objects with the left hand. The left hand is used for toileting; the right hand is used socially, for eating, and for purification before prayer.

Many religiously observant people, including some Muslims, Orthodox Jews, the Amish, and conservative Christians, do not touch people of the other sex who are not relatives. The interviewer who extends his or her arm to shake the hand of a person of the other sex may find that the overture is ignored or rejected. This should not be interpreted as a rejection of the interviewer's person. Many Muslims find casual touch by members of the opposite sex offensive, whatever the circumstances, but they might

welcome such a touch by someone of the same sex. There are great variations according to national origin and degree of orthodoxy. In this as in so
many areas, it helps to become truly familiar with people from the culture,
and to ask people from the culture to give you advice.

In many countries of the world, within-sex touching is quite common
and people of the same sex touch each other in intimate ways without sexual connotations. Boys will walk with their arms around other boys, and
men will sometimes walk with their elbows linked or holding hands, without any connotation of romance or sexuality. In Argentina, men who know
each other will sometimes greet each other with an air kiss to the cheek.
Women and girls in many nations also commonly walk with their arms
linked, holding hands, or with their arms around each other, and they may
play with or groom each other's hair. Sharing cars, rooms, beds, clothing,
and other personal items is not unusual for people from cultures where
space is at a premium and people need to pool their resources to survive.

If you are conducting a medical exam, request permission before you
touch the patient, and briefly explain the reason for each kind of contact.
For example, you can say, "Now I'd like to listen to your breathing to see if
your lungs are clear. . . . Now I'm going to feel your throat to check for
swollen glands." In most cultures, women would prefer to have their bodies examined by female providers, and this is particularly true for genital
and breast exams. Even discussing reproduction, sexuality, or menstruation
with a man may be acutely embarrassing to some women (Lipson & Dibble, 2005). Men would often rather have a prostate exam and other intimate exams conducted by a male provider. Men may also be unwilling to
discuss sexuality, and particularly issues of deviancy or potency, with a female provider. In situations in which it is impossible to match the patient
with a provider of the same sex, a careful explanation of the need for each
procedure may be sufficient to allay the patient's concerns, or those of her
husband or father. A female patient may be immensely comforted by the
presence of a female nurse in the room during an exam by a male physician.
Finally, some women will simply refuse to be examined by men, and these
wishes need to be respected.

Some cultures rely more on touch than on words for comfort. When
children are upset during interviews, they sometimes want a hug or they try
to sit on the interviewer's lap. Of course this can happen with children from
all cultural groups but may be especially common with children from cultures that tend to be physically close and demonstrative. Generally, interviewers should not have children sit on their lap during the interview—it is
especially important to keep boundaries clear with children who may have
had their own boundaries violated. I have found it works to say, simply,
"You can't sit in my lap, but why don't you pull your chair up right close to

mine?" Children seem to generally appreciate that I have recognized their desire to "get close" in this way, while still maintaining clear physical boundaries.

Depending on your context, you may choose to accept physical demonstrations of affection from a child, such as a hug at the end of an interview, or holding your hand as you walk from the interview room back out to the waiting room.

I tend to err on the side of caution. Parents who feel threatened by professionals—worried that I am trying to coopt a child's affections, or remove a child from their custody—are sometimes suspicious and resentful of even the slightest displays of affection or warmth between myself and a child. This can cause the parent to retaliate against the child. If I initiate a touch I make sure it is one (such as offering a high-five) that cannot be misinterpreted as sexual. If I have any concerns at all about the child's boundaries or if I have any concern that the caretaker is concerned about the child's physical boundaries, I refrain from touching the child and try to communicate my warmth and appreciation in other ways. For instance, I may get down to the child's level and thank the child sincerely for being willing to speak with me.

When interviewing or evaluating couples or parents, it is important to avoid attributing incorrect meanings to the presence or absence of physical affection. In traditional Japanese culture, for instance, affection is not expressed physically. Couples do not display physical intimacy toward each other in front of their children, and they are unlikely to caress, kiss, or demonstrate other forms of physical affection toward their children (Shibusawa, 2005).

PERSONAL SPACE

Cultures vary dramatically in how close to others people usually stand or sit, with people they know intimately, with acquaintances, and with strangers. The anthropologist Edward Hall (1959) identified four interpersonal distances—*public* (10 feet and beyond), *social–consultive* (4–10 feet), *personal–casual* (1.5–4 feet), and *intimate* (0–18 inches). (These are similar to the categories of touching noted in the previous section.) Hall noted that different cultures set distinctive norms for closeness for different occasions such as business, casual speaking, and courting. Standing or sitting too close or too far away can lead to misunderstandings.

In many parts of Africa, multiple families often live in large compounds. When Africans immigrate to Western industrialized countries they often move in with members of the extended family, friends, and acquaintances, to save expenses and pool resources (such as money, food, and babysitting). They may share living quarters, beds, cars, clothing, and other personal items—even shoes. Children may be very physical in their play, showing almost no sense of personal space. I have noticed this while working with Somali refugees, and it is sometimes a challenge for me. Once they get to know and trust me, the kids will often try to climb all over me and explore the contents of my purse. (A set of keys! A cell phone! Sunglasses! What great items to play with!). On one hand, I am happy they accept me enough to be physically close to me. On the other, I am concerned about my personal items, and I also know it is important for the children to learn appropriate boundaries.

If you are used to a greater interpersonal distance, you may experience someone from a culture where there is habitually less distance as being aggressive or overly intimate. You may experience their attempts to close the distance between you as a violation of your personal space. For instance, in general Brazilians, Cubans, Arabs, and Italians are used to a closer interpersonal distance than people from the dominant group in the United States and Canada. These have been called "elbow cultures" (Morris, 1994, p. 32). That is, they are most comfortable standing at an elbow's distance from their companions. If you are from a "fingertips" culture, such as the dominant groups in the United States, Britain, and Canada, where people are most comfortable standing about an arm's reach from conversation partners, you may find yourself continually backing up in small steps as a person from an elbow culture person moves in closer. The person who is speaking with you and who is accustomed to less interpersonal distance may experience you as cold and standoffish as you retreat. The converse is also true. Your attempts to stand or sit a little closer to someone who is not used to such short distances, such as many Native Americans, may make them feel crowded or make them feel their personal space is being invaded. Many Native American interviewees would prefer a greater amount of personal space between themselves and an interviewer, while sitting or standing. Japanese, Korean, Pakistani, and Irish people are apt to maintain a greater interpersonal distance from unfamiliar professionals than people from the dominant cultures in the United States and Canada.

What can you do about personal space? First, it helps just to be aware of this dynamic, so you can tune into the signals you are receiving at any point and adjust your distance to one that seems to feel comfortable to the person you are interviewing. Second, as you become familiar with people from a variety of cultures, watch their habitual use of personal space with people they know well and with relative strangers. This may give you clues as to how to behave with people from specific cultures. And, finally, remember that the relationship, genders, emotions, context, and discussion topics may supersede or offset broad cultural norms around interpersonal distance. As with all cultural generalizations, it is worth remembering that they may not hold true in any given circumstance with any particular person.

SMILING AND LAUGHING

A smile can stem from a variety of feelings in different cultures, including happiness, uncertainty, mockery, apology, confusion, humiliation, shame, and discomfort. People from the United States tend to smile for photographs, or to show gratitude, to make others feel welcome, or to acknowledge another's presence. In the United States smiling as a form of greeting is obligatory in all but the most solemn occasions, and even at funerals many people greet each other with smiles. In the United States, subordinates are expected to smile often at people in dominant positions, such as their professors and bosses, and women typically smile more than men when in mixed groups.

People don't smile as frequently or for the same reasons in all cultures. In Japan, for instance, people often smile and even laugh a bit if they are embarrassed, ashamed, or when a situation is uncomfortable, to relieve some of the tension. I was once friends with a Japanese woman who would habitually smile when I spoke to her about the saddest and most difficult material—which was disconcerting for me at first. A U.S. attorney has described taking depositions in Japan, and finding it easy to find the "tell" because the Japanese witnesses—and especially women—would giggle when he touched on a sensitive topic (the "tell" is the material they knew was problematic and were trying not to reveal) (Irving Levinson, personal communication, 2007). In various parts of Asia people smile to cover up humiliation, embarrassment, shame, or pain, especially when they have been made to "lose face." It is important to avoid feeling as if the person is trying to be a "smart aleck" or a showoff by smiling. On the contrary, in Asia the smile is often used to relieve tension or demonstrate submission. In Japan, Vietnam, and some other Asian countries women cover their mouth with their hands when they smile or laugh—it's considered inappropriate to let strangers see a woman's open mouth.

Smiling in Vietnamese culture has been explained in the following way:

> The smile, which is sometimes enigmatic to the American observer, is another nonverbal symbol conveying the feeling of respect in Vietnamese culture. It is used as an expression of apology for a minor offense, such as

being tardy to class, or as an expression of embarrassment when committing an innocent blunder. For the Vietnamese, the smile is a proper response
in most situations in which verbal expression is not needed or not appropriate. It is used as a substitute for "I'm sorry," "Thank you," or "Hi!" It is
used instead of a ready yes to avoid appearing over-enthusiastic. A smile is
also a proper response to scolding or harsh words [to show] that one does
not harbor any ill feelings toward the interlocutor or that one sincerely acknowledges the mistake or fault committed. (Nonverbal Communication
in the Vietnamese, Huynh Dinh Te, Massachusetts Legal Services Diversity
Coalition website).

The converse is also true. The serious expression on the face of an interviewer who is hearing about embarrassing material might be perplexing to
Japanese or Vietnamese interviewees who would expect the professional to
smile to put them at ease.

Like smiling, laughing also conveys different meanings across cultures.
Among Koreans, laughter is used to disguise many emotions, including
anger, frustration, and fear. Among Filipinos, laughter is used to convey
both enjoyment and pleasure but also to mask embarrassment over another
person's misfortune.

COMMUNICATING ABOUT COMMUNICATING

We communicate about communicating ("metacommunicating") through
nods, glances, raising our eyebrows, sharply taking in breath, and so on.
When people in the United States are ready to end a meeting, they frequently slap their leg with their palms, as if to say, "I'm ready to walk!"
(Givens, 2006). Children have to learn norms such as turn taking and
whom to look at during a discussion. Children often fumble with these customs, provoking adults to say "Don't interrupt" or "Did you hear me?"
when the youngsters commit conversational blunders. These conversational
norms also vary across cultures, contributing to the awkwardness one may
feel while speaking with someone from a different culture. The conversation may fail to proceed smoothly, and may be marked by awkward pauses
or interruptions, as each person searches in vain for habitual clues indicating when to speak, when to remain silent, and when to move on to a new
topic.

The absence of these nonverbal communications is also one reason
that communication on the phone can be especially difficult for people who
are using their second language. The absence of metacommunication also
contributes to misunderstanding the intention of e-mails, as people don't
have enough information to read the intention behind the others' words.

NONVERBAL SIGNS OF DISAGREEMENT AND AGREEMENT

Nodding to give assent and shaking my head to dissent feel so natural to me—they almost feel as if they are written into my genes. But these are culturally learned signals, as I discovered when traveling in Bulgaria once, where nodding signals disagreement, shaking one's head signals agreement, and bobbling the head in small circles shows that one is listening intently. I cannot describe how disconcerting it was for me to speak to a group of people and see them all shake or bobble their heads gently. I felt like stopping every sentence to ask, "What is it that you disagree with?" Nodding the head means "no" and shaking the head means "yes," in Greece, Yugoslavia, Turkey, Iran, and Bengal, as well.

"No" is signaled in a variety of other ways around the globe. Arabs from a variety of countries signal "no" by tipping the head backward and clicking the tongue. In Somalia, quickly twisting an open hand means "no" (Axtell, 1998).

In general, Chinese people like to avoid saying "no" because it is considered rude to be this direct with a negative response A gesture that is often used by Chinese to signal "no" or that "something is very difficult" (pausing to rethink) is to tip the head backward and audibly suck air in through the teeth. Another gesture that is used to indicate "no" in Taiwan and China is to lift your hand to face level with the palm facing outward and move it back and forth like a windshield wiper, sometimes with a smile, in a gesture that looks like the wave of a beauty pageant contestant. A gesture similar to one used to scold children in the United States, with the index finger pointing up and wagging side to side like a windshield wiper, means "no" or "You got it wrong," in much of Latin America.

Pursing the lips by pulling them inward or pushing them outward signals a *lack* of agreement in most cultures (Givens, 2006) and is often the first sign of discord. When you note a lip movement of this kind, you may want to ask interviewees to verbalize their response by saying, "How does this sound to you?" or "What do you think about this?" or "Please let me know what you're thinking."

Nodding may signal agreement or may mean the person has heard but does not understand or approve. If you have been giving an instruction or making a recommendation, it is a good idea to ask the person to verbalize or repeat what was said to check for understanding. If you are asking a question and want to make sure you are interpreting a head nod correctly as a sign of assent, you can ask something like, "Is that a 'yes'?" As mentioned earlier, in Chile, a wink of one eye in response to a question signals "yes." In Ethiopia, a sharp intake of breath signals "yes."

CLOTHING

How are you to understand interviewees' clothing, and how do they understand yours? Although we rarely think of it as such, clothing is a form of communication. Of course, the clothes we wear vary with our professional position and the circumstance of the interview. When given the choice, many young professionals like to dress informally in jeans and sneakers. While this may sometimes be appropriate, while working with children for instance, an adult may be so insulted by this perceived lack of professionalism that he or she will not return for a second appointment. It may appear to immigrant and ethnic minority interviewees, in particular, that the professional who has "dressed down" is not respectful and is not taking his or her job seriously, and therefore is not competent or trustworthy.

On the other hand, of course, it would not be appropriate to wear evening clothes or extremely formal or sexy clothes to traipse through mud to interview a victim at a crime scene! You would also call unwanted attention to yourself if you dressed in an overly formal way in low-income neighborhoods. Of course we want to wear comfortable clothes, and if we're interviewing in people's homes that are of questionable hygiene, we want to wear clothes that we can wash easily: But these should still look neat and professional. Try to tune into how your clothes affect interviewees, and adjust accordingly. While I would not cover myself with a burqa to interview even an observant Muslim family, I would choose to dress more modestly on the day I had such an interview scheduled, so my bare arms or legs would not be an insult or a distraction.

We must be careful about how we respond to (and report on) the interviewee's clothing. It is reasonable to notice whether an interviewee is clean or dirty, neat or disheveled. However, we must be cautious in drawing conclusions about the *meaning* of these observations. The fundamental attribution error, discussed in Chapter 3, involves attributing behaviors to internal characteristics rather than the circumstances. If I run to the store in grubby clothes I know that it's because I've just been scrubbing the kitchen floor, for instance, and it's not the way I usually dress. However, if I see someone else with dirty clothes I may jump to the conclusion that she is mentally ill or that he doesn't care about his appearance. I am attributing a temporary state (wearing dirty clothes) to an internal condition, when there are many other temporary explanations for the condition of the clothes.

People try to wear clothes that fit their images of themselves. But some people do not have access to the clothes they'd like to wear and are forced to accept the hand-me-downs that are given to them. I see this with the African refugees with whom I work. The young boys sometimes end up wearing pink sneakers or clothes that are way too big for them. When they first arrive they might wear red jackets or shirts which could lead to their being mistakenly viewed as affiliated with a gang, The Bloods, when this is not the case at all. The women might wear shirts with sequins, abundant frills, or gold trim, without a sense of how out of place these look in the morning at the local supermarket. In some countries breasts are not considered sexually provocative, and the women have not been accustomed to wearing bras. And so the women may nurse in public, or will often go braless. The men refugees' feet are sometimes smaller than the men's shoes that are given to them, and so they end up wearing women's shoes until they can afford replacements. All these predicaments around clothing increase the appearance of "difference" in the refugees and raise the likelihood that they will be frowned on by their neighbors and the professionals who meet them. It is important to remember, however, that these clothing choices are often not "choices" but, rather, constitute the best that can be done in difficult circumstances.

And, finally, just because a person chooses to dress a part, it doesn't mean the person's lifestyle corresponds to the part. A young girl can dress in a sexually enticing way without being sexually active, a young man can dress in "homey" clothes when he's from the suburbs, and so on. Clothes reveal something about us, but we should be careful not to overinterpret others' clothing. A psychology graduate student intern came to work on the first day she was going to see clients at a clinic wearing a long evening gown with a lot of cleavage showing. I asked her about this privately, and she said this was the dressiest outfit she owned, and she figured therefore it would be appropriate. She was from a farming family and had not learned the difference between dressy clothes and professional clothes.

Interviewees often wear clothing or especially jewelry with religious or spiritual significance. For example, Arabs from some countries wear a blue stone amulet to ward off the evil eye. Catholics often wear a cross, and/or a medallion of their patron saint. Some Native American groups tie a thread as a form of protection around their children's wrists (Joe & Malach, 2004). Many Jews wear a Mogen David (star of David) or a "chai" (the Hebrew letters signifying "life"). We may see the fringe of the tallis, or prayer shawl, peeking out from under the clothing of orthodox Jews. We may notice the special long underwear worn by Latter Day Saint interviewees, although this is unlikely to attract our attention unless we know what we are looking for. And, of course, head coverings ranging from yarmulkes on Jewish men to turbans on Sikh men to head scarves on Muslim women are all easily observed.

We cannot avoid responding emotionally to interviewees' clothing. It can be helpful to become overtly aware of our responses so we avoid the halo effect of letting a detail in the clothing overly influence our impression.

Do we feel curiosity? Disgust? Pity? Attraction? And how might these feelings impact the interview?

TATTOOS, PIERCINGS, AND OTHER FORMS OF BODY MODIFICATION

People in Western Industrialized societies throughout the world are increasingly modifying their bodies through tattoos, piercings, scarring, and branding. People engage in these forms of body modification for decorative reasons, to show their membership in a social group, out of boredom, as part of a BDSM (bondage, domination, sadomasochism) lifestyle, as a ritual in joining a gang or in prison, or because of the rush of endorphins or adrenaline that accompany the pain of the modification.

While some of these practices were once restricted to people from traditional societies or young people trying to make a statement, their use is spreading into groups of all ages and a variety of backgrounds. Although it can be hard, try to withhold judgment regarding body modification. It is better to note its presence and describe its nature than to pass judgment on the personality or lifestyle of an interviewee. If a tattoo is relevant and prominent, you may decide to ask about it.

CONCLUDING OBSERVATIONS

As much as an interview process is an exchange of words and rational information, it is also an exchange of nonverbal emotional cues. The nonverbal signals we give off to interviewees the first time we meet them set the tone for all future interactions. The nonverbal signals we convey provide interviewees with a sense of how they are doing, whether we like them, and whether we are on their side.

Across cultures, when there is harmony and understanding between conversation partners, they begin to mirror each other's body postures and movements. Some interviewers take advantage of this by deliberately falling into synchrony with the interviewee's movements—for instance, shifting position when the interviewee does. Many skilled and empathic interviewers do this instinctively without conscious awareness.

It is important to learn the cultural meaning of certain gestures so you can understand your interviewees better. However, trying to adopt the gestures of other cultures is a much trickier proposition. Often subtle rules based on age, gender, status, familiarity, circumstances, and so on dictate what should be communicated nonverbally with whom and when. A person who purposely tries to adapt the nonverbal communication of someone from another culture (for instance, bowing or kissing someone's cheek) without being intimately acquainted with that culture may risk being perceived as insincere or condescending.

I hope this chapter has raised your awareness of some of the intricacies and possible pitfalls of nonverbal communication. If these details have made you overly anxious about the possibility of making a nonverbal blunder, then I have failed in my intent. Rather, I hope you have learned about particular gestures to avoid and specific areas that require caution. Mostly, I hope you will be careful about interpreting the nonverbal behavior of your interviewees. If you are working with people from a given culture, try to learn more about nonverbal communication among those people by spending informal time with others in that culture. In this way, you will gain a sense of typical movements and gestures in their environment.

Uba (1994, cited in Sattler, 1998, p. 270) describes how difficult it is for interviewers to determine whether behaviors that suggest a personality or temperament problem in people from the dominant group reflect similar problems among members of ethnic minority groups:

> For example, when ethnic clients remain silent, speak softly, or avoid extended eye contact, are they revealing shyness, weakness, or reluctance to speak or are they exhibiting politeness and respect? Does expressing emotions in an indirect, understated way with little emotion suggest denial, lack of affect, lack of awareness of one's feelings, deceptiveness, or resistance, or do such expressions suggest a wish to sustain interpersonal harmony?

Misinterpretations of nonverbal behaviors such as these can lead to incorrect assessments and ineffective or even harmful interventions.

The most important attribute for an interviewer in a cross-cultural encounter is a friendly and open attitude. You convey this attitude through your body, through the way you use your voice, and through the words you choose. This attitude will go a long way to help you maintain the relationship and recover if you make a blunder, saying or doing something that you later discover was not culturally appropriate.

Questions to Think about and Discuss

1. Describe a situation in which you made a mistake or experienced confusion due to differences in nonverbal communication.
2. What would you tell a beginning interviewer in your field to keep in mind when greeting someone from another cultural group?
3. Describe how you would set up your interview room and hold your

body when interviewing a young child whom you want to help feel trusting and at ease.

4. A person you are interviewing is smiling and nodding. Name three different messages that these behaviors might be communicating.

5. A person you are interviewing is wearing clothing that is clearly worn out and old. How might this shape your perception of this person? What conclusions are reasonable and unreasonable to draw on the basis of your observation of the person's clothing?

RECOMMENDED ADDITIONAL READING

Givens, D. (2006). *The nonverbal dictionary of gestures, signs, and body language cues.* Available at *members.aol.com/nonverbal2/diction1.htm.*

6 Language Competence
Building Bridges with People Who Have a Different Native Language

The difference in languages is not a difference
in sound and signs, but a difference in
worldviews.
—WILHELM VON HUMBOLDT

Opportunities for misunderstandings abound when working
in English with someone who speaks a different native language, or who
speaks a different form of English from the interviewer. For example:

> A South Asian family turned up at a hospital to visit their uncle who was se-
> riously ill. On arrival a nurse informed them politely that their uncle was
> "sleeping now," so they went home. On their return the following morning
> for a visit, they discovered that uncle had in fact been "dead now," and that
> the nurse was using a euphemism in her effort to appear gentle and polite.
> The family's distress was exacerbated by the fact that they would have car-
> ried out the praying and washing ceremonies proper to their faith if they
> had known that their uncle had just died. They were denied this opportu-
> nity because of a linguistic misunderstanding. (J. Cambridge, personal
> communication, November 21, 2006)

Language differences and bilingualism are crucial but underestimated
and understudied factors in multicultural mental health, criminal justice,
social work, and medicine (Santiago-Rivera & Altarriba, 2002). In this

chapter we examine ways that language competence plays a key role in interviews. Topics include how to handle language differences between the interviewer and interviewee; how language affects memory, emotion, and personality; interviewing people who are bi- or multilingual; alternative forms of English; and, finally, language rights and the "state of the field" in assuring linguistically competent interviews. This chapter will help you understand better and work more effectively with interviewees who are multilingual, or with whom you don't share fluency in a common language.

ATTITUDE OF HUMILITY AND SUPPORT

I recommend an attitude of humility when interviewing people in a language that is not their native tongue. It's helpful if we first apologize for not speaking the interviewee's primary language, whether it's Polish, Spanish, Cantonese, or Swahili. People who are not fluent speakers of English, or who speak English with an accent, are often rejected and shamed by prejudices and serious problems related to their lack of English-language fluency. To be as welcoming as possible, I customarily declare that my lack of skills in the interviewee's language is *my* deficit rather than theirs. I might say:

> "Mr. Hubert, I am so sorry I don't speak Creole. I wish I could speak Creole so it would be easier for us to communicate. Today we're going to have the help of an interpreter, so we can understand each other. If I spoke Creole, I could speak with you directly in the language you prefer, and I'm sorry that isn't possible."

A Haitian interviewee who hears the foregoing kind of statement is apt to feel unexpectedly validated, predisposing him to trust me more readily.

Some interviewers are tempted to respond with frustration and impatience, rather than humility, when faced with an interviewee who doesn't speak English or doesn't speak it well. I know it can be tiresome to simplify our English or call in an interpreter to make sure we're understood. It can be difficult to plod our way through thick accents and incorrect phrasings. However, it's important for us to remember our ethical, moral, and legal obligation to conduct interviews to the best of our ability, regardless of the interviewees' English-language proficiency. People will stop speaking with us openly, or end an interview prematurely, if they sense that we are impatient with them. To avoid discrimination based on a lack of language competence, we must remain patient and supportive and take the extra step of calling in an interpreter whenever necessary (see Chapter 7 on interpreting).

In general, the more comfortable interviewees feel with us, the more they will be able to use all of their language skills. The more intimidating or impatient we seem, the more anxious our interviewees will feel. This stress will impede whatever English-speaking ability the interviewee may have. People's English also deteriorates if they are in pain, ill, intoxicated, in shock, fatigued, or frightened. Even if the interviewee does speak some English, we are still obligated to use an interpreter when the person asks for one, or when it would make communication easier.

Interviewing People with Limited English Language Proficiency

We need to make ourselves understood as clearly as possible, while at the same time making sure not to appear condescending or patronizing. This can be a tricky balance to achieve. Here are some tips for speaking with people who are less than fully fluent in the interviewer's language, but where an interpreter is not necessary or not available, or has been declined:

- Speak slowly and enunciate clearly (no mumbling). Monitor your speed to make sure you don't start speeding up as the interview progresses.
- Face the person and speak directly. Allow the person to see your lips and expression. Be careful to avoid covering your face with your hand or a clipboard. Facial cues facilitate communication.
- Do not insist on eye contact (see Chapter 5 on nonverbal communication).
- Avoid jargon, slang, abbreviations, and contractions (e.g., "the slammer," "gonna," 51A, CPS, EKG, and Ed Plan).
- Use active rather than passive verbs (e.g., "Please follow me," rather than "It would be helpful if you would head this way").
- Avoid complex verb constructions (e.g., "If you had sought help sooner, you might have found yourself in a better position . . . ").
- Repeat key issues and questions in different ways to ensure understanding.
- Avoid asking "yes" or "no" questions. It is too easy for people to answer one way or the other without really understanding your question.
- Use short, simple sentences with only one idea per sentence.
- Use widely known visual cues such as gestures, demonstrations, photographs, charts, objects, and brief written phrases when these seem to improve understanding. But remember, some people who are less literate may not know how to read graphs, maps, or charts, and gestures can be misinterpreted.
- Provide written materials in clients' native language for them to take home (Even if they cannot read, they may be able to have a friend or relative read the materials to them). If the materials are not available in their native language, provide these in English.
- Allow sufficient time. Give breaks. Pause frequently.
- Allow for silence to help people formulate their answers.
- Encourage the interviewee to ask you questions.

- Give supportive comments on the person's ability to communicate, such as "I know it's not easy to speak English. You're doing a great job."
- Listen attentively. People can detect when attention is really being paid to them.
- Do not speak abnormally loud unless the person is hearing impaired. It won't help comprehension, and it seems condescending.
- Clarify your limitations. Your willingness to talk about an issue may be viewed as evidence of "understanding it" or the ability to "fix it." It may be important to say, "I cannot help you with that housing problem, but let me give you the number of someone who can." If you fail to do this, interviewees may assume that they have resolved their housing problem because they spoke to you about it and you listened.
- Be patient. Remember, it is difficult to express oneself in a second language.
- Conduct the interview in a quiet room.

Note. Partially adapted from Shusta et al. (2005, p. 99).

I am often asked if it wouldn't be better for immigrants to learn English, and my response is, "absolutely." We should be subsidizing easily accessible English classes for anyone who wants to learn. It would benefit those individuals, their families, their community, and society as a whole. However, in many communities such helpful classes in English as a Second Language do not exist, are prohibitively expensive, or have waiting lists with hundreds or thousands of names.

In addition to these practical barriers, the task of learning a new language can be overwhelming—especially for older adults, for those who have had little formal schooling, for those who suffer from trauma and other major disruptions, and for those who are rejected by the community around them because of their race or culture or because they are in some other way "different" from the majority group. Learning English is just "too hard" for some people at certain times in their life.

Access to opportunities to learn English also vary among people and within a given person's life:

> When Sandra emigrated from Mexico to the United States in her early 50's, she worked in a university cafeteria for about a year. In this job she had opportunities to speak English with students and coworkers all day and her English improved tremendously. However, because this job did not include summer hours, she seized an opportunity to switch into janitorial services, where she enjoyed guaranteed summer employment but worked alone. In this new job, her English skills improved little for years on end; and perhaps they even deteriorated. Sandra's conservative husband discouraged her from taking English classes where she would be sitting in a classroom

beside male strangers. This deprived her of another opportunity to learn English.

Some immigrants' ability to learn English is inhibited by emotional conflicts. Perhaps they may believe that proficiency in the new language would in some way betray their ties to their country of origin. Others are afraid of sounding foolish or making mistakes as they try to function in a new language. Most immigrants yearn to be able to function easily and without embarrassment in the language of their new country, and they work hard to accomplish this.

When we interview a person who has a heavy accent or who does not speak English well, it is easy to view this as an indication that the person is not intelligent or educated, or to assume the person is foreign born or is un-documented. (Chapter 3 provides an example of the halo effect and discusses the fundamental attribution error biases.) We must conscientiously avoid rushing to judgments of this kind. As discussed previously, there are many different reasons why even the most educated and intelligent people may not speak English well.

In the next sections we examine the effects of using one language or the other on the recollection abilities of bilingual people.

TRYING TO REMEMBER

First we need to understand how memory works. Some memories come to us unbidden. For instance, I may be walking down the street and as I feel the first drop of rain I suddenly remember that I forgot to close the windows at home before stepping out. This is a spontaneous, effortless memory. In this chapter, we mainly address another kind of memory, those that people deliberately try to conjure up. These are the memories that would be accessed in response to questioning in an interview.

The process of trying to recall a specific memory has been described as "a stepwise procedure in which a chain of associations (imagery, language, feelings, concepts) is activated and the information matched to search requirements until a target memory is triggered. . . . A person uses whatever information is available to 'trigger' more information until the target information is itself activated" (Schrauf, 2003, p. 235). Our memories for events that have happened to us include a sense of reliving the event. In some way, we are imagining ourselves in the situation again as we conjure it up. And finally, we remember things that happened to us for particular purposes at particular times, related to our goals at the time of the remembering.

A memory may change somewhat as we retrieve it. After recalling and recounting the same event several times, we begin to form a "canonical account," which is the narrative that will become our "official memory" of the event and which may vary little in the retelling. For example, as I have recounted many times over the years the events surrounding the birth of my first child, I have developed a "standard" way of remembering and telling the story—this is my "canonical account" of the event. While I believe it is true, I have undoubtedly changed the emphasis at certain points for maximum effect, and there are some embarrassing details I probably neglect to tell, or don't even remember. I may have also incorporated details about that day into my story that I do not actually remember myself but which others have described to me, and which I now believe I remember. In fact, I may have even incorporated details from the births of my other children into that story, confused a bit as to which details belong to which story. Hence I tell the story in much the same way each time, leaving out certain parts, emphasizing others, and maybe even incorporating some details that are not truly part of my memory of that event. This is typical of "canonical accounts."

We experience distinct events differently, including how much of the experience is sensory and how much is mediated through language. Schrauf (2003) provides the example of jumping into a cold lake on a hot summer day. The sensory experience precedes and probably overshadows the linguistic experience, even though we may very well yell, "It's freezing!" However, we process most *social* experiences in our minds through words and the sensory element is typically less significant. For example, we may greet a coworker in passing and then say to ourselves, "Joan certainly seemed to be in a good mood today. I should have asked her about her weekend. I'll remember to do that at lunch." Even in stressful social situations where our bodies get "revved up," we are still apt to process the experience linguistically. For example, if I am driving and have a near miss with another car, I am apt to engage in a certain amount of self-talk afterward, such as "Wow that was close! Tomorrow I'll slow down at that intersection." In addition, if I tell friends about what happened, I add to the linguistic aspects of the memory.

We are able to remember details central to events that are somewhat stressful better than we are able to remember events that are not stressful at all, perhaps because we pay less attention to events that are stress free. However, events that are extremely traumatizing, terrorizing, or horrific, such as sexual assault, combat, accidents, or torture, may be difficult to remember in their entirety, or may come to us in fragments or unbidden in the form of flashbacks, nightmares, and emotional or sensory arousal (Pezdek & Taylor, 2002).

LANGUAGE AND MEMORY IN PEOPLE WHO ARE BILINGUAL

For a bilingual person, the linguistic processing that occurs during or after an event could be happening in either or both of the two languages, and the language and the words used will probably shape that person's memories of the event. However, we don't really know what factors lead bilingual people to encode events in one language or another, and what influence this encoding might have when they're interviewed about the event and try to retrieve the memory.

Linguists, cognitive psychologists, and anthropologists are just beginning to examine how choice of language, comfort with a language, and various emotions affect the ability to remember among people who are bi- or multilingual (Heredia & Brown, 2004; Altarriba & Morier, 2004). Most of this research has been conducted on simple tasks such as word or sentence retrieval and leaves open more complex questions such as:

• When an incident occurs in one language and people are asked about it in another, do they have more trouble remembering the incident?

• Do people usually remember an event in their first language or in the language in which it occurred, if these are different? Does it depend on the type of event?

• To obtain the most accurate information, should we interview in the language a person uses most, the language in which the target event occurred, or the person's first language?

• If an incident happens in one language, let's say English, and the person's first language is different, let's say Spanish, what will be gained and lost by asking about it in one or the other of these languages? Would the person be able to recall more if we inquired about it in both languages, one after the other? Will the memories themselves be different in each language? Will the recounting of the memories be different in each language (for instance, the number of details, or the order of the memories)?

• What is the cognitive process for bilingual people who are interviewed in their second language? Some respond automatically in that second language without translating to their first language. Others, who are less fluent in the second language, may translate questions into their native language, develop a response in that native language, and then translate the response for the interviewer. This is a cumbersome and exhausting process.

• What happens over time to memories that are initially coded in one language, if the person stops speaking that language? (This is of particular interest for people who have traumatic experiences in one language and then are adopted into a family that does not speak that language. How are these traumatic memories stored and do they manifest in some way?)

These questions become critically important in our interviewing work. Unfortunately, the answer to many of these questions is, "We still don't know for sure." Here I discuss some of the preliminary research and its implications for conducting interviews in English with people for whom it is not their native language. For simplicity's sake, here I talk about "bilingual" people—people who speak two languages, including English. Of course, many people are actually multilingual, speaking more than two languages in addition to the target language, in this case, English.

Not all bilingual people are alike. Some people are truly fluent in speaking, understanding, reading, and writing two languages, whereas others may speak both but read and write only one. Still other people—such as many refugees from Africa and Asia—are verbally fluent in a number of different languages but illiterate in all of them. (Indeed, some languages from Africa and India, and some Native American languages do not have a widely used written form.) Some people are *functional* bilinguals. This means they can function in their second language well enough to get by at work or school, but they have only a limited degree of fluency and a limited vocabulary in that second language (Baetens-Bearsmore, 1986).

Other differences among bilingual people stem from the age and the setting in which they've learned their two languages. People who learn two languages in one setting, such as in a home where they speak English with one parent and Mandarin with the other, are *compound* bilinguals. Compound bilinguals are more likely to encode experiences in two languages at the same time, and they learn to label their thoughts and emotions in the two language systems at the same time (Altarriba & Morier, 2004). Both languages are—in effect—their "native" or "first" language or their "mother tongue."

People who learn a first language in one setting, such as the home, and then a second language in another setting, such as in school or the workplace, are *coordinate* bilinguals. Coordinate bilinguals have learned each language in a different setting, taught by different people and with distinct feelings and associations in each setting. Therefore, coordinate bilinguals may have distinct "memory traces"—that is, different moods and environmental triggers associated with different words and concepts in each language (Heredia & Brown, 2004, p. 229). The immigrant clients we interview are more likely to be coordinate bilinguals who learned one language at home and then added English later in more formal settings. (In reality, these distinctions are somewhat blurred because most bilingual people have both coordinate and compound elements to their languages, as they continue to learn new words and concepts in each language throughout their life.)

Beyond differences among various bilingual people, there may be differences for a single person depending on the specific memory in question. That is, the same person could have easier access to certain memories in one language, to others in another language, and perhaps to still a third set of memories in both languages. Beyond the question of memory, bilingual people sometimes find it easier to recount a particular event in one language or the other. Specific occurrences seem to be better suited to explanation in a given language. Ideally, the interviewee can decide which language to use when over the course of an interview.

Finally, there is some evidence that the language in which we conduct an interview with a bilingual person will partially shape the memories that are elicited. In one study, fully bilingual participants were asked to describe an interesting or dramatic personal life experience for about 5 minutes. The same participants were later asked to discuss the same experience in their other language. The results were clear:

- The nature and quality of the reports given in the language in which the experience occurred was richer than in the second language of report.
- There was definite evidence of language-specific information, as individuals who recalled life experiences that were coded in a particular language produced more elaborate recall of that information when probed in the corresponding language. . . .
- Experiences appeared to be related more vividly when recounted in the language in which they had been experienced. (Javier et al., 1993, cited in Altarriba & Morier, 2004)

In a second study, researchers presented a specific word (e.g., "dream," "love," or "dog") to older Latinos who grew up speaking Spanish but who had been living in the United States at least 30 years and who were truly fluent in both languages. They then asked the participants, on alternate days, to associate that word with personal events from their past in either English or Spanish. They found that participants were more likely to recall memories in Spanish that occurred prior to their emigration, whereas memories recalled in English referred more often to events following immigration (Schrauf & Rubin, 1998, cited in Altarriba & Morier). This study suggests, but doesn't prove, that when an interview occurs in a particular language it calls forth memories of events that happened (and were encoded) in that language.

How are these studies relevant to our cross-cultural interviews? Let's look at an example:

Six-year-old Raquel, whose family comes from Mexico, speaks only Spanish in the home but is learning English in school. She is learning each language in a separate context and each has a distinct set of associations and emotions. (She is, therefore, a coordinate bilingual.) Raquel is sexually assaulted repeatedly over 2 years by her mother's boyfriend, Roberto. She encodes the assaults (puts them into memory) in Spanish because this is her dominant language and this is also the language in which the assaults occur. When she is 8, Roberto moves out of the home and Raquel feels safe enough to tell her mother what happened. Her mother contacts the police. Raquel is then interviewed in English by an investigator. Although Raquel has learned to speak English in school, she is still more comfortable in Spanish, and the assaults originally occurred in Spanish. Raquel may not be able to provide as much information about these memories in English as she would be able to provide in Spanish, and the interview is apt to be more stressful for her. Furthermore, if the interviewer asks a question trying to establish sexual intent, such as, "What did Roberto say to you while he was doing this?" Raquel probably will not be able to recount his remarks as precisely in English as she could have recounted them in the original Spanish.

The studies discussed above suggest that the choice of the language used in an interview may have a crucial impact on the quality and quantity of information obtained. Where precision and detail are important, such as in a forensic setting, the language chosen for the interview matters a great deal.

In the next section we examine numerous ways in which a people's language competency affects how they appear and how they feel—in short, their personality.

LANGUAGE AND PERSONALITY

Aside from memory, language competency also affects people's apparent personality—how they *seem* to others. As anyone knows who has ever traveled in a country where they speak another language, a person who is usually articulate, poised, and confident can feel like a blundering idiot while trying to be understood in another language. Our feelings about who we are, how competent we are, and even our feelings of being generally safe and able to take care of ourselves (and our families) are called into question when we lose our ability to communicate easily. Indeed, when people gain competence in a new language, it's a promising sign when they begin to "feel like themselves" in that language. In a variety of studies, bilingual people have been found to demonstrate different character traits in different languages (Perez Foster, 1999).

The author and poet Julia Álvarez (2004) writes of the alienation of speaking in a second language: "I didn't know if I could ever show genuine feeling in a borrowed tongue" (p. 29). Being allowed to speak in one's first language, the language of the heart, can allow a person's personality, mood, and even mental status to shine forth in a way that may be impossible while speaking a second language. For instance, a Brazilian mother may seem removed, disinterested, formal, and cold when interviewed in English, but she may brighten considerably and interact in a lively way with her children when speaking Portuguese. If she uses her English mostly in formal interactions, which she may experience as frightening, an assessment conducted solely in English will not tap into her true personality.

Research suggests that bilingual people who are interviewed and assessed in their second language are frequently misdiagnosed as more depressed than when they are interviewed in their native language (Perez Foster, 1999). Their concerns over choosing the right words make them appear more "down" than they would appear if freed of this burden. Perez Foster (1999) gives the example of a Yugoslavian man who was brought into the emergency room of a city hospital after threatening to kill himself:

> In a difficult interview, he finally said in his halting English, "You don't know me. The only thing you have to tell you whether I am crazy is my words, and I don't speak English that well. So why should I tell you all that I am thinking?" (p. 98)

Perez Foster then asks, "Do we assess this as paranoid suspicion or good reality testing?" After all, this man faced possible involuntary hospitalization as a result of the assessment. Fragmented speech, disorganized ideas, and flattened or inappropriate affect may be symptomatic of poor English skills under stress, and not indicative of psychopathology. People who are not that competent in English may appear passive, disorganized, simpleminded, or naive when interviewed in English only. They are often aware of this, which adds to their anxiety. For Koreans who are cognizant of their appearance and eager to "save face," for instance, being unable to express themselves adequately in English and be understood can be a blow to their self-esteem, and lead them to become defensive or ashamedly silent in an interview (Kim & Ryu, 2005).

Daily interactions with people outside the language group can be fraught with stress, anxiety, and bewilderment. Immigrants can be struck regularly with a sense of not belonging, as people around them easily converse in a code that they, themselves, cannot comprehend. Some emigrants lose self-confidence and remain silent and passive in public situations. As this state of affairs is prolonged over a period of years for people who are not successful in picking up the language of their new country, these ways of presenting themselves may become permanent personality traits. The discomfort may be relieved only when they mingle with a community of other people who speak their language, where they can speak more freely. Understandably, some immigrants prefer to spend as much time as possible in their own ethnic enclaves, in part because of this advantage of being able to be their "true selves" in their first language.

A Puerto Rican psychologist who speaks beautiful fluent English, Yolanda recently told me how she feels like a more quiet, less adequate person in English, and how this hinders her career advancement. Yolanda says that when she first moved to the mainland United States a decade ago she was unable to find employment in her field and ended up working in food service in the cafeteria of the university where she attended graduate school. She described the shame of not remembering the word for "broom," and her distress in having to ask a much younger student where she could find "the sweeper." More than 10 years later and with a doctorate and substantial professional achievements behind her, Yolanda still feels like a stumbling recent immigrant when she is required to assert herself publicly in English.

Another example:

> Derek was a graduate student in several of my classes. His written work was excellent; but he rarely said a word in class, despite my frequent encouragement. Finally, one day I asked him why he was so silent. He told me that before he moved to the United States from Jamaica at the age of 5 he was lively and talkative, but when he arrived at school in Boston his classmates mocked him mercilessly for his accent and his Jamaican expressions. He said he shut down then and became "a silent person." Now, 20 years later and speaking unaccented American English, Derek says he still cannot shake off this habit of silence around people who are not Jamaican.

I hope this section on how speaking one's non-native language can affect a person creates feelings of empathy in those who speak the dominant language. Sometimes English speakers grow impatient or angry when people with a different native language group speak that language around them. They may feel excluded or put out, irritated that they cannot understand what is being said. These reactions are normal but should also be tempered by knowledge of the difficulty of being forced to strain to express oneself on a daily basis.

LANGUAGE AND ABSTRACTIONS

Abstract words (such as "justice" and "truth") and emotion words (such as "fear" and "sadness") vary more across languages than words for concrete objects (such as "chair" and "wallet") (Ritchie & Bhatia, 2004). This suggests that in interviews where abstract concepts and emotions are central, people who are interviewed in a language other than their dominant language may be able only to approximate what they wish to say.

Abstract concepts such as trauma, mental health, developmental delay, depression, appropriateness, or anxiety might be confusing. These concepts are more apt to be understood if described in behavioral terms such as "not sleeping" "sighing all the time," and "behaving like a younger child" or in terms related to physical health such as "having a headache" or "heat in the chest."

I have seen this to be true in my own experience. I developed and implemented on several occasions a 5-day training for Spanish-language forensic interviewers. The interviewers (who were originally trained in English) reported great difficulty in translating abstract phrases and concepts, such as "You are not in trouble," "How did it feel?," "a hard time," and "date rape." This information is merely anecdotal, but it suggests that the people we interview may also have more difficulty articulating abstract concepts in interviews that are not conducted in their native language. These abstract concepts could include values, consent, power, truth, emotions, understanding, and many other topics that could be central to the interview, depending on the context. In addition, the interview conducted in English reflects the concepts and values of the English language and English or North American culture; this facilitates certain kinds of emotional expression and constrains others.

LANGUAGE AND EMOTION

Our emotions are influenced by the social context in which we experience them. For example, if we are in a solemn context such as an important business meeting we are not apt to respond to a funny thought that has occurred to us with the same feeling or expression of glee as we would in another setting. In addition, culture shapes how we experience our feelings in more of a long-lasting way. To give one example, people from India often express their grief in loud and dramatic ways at funerals, crying and weeping openly, but tend to show emotional restraint in other contexts, such as displaying romantic love. White middle-class people of Anglo-Saxon descent from the United States, on the other hand, tend to restrain their grief at funerals, making small talk and sometimes even laughing, whereas they often display romantic love openly in front of others.

In medical and mental health interviews, we are apt to ask interviewees about their feelings. Some languages do not have an easy way to differentiate between the constructs of "thinking" and "feeling" (Okawa, 2008). Even where the interpretation is good, or where the person we are interviewing understands English, it's all too easy to misinterpret an interviewee whose native language is not English. For example, being "happy" is highly valued in the United States and is seen not as merely a fleeting feeling but also as a measure of a person's psychological and social adjustment (Wilson, 2008). The word "happy"—used so frequently in the United States—does not even have an equivalent in most Slavic languages, where it is usually reserved for a rare feeling of deep bliss (Baranczak, 1990, cited in Wierzbicka, 1994). An interviewer or evaluator who expects interviewees from other cultures to feel "happy" and to say they are happy is imposing a U.S. worldview on others. "Happy" just isn't the same in all cultures.

Another emotion that is difficult to translate across cultures is the English concept of "anger." This is translated into Japanese as *ikari*. While this is technically the correct translation and *ikari* in many ways resembles the English concept of "anger," the exact components of each concept are different—and even the subjective feelings it describes are different (Kitayama & Markus, 1994). The two forms of anger are not identical, and so it is misleading for an interviewer to evaluate a Japanese person's anger in exactly the same way as a native speaker of English. Even if the Japanese person is speaking in English, he may retain the concept of *ikari* from his native culture.

To give another example of the importance of language in understanding emotion, in Spanish there are many ways to express the concept of anger and degrees of anger. These words include *enojado, enfadado, furioso, con ira,* and *con rabia*. The last two mean enraged or, literally, "with rage," but in certain countries the last one would only be used with animals, as in an animal with rabies, whereas in other countries it would be used to describe a very angry person. Woe to the interviewer who mistakenly says to an interviewee from the wrong country that he looks as if he is *con rabia*!

Languages prepare people for the cultures in which they live. In Western cultures with their emphasis on independence, anger is seen as a "natural" response to being treated unfairly or having one's individual rights and needs frustrated (Kitayama & Markus, 1994). In many Asian and Eastern cultures, the emphasis on interdependence and attending to one another's needs would seem to call for a distinct response—perhaps a different kind of anger or perhaps a completely different response such as a desire to meet the group expectations more seamlessly.

Amae, a key cultural concept in Japan, has been described as a "sense of being accepted and cared for by others in a passive relationship of reciprocal dependence" (Ellsworth, 1994, p. 38). This dynamic is thought to be modeled on the early mother–child bond and shows up in the relationship between employees and employers, students and teachers, and so on. Feelings of *amae* may be as "natural and basic" in Japanese culture as displays of anger are in Western cultures.

Language also shapes emotional life. Words sculpt our experience, rendering the raw and continuous material of our days into discreet moments, sensations, feelings, and thoughts. A given language enables certain emotions and inhibits others. Some emotions that are identifiable in a given language have no clear counterparts in others. For instance, the Korean word *han* refers to what is described as a "wrenching, incurable feeling of regret" (Lee, 2005, p. 231). To use another example, in Portuguese the word *saudades* describes a deep longing for a time, place, or relationship in the past. English translations such as "nostalgia" and "homesickness" cannot come close to capturing the feelings of the word. Without a word for it, I might ask if a person who does not speak Portuguese can even experience the exact feeling of *saudades*. At the very least, a Portuguese speaker who is trying to describe his feelings to a person who does not speak Portuguese has to use a series of other words to convey the feeling of *saudades*, a feeling that pervades a great deal of the artistic life of Portugal and—to a lesser extent—its former colonies of Brazil, Angola, Mozambique, and the Cape Verde Islands.

There is evidence that emotions receive a higher priority in some languages than in others. For example, the word "emotional" has a slightly negative connotation in English and the word "dispassionate" has a slightly positive one. In Polish, however, these terms do not have exact equivalents, but the words that most closely approximate them give a positive tinge to "emotional" and a negative tinge to "dispassionate," implying apathy, indifference, and coldness (Wierzbicka, 1994). The Polish are fond of overstatement, and frequently use modifiers such as "terribly," which may be contrasted with Australians who are fond of understatement, and frequently use modifiers such as "fairly" and "a bit."

The Rwandan language, Kinyarwanka, has a limited number of words for describing emotional states, as compared to English. The emotional states "tense," "jittery," and "worried" are all translated as "not calm" (Okawa, 2008). This lack of semantic equivalence makes it hard to determine how a Rwandan is feeling when interviewing in English, even if an interpreter is used.

There is also some evidence that some language and cultures simply *are more emotional* than others. For example, a study of people who were fluent in Spanish and English, half of whom had Spanish as their mother tongue and the other half English, found that all participants responded to measures assessing their mood state and anxiety with greater affect in Spanish, regardless of whether it was the first or second language they'd learned (Guttfreund, 1990, cited in Altarriba & Morier, 2004, p. 252). This suggests that bilingual people may present themselves differently in psychological and other assessments depending on the language used. We must use caution, therefore, before we ascribe meaning to expressions of emotion in other languages and compare them to English expectations or norms. In addition, interviewees' internal emotional life cannot always be easily "read" from their external displays, especially if we are not familiar with their culture (see Chapter 5 on nonverbal communication).

Many people learn their first language in the home, in a supportive and loving environment, and their second language in school or in the workplace, in a setting that provokes greater anxiety. Even for people who become truly bilingual, the first language may remain a language of human connection and warmth whereas the second language is a language of public performance and unease.

The distancing that bilinguals often experience in their second language has been called the *detachment* effect (Marcos, 1976, cited in Altarriba & Morier, 2004). Some psychologists have proposed that a person's first language allows greater access to emotional content, whereas the second language may offer a different advantage—it might afford people who have suffered traumatic experiences enough distance from them to begin discussing them (Altarriba & Morier, 2004). This increased emotional control in a second language can be an advantage or disadvantage, depending on the nature of the interview. I once reviewed a videotape of two Mexican girls who were interviewed in English about sexual abuse by their stepfather. They gave precise and clear information. However, the district attorney declined to prosecute, saying the girls looked stiff and formal, as if they had been rehearsed. I believe the girls would have expressed greater emotion and would have seemed more sincere if they had been interviewed in their native language.

A converse situation holds true with some people. Bridget told me about growing up in a home marked by paternal substance abuse and violence. She learned Spanish as an adult and currently speaks Spanish with her life partner. Bridget says she has less perspective on her childhood when she discusses it in English (her first language). When speaking about difficult topics in English, she feels like that vulnerable child again. When she discusses her childhood in Spanish, Bridget is able to see it more dispassionately, through the eyes of an adult. Spanish is both her second language and the language of her safe, adult self.

Perez Foster (1999), a bilingual psychoanalyst who has written extensively about psychotherapy with bilingual people, describes how she has learned to appreciate and make use of the dual language worlds of bilingual clients:

> I [became] willing to enter the fray of my own patients' dual-language worlds. I used Spanish and English alternately, wherever patients led me: sometimes to penetrate experience, sometimes to skim it, but always to glean new understanding of inner worlds that had been organized by two different types of culturally embedded language symbols. (p. 54)

For the deep levels of understanding required in psychoanalysis, Perez Foster advocates a dual-language approach to working with bilingual people. While this kind of understanding may not be needed or possible in many of our interviews, we should keep in mind that we are missing something when we interview bilingual people in one language only, particularly when it is not the language of their heart.

OPERATIONALIZING LANGUAGE COMPETENCE: U.S. GUIDELINES AND REQUIREMENTS

People from some immigrant groups, such as Cambodians, Russians, Poles, Sudanese, Somalis, Bosnians, and the Hmong, rarely have the opportunity to work with professionals who speak their language, virtually guaranteeing that the benefit they receive from services will be less than that received by native speakers of English.

In many settings, the serious shortage of bilingual personnel, interpreters, and translated material at public and private agencies can create severe barriers to quality services. Federal guidelines for health care settings mandate the following standards for linguistically competent services. Although many fields lag behind health care in terms of serving language minority clients, I believe the following standard should be adopted in other settings as well.

How Organizations Must Provide Language Access

- Organizations must offer and provide language assistance services, including bilingual staff and interpreter services, at no cost to each patient/consumer with limited English proficiency at all points of contact, in a timely manner during all hours of operation.
- Organizations must provide to patients/consumers in their preferred language both verbal offers and written notices informing them of their right to receive language assistance services.

- Organizations must ensure the competence of language assistance provided to limited English proficient patients/consumers by interpreters and bilingual staff. Family and friends should not be used to provide interpretation services (except on request by the patient/consumer).

- Organizations must make available easily understood patient-related materials and must post signage in the languages of the groups that are commonly encountered in the service area.

Note. Data from National Standards for Culturally and Linguistically Appropriate Services in Healthcare, U.S. Department of Health and Human Services (2001).

The Culturally and Linguistically Appropriate Services (CLAS) standards are based on Title VI of the Civil Rights Act of 1964, which forbids discrimination against any person on the basis of national origin in offering any services that receive federal financial assistance. This has been interpreted by the courts to require delivering adequate services to any individual who does not understand English, including arranging for interpreters, as well as informing clients or patients that interpreters are available. Options include hiring bilingual staff, hiring staff interpreters, using volunteer interpreters who are trained and bound by confidentiality agreements, contracting with an interpreting service, and/or partnering with language minority community-based agencies (Suleiman, 2003).

On August 11, 2000, President Bill Clinton signed an Executive Order stating that all agencies receiving federal assistance must provide services that are accessible to people with limited English proficiency. These stipulations apply to most health care, legal, criminal justice, education, and social welfare settings. Apart from the humanitarian and moral obligation to provide these services, agencies should be advised that they ignore these legal obligations at their own peril.

Immigrants deserve prompt access to high-quality interpreters; this is the law. Prohibited practices include:

1. Providing immigrants with services that are more limited in scope or of a lower quality. For instance, it's prohibited to offer a variety of treatment options for an English-speaking therapy client while offering only individual therapy for a client who speaks another language. An example of another prohibited practice in this category would be to offer weekly in-person visits by a social worker for clients who speak English but only phone check-ins for clients who speak another language.

2. Unreasonable delays, such as keeping someone in a holding cell or on an overly long waiting list because bilingual personnel are not available and/or interpreters have not been accessed.

3. Limited participation in a program or activity, such as having someone who does not speak English observe a group counseling session from behind a one-way mirror with an interpreter, but not being able to participate in that group directly.

4. Failure to inform people with limited English proficiency (LEP) of the right to an interpreter; and

5. Requiring people to provide their own interpreters.

Because this is a federal obligation, it remains in force even in those states that have English-only laws. The federal guidelines recommend balancing four factors in determining how far agencies need to go to provide language-competent services and in deciding which groups receive them. (See the U.S. Department of Justice websites for further information on obligations toward people with limited English proficiency.)

Generally, it is most important for an agency to do what is necessary to remove language barriers if a large number of people are affected by those barriers, if there is frequent contact with speakers of a given language, if the program is an essential one, and if resources are readily available to remove such barriers. An agency is permitted to take fewer steps to ensure language competence if it serves fewer people impacted by language barriers, has less essential programs, and has fewer resources. A small agency in a community that has over 99% English speakers may choose to rely on telephone interpreting services rather than hiring bilingual staff, for instance. However, *every* agency must have some plan in place for reducing language barriers.

The Department of Justice offers suggestions for improving agency language competence. The first step involves *assessment*: What are the language competence needs of your agency or program? Schools, faith-based organizations, census data, and Department of Labor Statistics may provide you with valuable information about the language needs in your community. Then your agency needs to determine the number or proportion of LEP persons eligible to be served or likely to be encountered and the frequency with which LEP individuals currently come into contact with your programs or activities. You will also want to assess the importance of your program, activity or service to people's lives and the potential to help LEP persons; the resources you have at your disposal; and the costs of implementation for meeting those needs that have been identified.

The second step involves *planning*: Your agency should come up with a careful plan as to the steps you will take in a wide variety of circumstances when encountering LEP people. How are interpreters to be chosen or called? Where can workers access translated documents? The more essential the service, the more important it is to have bilingual or interpretation services readily available. An agency may develop different plans for more common languages versus languages that are less commonly encountered.

Third, make sure *documents* are available to people who read other languages: All documents considered vital, and most documents routinely given to clients, must be available in languages that are commonly encountered by the agency. A document is considered "vital" if it contains information that is critical for obtaining federal services and/or benefits, or is required by law. Vital documents include intake forms, applications, notices, complaint forms, and so on. For many larger documents, it's sufficient to translate only the most vital information included in the document, and the large document does not need to be translated in its entirety. The mandate to provide translations applies to websites as well as printed documents.

Making Documents More Accessible to People with Limited Language Proficiency

Some people who are native speakers of other languages may prefer to read in the language of their host country. In addition to translating documents into a variety of written languages, agencies can help make their standard documents more easily accessible to native speakers of other languages by incorporating the following suggestions:

- Include pictures that illustrate or complement the written word (not just for decoration).
- Use simple vocabulary, where possible.
- Use short, active, and direct sentences. Include only one thought in each sentence.
- Avoid jargon, slang, colloquial expressions, and technical terms. If you must use technical terms, explain their meaning using simple words and expressions.
- Avoid or be cautious in your attempts to be funny or sarcastic: This tone may be misinterpreted by people who do not read your language well.
- Have people from the culture(s) you are targeting comment on drafts of your written materials while they are being prepared.
- Use bold print with high contrast between the print color and the paper color. It is harder for people who do not read a language well to "fill in" letters that are difficult to read because they are too small or faded.

DOCUMENTS IN DIVERSE LANGUAGES

I have conducted trainings in a large city where nearly 50% of the school population was Latino, but *none* of the current child protective services documents were available in Spanish. The workers told me they had some old forms in Spanish, but these did not include important changes that had been instituted 4 years earlier. Every day families were being asked to sign forms, including treatment plans, that they could not understand, and as a result of this oversight, if the families failed to comply, their parental rights could be terminated. Although the state agency serving this major city had apparently translated a limited number of forms a decade earlier, the newer computer-ready forms had not been translated.

Unfortunately, the serious lack of documents in needed languages is all too common throughout the United States, and it is especially drastic for families that speak languages that are less widespread than Spanish. Small agencies should not need to pay to translate similar documents. Often, several agencies can work together to develop standardized forms, and then pool their resources for translating these into a variety of languages. Or, generic forms can be translated and then the translations can be altered slightly according to each agency's needs.

We should also be making greater use of technology in this regard. I recommend that agencies make their translated documents available on the Internet, so other agencies can adapt and use them. Parent agencies should consider translating basic forms into a variety of languages and making these available to local affiliates. National Planned Parenthood, for instance, is considering doing just this for their forms, which could then be used or adapted by local reproductive health agencies throughout the United States (K. Anderson, personal communication, June 2006).

Bilingual professionals describe frustration when they must ask clients to sign documents that the clients cannot read themselves. Bilingual workers do their best to translate documents spontaneously at the moment, but the clients still have no opportunity to study the documents, examine the fine print, ponder possible consequences, or show the documents to trusted friends for advice. This kind of situation is far worse if the professional does not read English or speak the clients' language fluently, and therefore the verbal translation is a mere approximation.

Providing an interpreter to help with filling out forms, one client at a time, is time-consuming and expensive. (However, providing an interpreter is still more ethical than expecting nonnative speakers of English to fend for themselves.) Clients who have an opportunity to fill out paperwork in their own languages are apt to feel more empowered and welcomed than clients who have to seek others' help with basic forms.

Occasionally, written materials have been translated into a variety of languages, but no one has checked the quality of the translation. Much of the work I have seen translated into Spanish or Portuguese—intake forms, research surveys, flyers, even signs on buildings—has been poorly translated and is nearly incomprehensible. They are often full of spelling and grammatical errors and even an invented word or two, adapted from English. Sometimes they use colloquial words that are known to people from a certain country but are incomprehensible or even offensive to people from another country. Translations of official documents must be done by people who are fluent *writers* of the language in question and should then be checked by others. It is just as egregious to present immigrant families with materials full of errors as it would be to present English-speaking families with materials full of errors—this practice damages the agency's credibility and throws into question its commitment to reaching the minority language community.

One final note about written documents: They should be translated at the language level that is appropriate to the readers of that language in the community. For instance, while documents for university students can be translated at the university level, documents for migrant farmworkers will need to be written at a far lower level of reading comprehension.

LANGUAGE PREFERENCE

When working with immigrants, it is important to ask about the language(s) they prefer to speak and their language abilities in each. Some people who were born in other countries and speak English with a heavy accent are still more comfortable in English than in their first language, but the reverse could also be true. On the other hand, a mother of Puerto Rican descent, Gabriela, told me how angry she was that her son had been automatically placed in a bilingual classroom because he had a Latino last name. The boy in question was a native speaker of English, not Spanish.

Rich information can often be obtained by asking about the language(s) a family speaks. It may turn out that the father is from one ethnic group and speaks one language with his children, while the mother speaks another, and the entire family has learned to speak a third language that was used in public settings in their country of origin. Sometimes a family denies that it needs an interpreter, overlooking the fact that a key family member, such as the mother, may not speak English at all. They may be so accustomed to leaving the mother out of conversations, or having a child interpret for the mother, that they do not even realize the ways in which using an official interpreter could enhance her understanding and participation.

CHOOSING A LANGUAGE FOR THE INTERVIEW

Interviewers should not confuse language competence with competence to testify, or with general intelligence. A person may not be competent to testify in English but may be competent to testify in another language. A person who seems insecure, hesitant, and timid in English may radiate confidence in his or her native language.

There are four options for conducting interviews with people whose native language is not English: Conduct the interview in English only, conduct it in the person's first language only, have a bilingual interviewer conduct the interview, or use an interpreter. Let's examine the first three options. Using an interpreter is examined in Chapter 7.

Interviewing in English Only

If the person seems fluent enough in English, the interviewer may be able to proceed in English only. This is certainly the easiest option for interviewers who do not speak the person's first language, but it can cause problems. In workshops, sometimes I ask for a show of hands of people who have studied a language other than English. Usually almost everyone in a room raises their hand. Then I ask them to turn to someone they have never met and tell that person, in that other language, about the most embarrassing or frightening experience of their life. This notion is usually greeted with giggles. I point out that this exercise is what we are asking people to do when we subject them to sensitive interviews in a language that is not their first language. We are expecting too much of adults and children when we ask them to reveal sensitive information and overcome linguistic and intercultural challenges at the same time.

Interviewers sometimes tell me that the person they were about to interview seemed perfectly comfortable in English, and then "she just suddenly stopped speaking English and said she didn't understand." Too often, interviewers assume that immigrants are faking their limitations in speaking English, or they could really understand and make themselves understood if they "just tried harder." While this might occasionally be the case, I suggest that different processes are usually at work. Some people who are "functional bilinguals" are able to converse minimally on a regular basis in English in their schools or workplaces but have a surprisingly restricted general vocabulary and may be unable to discuss sexual, emotional, medical, legal, or personal matters in English. If the interview concerns a sensitive topic, the interviewee may grow nervous and become less fluent. Additionally, some people will smile and nod convincingly, leading us to believe they understand what is happening. But when they are queried directly, their lack of comprehension becomes all too clear. The following example illustrates some of these complexities:

> In a forensic interview, a teenager requested a Spanish-speaking interviewer. None was available, so she was interviewed in English with an inter-

preter present. The girl scoffed at the idea of needing an interpreter, because she spoke English in school every day. However, as the interview progressed the interviewer noticed that after the young woman gave an answer to a question in English, if the same question was repeated in Spanish, she'd supply a slightly different answer. In other words, her English was not as fluent as she wanted to believe. Her Spanish vocabulary was far more comprehensive than her English vocabulary, and so she was able to convey ideas more precisely and accurately in Spanish.

Even if an interviewer chooses to conduct an interview in English, if the client is bilingual, it would be best if the interviewer was bilingual also. If not, an interpreter should be on hand to fill in occasional words, as the need arises.

Bilingual people often engage in what linguists call code switching or code mixing, which means using words or phrases from one language while speaking another. Reasons for using terms from the other language include: an easier time remembering certain terms in one language than another, a preference for the terms in one language over another, and an effort to create an alliance with another bilingual person (Ritchie & Bhatia, 2004). Bilingual people who are being interviewed in English about difficult matters may feel stressed by the obligation to use English only.

Many people assume that teenagers will be able to handle themselves in English because of their age and physical maturity. I urge caution in making this assessment based on a teenager's maturity or apparent bravado. Some teenagers who look highly assimilated are recent immigrants or have had inadequate English-language instruction; their dress is typically more acculturated than their speech. Even people who are highly bilingual may grow tired as an interview progresses and lose some of their fluency in English if it is their second language.

Interviewing in the Person's First Language Only

People can be interviewed in their first language (other than English) only if the person conducting the interview speaks the person's first language fluently. For instance, a police officer who speaks Korean could interview a suspect in Korean. However, it is important that people with limited English proficiency receive the same quality interview as others. I have sometimes seen a two-tier system, where English-speaking clients are interviewed by professionals with advanced degrees and a great deal of training, while Spanish-speaking clients are passed on to a Spanish-speaking professional who may be much less qualified in their field. Clearly, the fact that a person speaks Spanish (or Mandarin or French) does *not* qualify that person to conduct a sensitive interview any more than simply speaking English qualifies someone to do that job. Interviewers who conduct their work in a language other than English should have the same kind of training and supervision as everyone else. For instance, if the police officers who conduct child interviews in English have been trained to work with children, then the officers who conduct these interviews in languages other than English should be similarly trained.[1]

When a person is interviewed in his or her first language only, the interviewer needs to have a clear plan about how to proceed. It is unrealistic to expect an interviewer to conduct an interview in Khmer, for instance, and then halt the proceedings to interpret everything into English for others who are sitting in the room or watching behind a one-way mirror. Rather, there should be a qualified interpreter behind the mirror to interpret for the observers, so the interviewer can concentrate on conducting the best possible interview.

If the interview is conducted in a jurisdiction in which video or audiotapes are admissible in court, there needs to be a plan as to how the documentation will be presented. Alternatives include transcribing the entire tape (or only important sections) and later translating the transcription, or placing English subtitles onto the tape, or having the tape interpreted simultaneously in court. Each of these options has advantages and disadvantages, including cost. An attorney might also choose to enter a summary of the evidence garnered during the interview, rather than submitting the entire tape.

The interviewer will need to make decisions about whether to take notes in English or in the language of the interview. Interviewers who choose to take notes in English may still want to record important quotes in the interview's actual language—so their essence can be more precisely preserved, and so the direct quotes can be entered into official documents where relevant. (More information on taking notes is contained in Chapter 10 on writing reports.)

---

[1]Some people recommend a cointerviewing or active interpreter model where native speakers of particular languages have been trained to conduct interviews accompanied by a professional who does not have the language skills (Burnard, 2004; Pitchforth & van Teijlingen, 2005). The cointerviewer does not have the professional qualifications to be an interviewer. In these circumstances, the cointerviewer is culturally and linguistically close to the interviewee and uses his or her language abilities and cultural knowledge to facilitate the interviewing process. This approach may not be without difficulties, however, including distortions in the asking of questions, improper communication of the purposes of the interview or the affiliations of the interviewers, deviating from interviewing norms, and the exclusion of the primary interviewer at times when his or her input could be crucial (Pitchforth & van Teijlingen, 2005).

Bilingual Interviews

The third option for interviewing non-native speakers is for a bilingual professional to conduct a bilingual interview, switching from one language to another as the interviewee does. This professional will be able to understand the cultural issues and nuances in the conversation, and will be able to help out if the interviewee says, "How do you say _____?" in one language or the other. This professional may also be able to offer assurances in the interviewee's native language, such as, "You're doing fine. It's okay." In my opinion, bilingual interviewers for bilingual clients are clearly the best choice, and all our agencies and practices should employ qualified multilingual people whenever possible. Some bilingual interviewees prefer to speak about events in the language in which they occurred. Others prefer to use a different language, to distance themselves from it, at least as a stepping-stone until they become less distressed by the memory (Altarriba & Morier, 2004; Javier, 1995). Still others use both. Some bilingual people say they are comfortable being interviewed in English, and they begin in this language. As they enter the more emotionally laden content of the interview, they begin responding in their native language, or use words from their native language, without even realizing it (code switching). A bilingual interviewer can follow the person's lead.

A bilingual, bicultural[2] professional will be able to detect and interpret cultural cues as they emerge in an interview and identify those concepts that cannot be easily translated from one culture to another. A bilingual professional can also more effectively communicate with the family or community members who do not speak English but still need to be included.

ALTERNATIVE FORMS OF ENGLISH

Interviews have an extra layer of tension for people who are unaccustomed to speaking the form of English that is most common in your specific region. Can you imagine how hard it is for children or adults who are accus-

---

[2] "Bicultural" is usually used to describe a person from a given minority cultural group who is also comfortable in the dominant culture. I would like to point out that people who were born into the dominant group or a different minority group but who have intimate personal and professional contacts with members of a particular minority group may also be bicultural. "Bicultural" describes people who can feel and act like a native in two cultures, regardless of their place of birth or their genetic background.

tomed to speaking African American Vernacular English (formerly called Black English) or Jamaican, British, South African, or Kenyan English being interviewed by an authority in an English that sounds strange to them and in which they feel inadequate? Trinidadian scholar Dowdy (2002) writes about the difficulty of having to speak in the "master discourse" rather than "the language of personal expression" (p. 4):

> At a loss for words really describes the feeling of the soul in the "White" language world. Thoughts come into her head in her family's intimate vocabulary, and she strains to translate those ideas into the accepted form expected in public conversation. She expects that her usual facility with language will be available to her when she begins to speak in public. Instead, there are cold, metal sounds bouncing off her teeth, the act of translation cooling the passion of the thought. . . . The continual disappointment with the master discourse creates a shroud that covers every utterance with a doubt about its worthiness. The voice in her head does not match the tone in her throat. She sees and hears herself becoming a tape played at the wrong speed. (p. 12)

Our interviews should not cause this unhappy situation. With an open and warm attitude, we should convey that however the interviewee speaks is just fine—we will listen, and we will do our best to understand.

Small rejections of their language can seriously hinder our ability to set up a trusting relationship with people from a different cultural group. Delpit (2002) describes this eloquently: "Since language is one of the most intimate expressions of identity, indeed, 'the skin that we speak,' then to reject a person's language can only feel as if we are rejecting him" (p. 47). We must be careful not to correct our interviewees' English and not to show impatience if we are having trouble understanding them. Our responses to people who use different dialects of English are more than just responses to "difference"; they are responses to foreignness or poverty. Purcell-Gates (2002) discusses how the language a person speaks "is the clearest and most stable marker of class membership" (p. 133). She continues:

> [The] dialects of those in power do not elicit the same knee-jerk disdain and assumptions of deficit as do the dialects of the sociopolitically marginalized. For example, the Boston dialect of the Kennedys or the Southern dialect of Jimmy Carter are never pointed to as evidence of cognitive and linguistic deficit. But let a poor, urban, Appalachian woman speak for only a few minutes and powerful attitudes of prejudice and assumptions of inferiority are elicited. (pp. 133–134)

Some interviewers hear people's speech and—on a gut level—assume that the way they talk marks them as uneducated or stupid. This can be true for White people who might be considered "hillbillies" or "White trash" as well as immigrants, African Americans from the rural South, and Native Americans who might speak with a slightly different syntax and intonation. We must guard against these responses, and know they are ingrained stereotypes based on perceptions of social class and difference.

CONCLUDING OBSERVATIONS

If the interviewee does not speak English fluently, for many kinds of interviews we should call in a qualified interpreter immediately (see Chapter 7, "The Interpreted Interview"). However, we still frequently need to converse with people who are not native speakers of English, who speak with a heavy accent, or who speak a form of English that is not familiar to us. In these encounters we must be supportive and understanding and make a concerted effort to understand people's speech without shaming them.

Language competence may be the great new frontier in cultural competence. While ethical guidelines are clear and unequivocal, many of our agencies remain in violation of those guidelines. If we want our interviews to be successful—so we can obtain accurate information, understand our clients' full personalities and emotions, and help them access their memories— we need to be able to speak with them in their preferred language (which may reflect their preferred culture). In some cases, we can do this directly, if we are bilingual in the client's language. In other cases, we need to enlist the help of an interpreter.

Questions to Think about and Discuss

1. You are about to start an interview and you realize the interviewee speaks English only haltingly. What do you do and what do you say? (This will vary with your context.)
2. You are interviewing a person in English whose first language is Spanish. Discuss some of the drawbacks of conducting the interview in English.
3. Discuss three steps you can take to improve the language competence of your practice or agency.
4. Describe an interview or a conversation that you conducted in English with someone whose English was not fluent. How did the language gap affect the understanding? Did you become aware later that you may have misinterpreted something, or been misunderstood?

RECOMMENDED ADDITIONAL READING

Bhatia, T., & Ritchie, W. C. (Eds.). (2004). *The bilingual handbook*. Malden, MA: Blackwell.

Delpit, L., & Dowdy, J. K. (2002). *The skin that we speak: Thoughts on language and culture in the classroom*. New York: New Press.

Perez Foster, R. (1999). *The power of language in the clinical process: Assessing and treating the bilingual person*. New York: Jason Aronson.

U.S. Department of Health and Human Services, Office of Minority Health. (2001, March). *National Standards for Culturally and Linguistically Appropriate Services in Health Care* [Final report]. Washington, DC: Author.

1 The Interpreted Interview

Interpreters make it possible to listen to people who otherwise would be voiceless in our interviews. High-quality interpretation allows us to obtain information, gain interviewees' confidence, reduce their isolation, understand their worldview, and convey information as needed. Poor-quality interpretation leads to frustration for all involved, and it can leave clients even more vulnerable than before we interviewed them. Similarly, when interpreters are used inappropriately, problems abound.

This chapter provides an improved understanding of when and how to use interpreters, and your options in this regard. You are also invited to consider some of the subtleties in the interpreting process. This chapter will help you make optimum use of interpreting services in interviews, to improve your relationship with the interviewee, and to gain the most accurate information possible.

THE INTERPRETER'S POWER

We cannot underestimate the power of the interpreter in an interview. The head of interpreting services at a major private U.S. hospital said the following: "Interpreters are the most powerful people in a medical conversation" (Davidson, 2000, p. 379). I believe interpreters are equally important in nonmedical settings, too.

Interpreters do not simply convey the spoken word from both sides, although this is their primary stated function. They also serve as the agent of exchange and negotiation between the worlds of the interviewer and the interviewee (Davidson, 2000). Unfortunately, it is not possible to receive an absolutely perfect interpretation because subtleties of meaning and context differ across cultures. At best, an interpreter can convey what each party says and means in a "good enough" fashion to facilitate mutual understanding.

All participants in an interview have a goal. Sometimes, the goals of the interviewer and interviewee may not simply differ; they may also be in opposition. While interpreters should maintain neutrality in this kind of situation, often they ally themselves with the institution that is paying them. For instance, perhaps a woman is being evaluated to see if she qualifies for disability services. The woman hopes to qualify for the support, whereas the evaluator may have been told to cut down on the number of new enrollees. The interpreter might try to support the institutional goals of limiting access to services, which is far from a neutral stance.

To use another example, interpreters employed in a medical environment may see their role as assuring speedy appointments to ensure the efficient use of the doctors' time. Other interpreters who identify closely with members of their ethnic community may see their role as protecting the community's reputation and may tell an accused person, "Don't worry! Let me handle it," providing what they think is the least damaging version of a story rather than interpreting accurately.

We usually think of interpreters as conduits rather than participants in conversations. However, research shows that interpreters regularly edit, delete, emphasize, deemphasize, and embellish statements from both parties. "Interpreters do not merely convey messages; they shape and, in some real sense, create those messages in the name of those for whom they speak" (Davidson, 2000, p. 382). Interpreters not only shape the content that is conveyed but also make choices about when to speak, whom to interrupt when they speak, and which comments they will "let pass" without interpreting.

Interviews occur between people of unequal status. Usually the interviewee is either seeking a service or position or seeking to avoid an unfavorable outcome that might result from the interview. The interviewee is usually dependent on the interviewer's judgment and goodwill to obtain the best possible outcome. An interviewee who is also forced to depend on an interpreter is even more disempowered. The clients for whom the interpreter is speaking are usually immigrants, often from developing countries, who may feel insecure in their new land. This insecurity increases even further the interviewees' feelings of vulnerability and the interpreters' consequent power.

Indeed, those who are dependent on interpreters have good reason to feel vulnerable. In a study of Spanish-language interpreters in a city hospital, Davidson (2000) found that when the patient and physician speak the same language, almost all the patient's questions are answered by the physician. But when an interpreter is involved, more than half the questions are not even passed on to the physician. In some cases, the interpreter answers the questions him- or herself. In other cases, the interpreter simply ignores the questions. Because all too many interpreters fail to give patients an opportunity to explain their concerns adequately, physicians often see their immigrant patients as overly passive, or believe the patients are complaining about nonexistent problems.

Perez Foster (1999) offers us the example of a Dominican doorman who was occasionally enlisted to serve as an interpreter in clinical interviews. Over time the clinicians discovered that he was exaggerating the promiscuity and drug use of the clients in an attempt to feel himself separate from and superior to those more recent immigrants. Acknowledging the potential power of interpreters, we become aware of the need to be careful in their selection, training, and supervision.

WHEN TO USE AN INTERPRETER

Professionals who speak a bit of a second language may be tempted to conduct interviews in the interviewee's language, thus obviating the need for an interpreter. While this may save time and money, it is not advisable unless the interviewer is truly proficient in the language and culture of the interviewee. Clearly, conducting an important interview without thoroughly dominating the language increases the likelihood of miscommunication. Knowing "restaurant French" or "street Spanish" or even "a bit of Creole" is not adequate to conducting an important and sensitive interview in this language. If an interviewer begins using the interviewee's language but does not speak it adequately, it places the interviewee in the awkward position of not wanting to insult the interviewer by requesting an interpreter.

Interpreters may be needed at various stages of the interview process, from setting an appointment to interviewing to presenting the report to pursuing follow-up contacts. People with limited English proficiency need to be informed of their right to an interpreter. They need to be told that they may request an interpreter at any point in the provision of services, even if they have initially declined one. Some clients refuse an interpreter's services out of pride or out of a fear that they will not be taken seriously if they do not speak directly in English. Sometimes they decline because they do not understand the offer, they are afraid of breaches in confidentiality, or they are concerned that they may be charged for the interpreter's services. Often, people who "get by" in English in most situations are putting themselves at a great disadvantage if they do not avail themselves of an interpreter in important official interviews, where even the slightest misunderstanding could have life-changing repercussions. This potential hazard should be explained to them carefully.

Professionals might fail to access an interpreter because of the costs, delays, and complications involved. Often an interviewer assumes that clients do not need an interpreter because they seem able to express themselves well enough in English. However, as the conversations proceed and become more precise and emotionally laden, and as the clients become tired and stressed, their English often deteriorates. It is one thing to be able to make small talk or buy groceries in a second language; it is quite another to give and receive complex information with tremendous consequences in that second language (see Chapter 6 on language competence).

FINDING AN INTERPRETER

When an interpreter is needed, agencies should try to obtain the services of a professionally trained interpreter. Some jurisdictions have court certification, medical certification, or other official certifications for interpreters, while others do not. In most situations that do not take place in court, a court-certified interpreter may not be necessary and may be prohibitively expensive. However, if the material is going to be used in court, professionals should check to determine the exact requirements in their jurisdiction. In some areas, unfortunately, even court certification is not a guarantee that the interpreter is qualified and well trained. For example, when Texas began licensing its court interpreters in 2001 and judges were authorized to write a letter declaring that someone they knew was qualified to be a court interpreter, unqualified people were grandfathered in under this program.

Even if a court-certified interpreter is not legally required in a given interview, interpreters used for important interviews should be professionally trained. Agencies need to maintain a list of professionally trained interpreters to achieve coverage in a variety of languages; they should not wait until the middle of a crisis before they scramble to find an interpreter in a language that might be less common in their area.

The federal order on serving people with Limited English Proficiency allows for agencies to rely on qualified voluntary community interpreters who are bound by confidentiality agreements.[1] Several women's crisis centers in my area have banded together to establish an intensive training pro-

---

[1]See the U.S. Department of Health and Human Services Office of Civil Rights Guidance Memorandum on Prohibition Against National Origin Discrimination: Persons with Limited English Proficiency.

gram for bilingual volunteers who are taught to serve as interpreters. Many of these bilingual volunteers end up taking further training to learn to work on the hotline and attend to crises. Volunteers from dozens of languages have been trained and are available within 24 hours. Not only does this increase the centers' ability to serve immigrant communities—it also increases knowledge of the centers' services within those communities. The bilingual volunteer training program serves as a form of outreach.

Baker (1981) urges us to be especially cautious when employing interpreters who claim fluency in a variety of languages and may exaggerate their fluency in their eagerness to obtain work. For instance, a Polish immigrant may claim to be able to interpret in Russian *and* Polish although he possesses only rudimentary abilities in Russian. Or a Somali interpreter may say he speaks Arabic although he has only used Arabic in the mosque to pray and does not speak everyday Arabic. Interpreters should be able to demonstrate certification or training in the specific language that they are going to interpret. Where a certified interpreter cannot be found and a noncertified interpreter is necessary, another interpreter or a bilingual professional should first interview the would-be interpreter in the language required, to avoid later embarrassment and problems. This interview should not focus simply on language competence; it should also assess for the interpreter's interpersonal sensitivity, knowledge of the cultural issues of the target population, and some of the difficulties that might emerge in the interpreted conversation.

Agency officials need to think carefully before asking their multilingual staff to take on interpreting duties without additional training or compensation. For instance, in some police, social work, educational and medical settings, multilingual professionals are asked to interpret for their colleagues in addition to carrying a full workload. This is an unfair burden and may hinder the quality of the work. First of all, these professionals have not usually been trained in interpreting—which is its own professional field. They may make crucial errors because of their lack of interpreter training. Second, unless interpreting is part of their job description and they have a reduced caseload to compensate for the time they spend interpreting, bilingual professionals who are asked to interpret in addition to fulfilling their regular responsibilities are being forced to perform two jobs. This is a recipe for burnout and a poor outcome. Third, although their language skills may be good enough to work in a bilingual context, they may not have enough skills in English or the target language to be able to interpret. For instance, I know a Mexican American police officer whose Spanish certainly helps him communicate with Latinos in his work. He dreads being asked to interpret for his colleagues, however, because his Spanish is only mediocre. He does not want to tell his sergeant that he is unqualified to interpret or that he needs to take a Spanish-language class. He believes that this kind of disclosure would make him lose status in the department.

Finding the right interpreter also means finding someone who can understand the interviewee's dialect. For instance, many Native American languages have different dialects, so the interpretation may differ if the interpreter speaks a different dialect. People from many Apache bands speak Athebascan, but the dialects are so different that one Apache band may not be able to speak comfortably with members of another. The same may be said of speakers of many other languages, from Mandarin to Arabic to Quechua. The differences in the various dialects may be so broad as to make mutual understanding impossible, or may be relatively minor. Spanish has many words that vary from country to country and region to region. I first learned to speak Spanish in Ecuador, where the language is infused with many words from Quechua. I didn't even know that these words were not Spanish until I traveled in Spain and was met with blank stares when I used the word *ñaño* for brother, for instance, or *chompa* for sweater. However, a professionally trained interpreter should have enough flexibility to be able to understand a variety of dialects, to be able to express him- or herself in a "standard" form of the language, and enough confidence to make an inquiry when he or she does not understand a specific word or term.

It can be difficult or virtually impossible to find a "professionally trained interpreter" in some languages, particularly in smaller communities, or where people who speak a given language are uncommon. For instance, trained interpreters in many indigenous languages of the Americas, African languages, and Asian languages that are less common in your community may be hard to come by. To interpret an important Tennessee court case in the Mexican language Mixtec, the Southern Poverty Law Center flew in a trained interpreter from California (Samuels, González, & Lockett, 2006). Clearly this is going to be beyond most of our means in most situations. When a trained interpreter is not available, you will need to be extremely judicious in how you choose an interpreter. The next two sections provide several suggestions.

Telephone Interpreting Services

Some agencies rely on companies that provide telephone interpreting services. These services can either be contracted on a monthly basis or used spontaneously and paid for by the minute. Typically, the agency calls the service and asks for an interpreter who closely matches the client's needs (e.g., an interpreter who speaks Egyptian Arabic or Dominican Spanish).

The telephone interpreters can be patched in to interpret phone calls or can be used through the telephone for in-person interviews and sessions. For these in-person interviews, the interviewer sits with the interviewee but speaks into a telephone in English. The interpreter then provides the interpretation through a telephone held by the interviewee, and vice versa. While this arrangement is far better than *no* interpreting, it can be confusing and alienating (particularly for children) and should be used only as a last resort. It can be hard for people to trust the confidentiality of interpreters whom they cannot even see, and the conversation becomes highly unnatural. The nonverbal communication is stilted and is completely unseen by the interpreter.

Telephone interpreting is used in some hospitals for medical consultations. Although I have not seen a formal evaluation of this procedure, I am skeptical about its effectiveness in medical interviews, where patients so often point to parts of their body and want to show things visually to the medical provider. The interpreters' inability to see patients hinders their effectiveness. Additionally, if the telephone interpreters have not received specific preparation in medical interpreting, they are unlikely to know the appropriate translations of medical terminology. If they use words that are not sufficiently specific, the patient is not being truly informed. On the other hand, if they use an overly technical term, the patient is unlikely to understand. While this is true of all interpreting, the telephone interpreter is hindered by being unable to check the patient's expression for understanding.

Computer Translations

Some midwives in London have begun carrying laptops equipped with translating software on their visits to immigrant pregnant and postpartum patients. They find this is better than not having any interpreting ability at all, and their agencies simply do not have the money for regular interpreters. By mediating their conversation through a computer, they believe the woman's confidentiality is better preserved than requesting that she provide an interpreter of her own, who is most likely to be a family member. However, this method of communicating is clumsy and often inaccurate. Computer translating programs make numerous errors and cannot tell the difference between homonyms such as "bear" meaning the animal and "bear" meaning to carry a burden or tolerate or "bear" as in bear a child. They also cannot interpret the woman's speech if the woman is illiterate or does not know how to spell properly, and they are generally unusable for translating words into English from another language that uses a different alphabet, such as Chinese, Arabic, or Russian.

Selecting an Interpreter

Try to keep in mind the following areas when choosing an interpreter Some of these issues are more important than others, depending on your context and the particular interviewee:

- Proficiency in the two languages
- Interpreter training and certification/licensing, where applicable (with proof)
- Interpreting experience (with proof or references, where possible)
- Knowledge of the topics to be discussed and comfort with them
- Ability to maintain confidentiality
- Familiarity with the interviewee's dialect/national origin
- Willingness to work as part of a team
- Sufficient self-awareness so as not to impose his or her own issues on the interviewee
- Willingness to treat all interviewees with respect regardless of gender, sexual orientation, marital status, political beliefs, religion, caste, socioeconomic status, disease status, mental health issues, and so on
- Professionalism and willingness to observe professional boundaries
- An understanding of the appropriate role of the interpreter

INFORMAL INTERPRETERS

Avoid informal ad hoc interpreters—people from the interviewee's family, friends, office workers, and others. As agencies scramble at the last minute to meet the needs of the linguistically diverse families in their areas, sometimes they rely on secretaries, janitors, siblings, and others to interpret for interviews. Even battering men have been asked to interpret for their victimized wives and children—an obvious conflict of interest. I have heard of the local Spanish teacher—known to virtually everyone in the school system—being asked to interpret child abuse interviews in Spanish.

When an interpreter is used, children and families have the sense that the ears that are *really* hearing them are those of the interpreter. Clients may decline to speak openly when a local teacher, member of the clergy, or other well-known community member is interpreting, because of concern that everyone in the community would end up knowing their business.

It is problematic to use untrained interpreters for a variety of reasons. An untrained interpreter might be too embarrassed or disturbed by the material to interpret accurately. (Recently, when a victim began revealing the sexual part of an assault, the Portuguese interpreter in my area blushed, shook his head, and said he could not repeat what the victim had said.)

An untrained interpreter may want to help the interviewee or the interviewee's family or their community to save face, thereby failing to interpret some of the more problematic or incriminating information. This may be just the information that we need most. For instance, a young Puerto Rican girl disclosed that the uncle with whom she was living had sexually molested her. In the interview with the detective, the interpreter said to the girl in Spanish, "Why don't you say it was just physical abuse and not sexual abuse? You can get out of his home that way and he won't get into so much trouble."

An untrained interpreter is more likely to embellish or delete information, which could impede the success of an interview. These deletions and embellishments are particularly problematic in legal settings where inconsistencies in testimony (which actually result from faulty interpretation) might seriously jeopardize a case.

Untrained, informal interpreters are likely to be familiar only with their own dialect of the language. A trained interpreter should be familiar with the way the language is spoken in a variety of countries. (For example, *coger* is a common word in Spanish but means different things throughout the world. In some countries it is an everyday word meaning "to get," and in others it is a particularly crude word for sexual intercourse. A trained interpreter should not stumble over a word like this and should know its multiple meanings.)

An untrained interpreter might unknowingly use regionally specific words or English words that would not be understandable to the client. For example, I witnessed an interview that was interpreted by a Puerto Rican social worker who had no training in interpreting and who used Spanglish throughout the interview. (Spanglish, used by many Latinos in English-speaking countries, is a form of Spanish that includes a large number of words that have been "borrowed" from English and sometimes transformed into Spanish by adding on Spanish endings or pronunciation.) This interpreter asked the child what she did for *el Easter* and instructed her to *eskipear* (skip) an item on a checklist. The child—who had recently emigrated from Central America—did not understand these words, which were actually adaptations of English. This same social worker interpreted the interviewer's question, "Can you tell me the difference between the truth and a lie," using the Puerto Rican word for fib, *un embuste*. When the girl looked back blankly, the interpreter said she did *not* know the difference, which was not the case at all. Rather, the girl did not recognize the Puerto Rican slang word. The child's supposed inability to differentiate between truth and a lie then tainted the rest of the interview.

When an interviewee makes a statement that is disjointed or doesn't make sense, an untrained interpreter may try to read the client's mind and piece together incoherent statements into a coherent whole, "cleaning up" the confused statements. This is called overinterpreting, when an interpreter tries to convey what interviewees *mean* rather than what they *say*. A trained interpreter would be able to convey the competency and form of the original statement—in addition to the content.

An untrained interpreter may not know or follow the rules of keeping confidential what happens in the interview. Nothing makes people clam up faster than the perception that their private business is going to become common knowledge. A Chinese-language interpreter in a hospital near me used to betray confidences in this way, saying to a patient in the emergency room, for instance, "You should stop by to see Wang on the third floor. He's in for a bad liver." The hospital could not understand why the Chinese patients would not talk freely, until a Chinese-speaking nurse sat in on a conversation and found out that the interpreter could not be trusted.

An untrained interpreter who knows the interviewee or his family, or who is a member of the family's place of worship or community, might want to control what the interviewee says or might report it back to others. One would hope that a trained interpreter would be professional enough to understand and respect the ethical mandates of accuracy and confidentiality. After all, his or her livelihood depends on it.

There can also be problems of *perceived* lack of confidentiality and multiple relationships. Even if the person interpreting does not actually betray confidences, interviewees will worry about this. Everyone knows one another in some small ethnic communities, and secrets are hard to keep. Trained interpreters will be able to explain their role and the concept of confidentiality and then briefly explain their professional commitment to confidentiality.

Family members should not be allowed to act as interpreters or be involved in interpreting sessions, except at the explicit direct request of the interviewee. Even in these situations, it behooves the professional to make sure the interpreter is serving the client's best interests. Sometimes family members deliberately distort the statement of the individual interviewee or interviewer to serve the family's perceived interests. For instance, if a child being assessed tells an interviewer that he does not do his homework because he has to care for his four siblings every day after school, the interpreter might choose, instead, to say that he doesn't do his homework because he doesn't feel like it, because the interpreter believes this response will be less damaging to the family. The informal interpreter might also invent or hide information to try to protect the interviewee from being sanctioned or punished.

Using Children as Interpreters

Minor children should not be asked to interpret in interviews. In children's presence, interviewees will often refrain from conveying their true level of distress or will pass over the disturbing details of an event. Equally damaging, a child may be exposed to information from which he or she should be protected.

Interpreting also puts inappropriate pressure on a child, who then feels responsible for the outcome of the interview and might—indeed—be blamed by the family if the outcome was not to their liking. In addition, the child might not have adequate vocabulary or understanding to convey sexual detail or legal or medical information. Imagine the anguish a child feels when asked to interpret the results of medical tests for a parent, or the pressure the child feels when asked to convey personal information to someone in law enforcement! To protect their loved ones, children may fail to interpret correctly.[2] Adults may also ask children who are interpreting for them to give "the best answer," and so the child is put into the position of having to try to figure out what the best answer might be.

So much is missed when a child is used as an interpreter. Some issues cannot or should not be explained in front of a child and therefore are skipped over entirely. Other concepts will be misunderstood or misinterpreted by a child. Sometimes parents will grow angry at a child who is struggling or hesitating while interpreting, thinking the child is being recalcitrant or willfully introducing delays.

With all of these admonitions against using children as interpreters, I have found myself in situations where I had to do just that:

> Late one summer I arrived at the apartment of a Somali woman who was home alone with her two school-age children, her preschooler, her toddler, and her infant. The father, who spoke some English and had said he would be home, was not there when I arrived. We were in a time crunch. The mother and I packed up the children and walked over to the school, where she had an intake appointment with a Headstart Center (federally sponsored preschool program). The Center had not scheduled an interpreter, despite my request. I was unable to reach Somali social workers on the telephone. It was crucial to get

---

[2]In 2005 the California State Assembly approved Bill (AB) 775 that prohibits interpreting by children under the age of 15 in hospitals, clinics, and doctors' offices. The bill does not affect casual interpretation by a child, such as the transmission of the time of the next appointment, but rather focuses on discussions of substantive medical concerns between a medical provider and a patient.

the preschooler enrolled in the Center, so we proceeded with the two school-age boys interpreting. This was not without its complications.

The Headstart intake interviewer wanted to know the following: At what age did the preschooler first sit up? What were the mother's goals for him? What were the boy's areas of strength and weakness? How would she describe his social skills? What activities did he prefer? How should they help him fall asleep at nap time? Admittedly, much information was lost and undoubtedly some information was misconstrued, as these two young boys who had minimal English themselves struggled to make bridges between their mother and the interviewer. Not only did the boys not recognize words like "goals" in English, I am not sure whether they knew them in Somali, if indeed the same concept exists. This was far from an ideal interview, but the boy was enrolled in preschool, the emergency contact information and medical information was conveyed, and—in the real world—this was the best we could do, balancing the competing needs for accuracy and timeliness. I asked a Somali social worker to schedule a meeting between the parents and the Headstart director on a later day to facilitate the relationship between the family and the Center, and to make sure any inaccuracies conveyed in this initial interview would not be perpetuated throughout the boy's school career.

PREPARING INTERPRETERS

Ideally, the interpreters we use are professionally trained and certified and familiar with our setting. In practice, today, this is often not the case, as agencies scramble to get conversations interpreted using the resources they have on hand. This section describes some of the orientation that nonprofessional interpreters may need before working on sensitive issues. Much of this advice would be unnecessary to convey to a professional interpreter, and it might even seem insulting. Readers need to use their judgment with each interpreter, to decide how much advice and guidance is necessary.

A New York City health center recently assessed all the people who they used as Spanish-language interpreters. Only half were found to have the requisite language skills in both languages to interpret accurately. These people were then given some training in interpreting, for which they expressed gratitude. At last, this aspect of their work was being recognized! They were eager to improve their interpreting skills.

While it is ideal to assess and provide formal training for interpreters at your agency, until such a program is established you may at least want to prepare a checklist that you can review with interpreters before using their services, to make sure you have discussed all relevant information.

Preparing the Interpreter for Your Interview

Professionally trained interpreters should already be familiar with guidelines on how to interpret for an interview. However, even people who work for interpreting agencies may not have received professional interpreter training.

- Inform the interpreter of any special circumstances surrounding the interview, such as audio- or videotaping or a one-way mirror.
- Record the interpreter's name, qualifications, and contact information.
- Remind the interpreter that confidentiality is of the utmost importance. Interpreters must not discuss the interviewee, the interview, or any personal information learned in the interpreted conversation with anyone else. Ask the interpreter to read carefully and sign a pledge of confidentiality in which he or she promises not to speak about the interview or reveal the identity of the participants. Ask the interpreter to discuss questions about confidentiality with you before the interview begins and after, as necessary.
- Where relevant, inform the interpreter of the possibility that he or she might be asked to testify in court.
- Tell the interpreter that if he or she knows the interviewee or the interviewee's family, which might jeopardize the client's sense of confidentiality, he or she should not take the interpreting assignment. If the interpreter discovers a connection to the client's family after the interview has begun, the interpreter should ask for a pause and inform you of the dual relationship so you can decide how to proceed. (In some cases, even where the interpreter has had prior contact with the interviewee, an explanation of the interpreter's role and pledge of confidentiality will be sufficient to allay concerns and the interview can proceed. In other situations, another interpreter would be preferable.) Interviewees who have had prior social contact with the interpreter are often evasive or overly polite, or they deny problems, difficult feelings, or sensitive issues.
- Tell the interpreter about the nature of the interview you are undertaking and explain the level of precision that is needed. For instance, interpreting for a standard medical exam might not require the same attention to careful phrasing as a forensic interview, because concerns about leading the interviewee would not have the same legal importance. However, subtle differences between words such as "hurt," "sting," "ache," "itch," "throb," and so on, may be important in a medical interview.
- For forensic interviews, inform the interpreter in advance that you have to be careful about how you phrase questions, and that you may sometimes ask questions in a way that seems funny, awkward, or indirect. It's important to instruct the interpreter not to rephrase any questions but still to speak in a way that the interviewee will be able to understand.
- Ask interpreters to assure the accuracy of their work—without embellishments, omissions, or editing. The interpreter should not leave out details that may seem unimportant. Ask the interpreter to translate word for word and not infer or summarize. If the interpreter does not understand terms or expressions that need translating, he or she should ask for an explanation.
- Ask the interpreter to translate at the same level of language skills as the client.

Words that may not translate exactly, such as medical or legal terminology, may need to be defined and conveyed in a more easily understandable way.

- Inform the interpreter that if the client answers in partial sentences, in a confusing way, or in baby talk—these answers should be communicated as they were stated, and not changed, clarified, or improved. Ask the interpreter not to guess what the client meant but rather to repeat in English precisely what the client said. Let the interpreter know that you are not interested merely in what the client says, but also in how he or she says it. Ask the interpreter to tell you if the interviewee's speech is confusing in some way. (A good interpreter will ask for a moment to give an "aside" during an interview, to inform you of some irregularity in the interviewee's speech that otherwise may not be evident. For example, if the client has a notable stutter, articulation difficulties due to overmedication or another problem, or appears to be in an altered state, or has other peculiarities that may be lost in the interpretation, the interpreter should convey this information to you because it might affect both the quality of the interpretation and the line of questioning.)

- Where applicable, tell the interpreter that sometimes during interviews people will discuss mundane matters and conversely that sometimes they talk about acts that will be painful for the interpreter to hear about and repeat. They may talk about suffering and acts of violence that are hard for the interpreter to imagine or believe, and that might make the interpreter feel sad, repulsed, or angry. Instruct the interpreter to stay as neutral as possible and avoid showing through manner or facial expressions that he or she disbelieves the interviewee or is upset, angry, or disgusted.

- Let the interpreter know that the interviewer or client (even a child) might use words that the interpreter is uncomfortable saying—slang words or sexual words, for instance. Ask the interpreter to stick closely to the words that are used and try to put aside feelings of embarrassment. Ask the interpreter to try to use the same kind of words that you and the interviewee use. That is, if the interviewee uses a word like "dick" in his or her first language, the interpreter should not substitute the more formal word "penis" but should try to use a similar kind of slang term.

- Ask the interpreter to convey the affective (feeling) tone of the interviewee's statements and not just the literal content.

- Let interpreters know that their own opinions on issues such as sexuality, politics, abortion rights, family violence, drug use, and so on must be kept out of the interpretation work.

- Ask the interpreter to try to remain impartial at all times. The interpreter should not lean toward any outcome other than the accurate transmission of information.

- Ask the interpreter to show sensitivity to the anxieties and difficulties that the client may be experiencing in the interview.

- Interpreters need to be aware of and sensitive to cultural beliefs and rules of behavior of other cultures. Ask the interpreter to explain these to the interviewer, when appropriate.

- Let the interpreter know if you want help understanding relevant cultural issues (see the next section of this chapter).

- Ask the interpreter if he or she has any questions.

Baker (1981) cautions against interpretation that overemphasizes exactness over understanding, in describing a court hearing:

> The judge asked the [unaccompanied refugee minor] youths through an interpreter if they "agreed to being placed under the custody and guardianship of the agency and to follow the reasonable directions thereof." It was later discovered that the interpreter's close translation of this question had led the youths to believe they had been placed into slavery. (p. 392)

In other words, interpreters should stick closely to the language used, and at the same time ensure that the *meaning* of the statements is conveyed.

CULTURAL ASIDES AND OTHER REASONS TO PAUSE AN INTERVIEW

In some kinds of interviews you may want the interpreter to serve as a cultural bridge from the interviewer to the interviewee and back. For instance, if a Muslim interviewee says something about being hungry, it may be helpful for the interpreter to inform the interviewer that the client is fasting from sunrise to sunset because he is celebrating the holiday of Ramadan. Failure to understand this cultural information might lead an interviewer to assume the interviewee is hungry because he cannot afford to buy food.

On the other hand, in some interviews you may be quite familiar with the interviewee's culture, although you still need to rely on an interpreter for language interpreting, and you may therefore tell the interpreter not to explain cultural material but rather just to convey words. Perez Foster (1999), who is a psychoanalyst, believes the exact words used are important in psychoanalysis; thus she asks interpreters to be *translators* only, not interpreters, conveying the exact words used, word for word, as much as possible, rather than meanings. This is not the usual stance.

In the course of an interview or other intervention, the professional may ask questions or make statements that could be offensive. Most professionals appreciate it when an interpreter informs them if this is a problem, in what's called a cultural aside. For instance, in trying to learn about a Japanese family, an interviewer might ask a parent questions about abuse in his or her own childhood. It might be helpful for the interpreter to tell the interviewer that the parent is not likely to answer this question truthfully before a relationship and context have been established, rather than allowing the interviewer to proceed with offensive questioning. This added cultural information is far preferable over what often occurs—the interpreter decides not to ask the potentially offensive questions and then fails to inform the interviewer of this omission. Or, alternatively, the interpreter asks the question and the interviewees are offended and refuse to reveal themselves further throughout the course of the meeting. The interviewer may never even become aware of the insult and its affect on the interview.

The interpreter should be instructed to stop the interview if he or she needs to ask a question or clarify a concept. If there is a concept that cannot be translated easily into English, or into the other language, the interpreter should inform the interviewer. Similarly, if the interpreter does not understand a word because it is in a different dialect or for some other reason, the interviewer should be informed promptly.

Interpreters often need to give their best guess as to the meaning of a word as used by a particular person in a particular context. For instance, if a person mentions the word *salsa* in Spanish, this could mean a sauce, a dance, sexual intercourse, or, in Puerto Rico, a beating. Or, to use another example, in recounting sexual abuse in Spanish, a person who uses the word *leche*, which literally means "milk," is apt to mean "ejaculate" or "cum" rather than the dairy product.

Even when using his or her best professional judgment, the interpreter can still make mistakes. It is better to err on the side of caution. If the client uses a word that is unfamiliar to the interpreter (a special word for a body part or a kind of food, for instance), the interpreter can give the word in its original form to the interviewer and explain that he or she is not sure of its meaning. Then the interviewer can ask the client for clarification.

Also, if the interpreter believes there is something wrong with the quality of the interpretation—and this is such a big problem that the interview will not be accurate—the interviewer should be informed right away. Sometimes an interviewee is not verbal in any language because of a hearing, speech, or cognitive impairment and this may not become apparent until the client is approached in his or her first language. Other communication barriers include incorrect assumptions about the client's language. For instance, sometimes Portuguese speakers are asked to interpret for interviews with Cape Verdeans (or French speakers with Haitians, or Spanish speakers with indigenous people of the Americas who do not speak Spanish). As the interview begins, the interpreter may discover that the client speaks only a little Portuguese but mostly speaks Krioulu. Cape Verdean Krioulu contains some Portuguese words, but not enough to render an entire interview.

If the interview is truly urgent, for instance, the person needs to establish an urgent safety plan for that day because he or she is at immediate risk, then a less than ideally interpreted interview may be adequate for that day while a more appropriate interpreter is recruited for a later date. However, in the case of a formal forensic interview necessary to gather complete information for court, a less than ideal interpretation should be rejected and the interview delayed until an interpreter who is better suited to the circumstances can be found.

THE INTERPRETER'S ROLE

Some interpreters hope to establish an intimate and supportive relationship with an interviewee and his or her family, and they serve almost as cultural brokers or mediators. If the interpreter serves in some ways as a cultural broker, it is important to remember that the interpreter's portrayal of the culture is just one perspective. It may not be typical, correct, or unbiased.

It is common for experienced interpreters to meet briefly with clients before the interview begins to say, essentially:

> "I am so-and-so. I will be interpreting for you today during this interview. Anything you say to me I will be repeating in English to the person who is interviewing you. If you try to ask me something directly, I will repeat it to the person who is interviewing you. Please do not think I am being unfriendly if I do not respond to you directly. My job here is to help you understand everything that is being said to you, and help the person who is speaking to you understand everything you say. I am also going to ask that only one person speak at a time, so I can make sure I can hear each person clearly. I have promised confidentiality. That means that I will not repeat what you tell me to anyone who is not involved in your case. If we see each other in another situation sometime, you don't have to worry. I am a professional interpreter and will keep secret what you say. Do you have any questions?"

This kind of brief introduction helps the client understand the interpreting process. Forensic interviewers sometimes prefer to have this introduction take place in the official interview room, so it becomes part of the record.

Interpreters advocate for both interviewees and interviewers through their commitment to the communication process and the complete accuracy of their interpretation. Interpreters must not advise, counsel, make judgments, or interject their opinions when in the role of interpreter. However, interpreters may bring up nonverbal cues or contextual, social, or cultural issues that clarify the intent of the speakers.

Apart from the brief introduction, the interpreter should not say anything to the client that the interviewer has not said. The interpreter should not reassure the client, ask the client if he or she is telling the truth, or give an opinion about what may have happened. The interpreter should not influence the interviewee by suggesting an action to take or what to say. If the interviewee asks the interpreter a question, the interpreter should convey that question to the interviewer so he or she can reply.

Interpreters should be as unobtrusive as possible. While interpreters can be friendly, they should not try to make strong connections with interviewees—that is the interviewer's job. In general, during an interview the interpreter *should not* seek out eye contact with the interviewee. The interpreter's job is just to help the client and interviewer communicate successfully.

Interpreters should maintain a professional demeanor at all times. Unless they explicitly have a dual role with clients—for instance, if they serve as both advocates and interpreters—they should not give out their phone numbers to clients, establish a relationship with a client outside the professional situation, provide transportation, or accept gifts from clients. Any of these actions could compromise their neutrality. These informal contacts could also make the interpreter aware of personal information relevant to a client's case—information that had not been revealed in the professional setting—which could be extremely awkward. For instance, Baker (1981) describes an interview in which a Vietnamese youth swore an interpreter to secrecy before revealing that he was planning to run away from his guardian. How awkward it would be for an interpreter to drive an interviewee home after an interview and discover that the interviewee had been lying about some crucial information! The clearer the professional boundaries, the less likely this is to occur.

In some ethnic communities a small cadre of bilingual people meet virtually all of the needs of their community members who do not speak English. Formally and informally, for pay and on their own time, they may serve as cultural brokers with the schools, government agencies, and medical providers. They may serve as interpreters, translators of documents, drivers, and chaperones. They may fill out forms, make phone calls, and accompany people to important events. They may be paid by official agencies for some functions, paid by individuals for others, and perform others on a volunteer basis. These people may be ethical and community minded, or they may be unethical and demand sexual favors or a share of financial benefits in exchange for the assistance they offer. Interpreters who are paid by official agencies sometimes also demand pay, under the table, from the interviewees. Because these cultural brokers often come from the same background as the people with whom they are working, they are vulnerable to similar trauma, privations, and pressures. This is one more reason, I believe, why it is important to pay for the services of interpreters and cultural brokers. If the pay is adequate, qualified people are more likely to assume this role and they may be less inclined to put their position at risk by behaving unethically.

THE INTERPRETED CONVERSATION

Interpreting between languages is more difficult when the languages and cultures are especially far apart in their concepts, structure, and origin. For example, Cantonese and English share fewer concepts than do German and English. But even in the case of languages that share similar origins, misunderstandings occur frequently. Sometimes bilingual speakers "code switch" or use words and concepts from one language in another (see Chapter 6 on language competence). This can make interpreting extremely difficult. For instance, when asked what happened, a young Chicana girl might respond, *Mi hermano me molestó*. In Spanish, this means "My brother bothered me." However, if the girl speaks some English she might be using the word *molestar* in the English sense, meaning, "to molest," meaning "my brother *molested* me." (In this case molestar/ molest is a false cognate, a word that *sounds like* a word in the other language, but has a different meaning.) An interpreter must make a multitude of fast-paced decisions to render accurately this seemingly simple sentence of just four words.

Interviewers need to try to avoid ambiguity in their phrasing of questions, so the question that is being interpreted is the one the interviewer originally intended. For example, an oncologist asked a South American patient, "Mrs. Gomez, is your family complete?" The patient thought this question referred to whether her nuclear family was intact, and so she replied affirmatively. The physician actually meant, "Do you have all the children you want to complete your family?" (In both English and Spanish, the word "complete" could be interpreted either way.) The oncologist then chose a course of treatment which—as a side effect—rendered the patient infertile. This misunderstanding had heartbreaking consequences for the patient when she later tried to conceive (J. Cambridge, personal communication, November 21, 2006).

Semantic Equivalence

Careful interpretation may require using long explanatory phrases to convey an idea that is a much simpler concept in English. For instance, there is no exact equivalent in Spanish for the concept of "foster care" or "foster family," and there is no exact equivalent in Russian for "wife battering." Each time these concepts are conveyed, the interpreter must use a longer phrase and explanation than the simple English words. (Of course, the converse is also true. Some concepts that are conveyed in one word in other languages require a longer phrase and explanation in English.)

An interpreter might seem to take an inordinately long time to convey

a brief statement to a client who is unfamiliar with Western medical or social work concepts. For instance, a social worker might say to a client, "I'd
like to ask your permission to speak with your doctor." This might seem
like a fairly straightforward statement to interpret. However, the interpreter must first explain to the client what confidentiality is, and that she
ordinarily has the right to expect it. Then the interpreter must explain that
the social worker is seeking an exception to the expectation of confidentiality. The interpreter must then indicate that the client can grant or deny this
permission through signing a form. A short statement has been considerably lengthened into a cultural lesson.

The lack of semantic equivalence, an exact correspondence from one
language to another, ensures that something is inevitably lost in interpreted
interviews. Okawa (2008) describes how the word for "torture" in some
languages is translated simply as "beatings." An interviewee who was sub-
jected to other forms of torture might then deny having been tortured because he or she was not beaten.

Sometimes the words chosen by an interviewee or the interpreter do
not fully convey what the interviewee is trying to say. For instance, an Ethiopian survivor of torture described being beaten by "sticks." Upon inquiry,
she revealed that these sticks were heavy clubs (Okawa, 2008). If the asylum evaluation had included only the word "sticks," it would not have accurately conveyed what this torture survivor had endured.

Languages are filled with metaphoric speech, which can sometimes
lead to cross-cultural misinterpretation. In general, interpreters are trained
to find an equivalent English-language expression for the expression in the
original language. That is, if a client says in Spanish, *Me costó un ojo de la
cara* (literally, "it cost me an eye from my face") that could be interpreted
in English as "It cost me an arm and a leg." In practice, many metaphoric
expressions do not have an exact equivalent in both languages, and these
are often hard to think of in the moment. Interpreters typically say, "She
used a metaphoric expression meaning that it was very expensive" to interpret the above expression.

Practical Considerations

Conducting an interview through an interpreter will take considerably longer than conducting an interview directly in one language only. We should
schedule longer blocks of time (if the client can tolerate it) for those sessions that are interpreted. Nevertheless, if the interviewer and interpreter
work well together, they can pick up a good rhythm.

Interviewers should do their best to ensure acoustics in the interview
room that are conducive to interpreting. Hearing well is key to being able

to interpret. Professionals should do their best to eliminate extraneous noises such as fans or background music.

In adversarial situations, such as when an accusation is made against an alleged perpetrator of violence, different people should interpret for the victim and for the accused, to keep each testimony as "pure" as possible. Most especially, a child who sees a person interpreting for the accused, thereby speaking "in the voice" of the accused, may be inhibited about speaking freely with that interpreter present.

The interviewer should speak as if he or she is talking directly to the interviewee. For example, say, "What did you have for breakfast this morning?" directly to the interviewee, rather than saying to the interpreter, "Ask her what she had for breakfast this morning." And when the interviewee speaks, the interpreter should speak in the interviewee's voice also using the first person, as in, "I ate toast" rather than, "She says she ate toast." This preserves the immediacy of the relationship and avoids confusion (Bradford & Muñoz, 1993).

Rather than working as cointerviewers, the interviewer and the interpreter should try to work as one person, with the interpreter conveying the personal style and approach of the interviewer as well as the interviewee: "A gentle statement must be translated gently, for example; a confrontation must be translated as such; and a supportive statement must reflect warmth in its content" (Baker, 1981, p. 393). Studies have found, however, that some interpreters in medical settings are so eager to get down to business that they fail to interpret the pleasantries that physicians use to greet patients, thereby inhibiting the building of rapport (Davidson, 2000).

In an interview, the participants should be positioned so the interviewer can establish a connection with the interviewee. The interviewer should sit closer to the interviewee than the interpreter does. The interpreter should probably sit to the side of, and slightly behind, the interviewee. The interviewer should look at the interviewee, not at the interpreter, and should communicate as much as possible that it is a dyadic—not a triadic— conversation. Although it may seem funny at first, the interviewer should hear the interpreter without looking at him or her. If the interviewer focuses on and smiles at interviewees, speaks to them directly, and makes occasional eye contact with them, it will be easier for them to feel connected than if the interviewer's focus waivers between the interviewee and the interpreter.

If an agency relies on the same interpreter regularly, this interpreter should have the opportunity to benefit from technical, not just administrative, supervision. If the interview is recorded electronically, it would be helpful for another professional interpreter to review the quality of a recorded interpretation occasionally (respecting the confidentiality of the original interview, or course). Or, another interpreter could be asked to sit in on the interpreting from time to time. This peer supervision is similar to that received by all professionals and should be conducted in a spirit of co-operation and helpfulness. Formal or informal peer supervision of this kind helps interpreters keep their skills honed and also helps prevent burnout.

Simultaneous versus Consecutive Interpreting

In simultaneous interpretation, the interpreter listens and speaks at virtually the same time rather than waiting for pauses to repeat what he or she remembers. Some writers suggest that simultaneous interpretation improves the accuracy, speed, and naturalness of interpretations (Bradford & Muñoz, 1993). Some psychotherapists prefer simultaneous interpretation for clinical work (Perez Foster, 1999). However, simultaneous interpretation probably is not the best approach for an interview. Simultaneous interpretation requires that two people speak at the same time (the interpreter and the interviewee, for instance). This produces a confusing record and makes it virtually impossible for a stenographer or video camera to record the conversation, or to produce a written transcript of a recorded conversation.

In general, in question-and-answer situations where the conversation is either recorded or documented (as is usually the case in interviews), consecutive interpretation is preferred. In consecutive interpretation, the interviewee and interviewer are asked to speak clearly in relatively short utterances, pausing between each utterance to allow the interpreter to render the speech into the other language. Only one person speaks at a time. While this is slower than simultaneous interpretation, it may be less confusing to all parties—as only one voice is heard at a time. Information is less apt to be lost when you use consecutive interpreting, and so I recommend using consecutive interpreting in interviews when possible.

Interpreting for Children and People with Developmental Delays

Interpreters may need to adjust their practice when interpreting for a young child or a person with developmental delays or certain kinds of mental illness. A 5-year-old, for instance, may become confused by an interpreter who has just introduced herself as "Ms. Jones, the interpreter," and then immediately interprets the interviewer's speech (in the first person), saying, "I'm Caroline Thomas, I'm a doctor and I have a few questions for you today." When working with people who would be confused by this constant switching of person, interpreters may choose, instead, to say, "The doctor wants to know. . . . " In other words, the interpreter's goal is to convey conversation in the clearest way possible. Occasionally this demands straying from standard interpreting practice.

Additionally, to gain the trust of a young child, the interpreter needs to act authentically. The child may feel as if he or she is truly speaking to the interpreter—who is likely to be from the same ethnic group and is more likely to understand the cultural norms than the interviewer. When working with a young child, the interpreter will probably want to be warm and affectionate and inspire the child's trust, rather than coolly withholding warmth and eye contact:

> An experienced court interpreter described interpreting for a young child, Billy, in a brutal rape case in superior court. When she met Billy, she asked him where he wanted her to sit. Billy asked her to sit with him in the witness box, which the judge allowed. By the end of his testimony, Billy had crawled into her lap for security. In this case the judge saw the child request the physical closeness from the interpreter and permitted it. (I. Cornier, personal communication, March 22, 2004)

INTERPRETER VULNERABILITIES

Interpreting well is hard work. The interpreter must be completely fluent in both languages. The interpreter must tune in to differences in word usage and must listen, speak, and translate all at once. Additionally, because emotional rapport and empathy are crucial, the skilled interpreter tries to convey the same feelings and use the same intonation as the people being interpreted. This requires not just linguistic dexterity but emotional dexterity as well.

Interpreting in interviews about interpersonal violence and other kinds of trauma can be especially grueling emotionally. A highly experienced court interpreter told me the following story:

> The worst time for me was when I was interpreting the victim impact statement of a sadistic rape. This young girl read page after page about how awful her life had been since the rape. She was weeping while she was reading the statement and I was repeating everything, speaking in the first person and using the word "I," as if it had happened to me. I was trying to put emphasis where she put emphasis and convey in my speech, as much as I could, the feelings she was conveying as she spoke. Then at the end, the court took a recess and I went to the bathroom, splashed water on my face, and I was supposed to walk right into the next courtroom and begin working on the next case. I was shaking like a leaf. Sometimes I have to interpret for defen-

dants who have done awful things and they might speak about them coldly or even cruelly, and that's hard, too, because again I'm using the first person and trying to convey the feeling in their voices. I hear myself speak and I almost feel like I'm talking about *me*, since I'm using the first person. It can be overwhelming. (I. Cornier, personal communication, February 2004)

The interpreter is expected to stay neutral and therefore must constantly repress any sign of partiality to one side or the other. The interpreter may be aware that certain unstated bits of information would be helpful, and yet it is not his or her role to seek out or convey this extra information. Typically, court interpreters do not have mental health training and do not belong to a supportive team with whom they can debrief. They are isolated with their reactions to their work.

Interpreters are usually drawn from the same ethnic communities as the clients for whom they are interpreting, and therefore they may share similar trauma histories. If a person interpreting for an interview with a victim of torture or a witness to war, for example, has had similar experiences, the interview could stimulate the interpreter's own memories. Interpreters should be trained to set their own boundaries in this regard, perhaps declining to interpret for certain kinds of interviews. Supervision around these issues would also be helpful. Interpreters who feel moved to talk about their own traumatic experiences may need to be reminded to focus on the interviewee's issues during the interview.

Children's advocacy centers, child protective services agencies, women's crisis centers, police departments, mental health centers, attorneys, and others who frequently rely on interpreters for help with sensitive and painful material should try to cultivate a group of interpreters with whom they work regularly, who are familiar with the system. It may be important to hold a short debriefing with the interpreter after a particularly difficult session. This will provide humane relief for the interpreter and make him or her less likely to discuss the case with friends or coworkers. The interpreter who feels like a valued part of a team will be more likely to return on future days to interpret other difficult interviews. The debriefing will also serve as a forum to check the accuracy of the interpretation. Although the interpreter may be eager to learn more about the case, it would be inappropriate for the professional to discuss case information beyond the specifics that were mentioned during the interpreted interview.

This postinterview discussion can also afford an opportunity for the interpreter to convey information that may not have been conveyed during the interview regarding peculiarities of the client's accent, articulation, affect, or other meaningful details that might have been overlooked. For instance, an interpreter might mention that although a client claims to be Mexican, his slang and accent sound more Colombian.

Interviewers are entirely dependent on interpreters in situations in which their services are used. If a conversation is interpreted inaccurately—either intentionally or unintentionally—the interviewer is unlikely to find out. It is crucial, therefore, that we find, train, and cultivate relationships with competent interpreters who understand and respect the boundaries of their role.

Conducting Interviews Using Interpreters

- **Address the interviewee directly.** That is, say, "How are you feeling?" rather than "Ask her how she is feeling." Avoid directing your comments to the interpreter.
- **Connect with the interviewee.** Establish your usual warm, personal relationship with the interviewee directly. Only your words are being channeled through the interpreter. Your relationship is established directly with the interviewee. Look at the interviewee rather than at the interpreter.
- **Avoid technical jargon and abbreviations.** These may be unfamiliar to the interpreter and the interviewee. Avoid using technical or legal jargon such as "lascivious intent" or abbreviations, such as "perp" or "CPS" in conversations that are being interpreted, unless there is some particular reason why the technical term is required (e.g., if someone is being charged, he or she should know the particular charge and an explanation of that charge should be given).
- **Speak loudly enough but don't yell.** Sometimes people think if they raise their voice loud enough, even nonnative speakers of English will understand them. This can be intimidating. On the other hand, it is also important to avoid mumbling. The interpreter must be able to hear you well.
- **Speak slowly, using short phrases, and pause for interpretation.** Interpreted conversations take longer. This is unavoidable.
- **Invite correction and discussion of alternatives.** Say, "Correct me if I'm wrong, I understood . . . " and "Do you see it another way?"
- **Explore the issues that the interviewee raises.** According to their speaking style, interviewees will sometimes answer in a roundabout way that may seem irrelevant. However, issues that seem like distractions may lead to crucial information or may reveal difficulties with the interpretation. In many cultures people answer questions indirectly, through storytelling. You may need to learn to be patient when interviewing someone who follows this style.
- **Pursue concerns.** Return to an issue if you suspect a problem and at first you get a negative response. Make sure the interpreter knows what you want. Use related questions, change the wording, and come at the issue indirectly if somehow the response does not seem right.
- **Provide written instructions.** If your interview results in a plan of action or treatment plan, have interviewees outline the plan themselves so you can check for understanding.
- **If alternatives exist,** spell out each one.

- **Emphasize by repetition.**
- **Address concerns about confidentiality.** Rumors, jealousy, privacy, and reputation are crucial issues in close-knit ethnic communities. Acknowledge the problem and explain the degree of confidentiality that you and the interpreter can ensure.
- **Gender may matter.** Male interpreters may make some women extremely uncomfortable and unwilling to talk about sexual, marital, physical, or reproductive issues, and they may inhibit the women from consenting to a physical exam. While female interpreters are apt to be more appropriate in much work with women, the converse is not necessarily true. That is, some men would rather have women interpreters, depending on the issue, because they may be hesitant to appear weak or vulnerable in front of other men. True familiarity with the culture will help the interviewer determine the importance of the interpreter's gender in a given interview. If there is an opportunity to choose an interpreter of either sex, the interviewer should ask the client about his or her preference.
- **Debrief.** Whenever possible, and especially when you will be working with an interpreter on an ongoing basis, check in with the interpreter briefly after the interview to see if there are any concerns that the interpreter would like to share with you.
- **Convey concerns.** If you are concerned about the quality of the interpretation, you should advocate on your clients' behalf by speaking with the director of interpreting services, finding better trained interpreters, or discussing your concerns with colleagues until a solution emerges. Some interpreters are inadequately trained, don't understand or follow the rules of confidentiality, or censor what an interviewee says in order to help the ethnic community "save face."

CONCLUDING OBSERVATIONS

Interpreters are essential figures in interviews where bilingual interviewers are not available in the clients' language. Interpreters have a great deal of power to determine the success of an interview, and therefore great care should be taken in finding and using qualified interpreters, letting them know about your needs, providing them with quiet rooms in which to work, and making the best use of their skills. Interviewing with the help of an interpreter requires patience and practice.

Using an interpreter with someone who does not speak English is really a question of providing language access. Most of us are required by law to serve all people in our communities, regardless of their language background. Clearly, as Western industrialized countries continue to be nations of immigrants, and as immigrants move throughout these countries from large cities into towns and rural areas, we will all become more accustomed to making use of interpreters in some of our interviews.

Questions to Think about and Discuss

1. Discuss ways the agencies in your area can improve their access to competent interpreters. Which immigrant communities are currently best served and which are most in need of services?
2. Is your organization providing the same quality services to people who have limited English proficiency as they are to others? If not, what else should be done?
3. If you have worked with an interpreter, describe a time when it was particularly successful. What helped the process work well?
4. If you have worked with an interpreter, describe a time when it was frustrating. What was problematic about it?
5. What would it feel like to be 8 years old and be asked a lot of personal questions by an adult in a language you don't understand, and then hear the questions again in your own language? What might make this process easier?

RECOMMENDED ADDITIONAL READING

Fontes, L. A. (2005). Working with interpreters in child maltreatment. In *Child abuse and culture: Working with diverse families* (pp. 159–175). New York: Guilford Press.
Pochhacker, F. (2001). *Interpreting studies reader.* New York: Routledge.

8 Understanding and Addressing Reluctance to Divulge Information

> If you keep your mouth closed you cannot bite
> yourself.
>
> —KOREAN PROVERB

As interviewers we often feel we have a right to information because we have the interviewee's best interests at heart, because of the power our organization represents, or because speaking openly with us just seems like "the right thing to do." It may seem self-evident to us that the interviewee should be willing to divulge sensitive personal information, and that this revelation will lead to helpful interventions. We may believe that talking about a difficult experience will bring relief. Or, the consequences of *not* speaking with us may seem like sufficient reason for interviewees to reveal themselves. However, interviewees may not agree with these assumptions. Even if we are expert at building rapport, we may encounter hurdles and barriers when seeking the information we need to do our jobs.

It is absolutely imperative, therefore, that we understand the reasons why people hesitate to speak with us. Then we must learn ways to handle their reluctance. When interviewing children, teens, or adults in a variety of settings, this knowledge will improve the value and quantity of the information we obtain, the speed with which we obtain it, and the quality of the relationship formed during the interview. And, finally, we must develop an ethical compass that tells us when to press forward and when to suspend our inquiries.

This chapter discusses some of the cultural reasons interviewees may be reluctant to confide in us in general, or hesitant to address certain topics in particular. It describes ways to address sensitive topics and to overcome reluctance when necessary. It explores in somewhat greater depth four of the most difficult yet most important subjects to discuss in many interviews: substance abuse, child abuse, intimate partner violence, and sexual assault. The chapter concludes with a discussion of when and how to respect people's right to remain silent.

ATTITUDES TOWARD SPEAKING OUT

People who are hesitant to respond to an interviewer or who respond in monosyllables may appear to be evidencing pathology, when in fact they are displaying a culturally appropriate hesitancy to speak too much. In her memoir on growing up in the Kashmir region of India, Koul (2002) describes attitudes towards the act of speaking:

> Much is left unspoken. The spoken word is a force to be reckoned with, reverberating forever in the cosmos, causing all kinds of repercussions. This is because words have a deity all their own, an unrelenting goddess under whose regime a sound once uttered, cannot die but goes around and around, doing good or bad, depending on its nature. (pp. 81–82)

On the other side of the planet, the Navajo people in the United States share a somewhat similar belief, that if you talk about something you bring it to you. When hearing bad news such as a physician revealing a negative prognosis, Navajo family members sometimes turn their back on the bringer of bad news during the discussion. In interviews about sexual abuse, children and family members are sometimes hesitant to discuss what happened; they feel somehow that discussing sexual abuse will attract more of it (Steele, 2007). This is radically different from the typical Western psychological view that talking about something will "get it off your chest" and make you feel better.

A wide variety of beliefs restrain interviewees from speaking with us freely. For instance, Vietnamese people may be hesitant to divulge personal information because they believe it could jeopardize their legal rights (Novak, 2005). West Indians and immigrants from the English-speaking Caribbean value "not telling people your business" and "not putting your business on the street." This inhibition may be even more pronounced if a family member is present who is unaware of the problem (St. Hill, 2005). Many Latino cultures use the expression *la ropa sucia se lava en casa*, which is an admonishment to wash one's dirty laundry at home. The Korean language has a comparable phrase, *jip-an*, which means "within the house." Korean families hesitate to reveal a wide range of issues to people who are not jip-an, to preserve the family reputation and protect the family from shame (Kim & Ryu, 2005, p. 352). Jews' hesitation to reveal problems to people from outside the culture is revealed in the Yiddish expression *shandeh fur die Goyim*, which roughly means a shameful situation that non-Jews might use as a weapon against Jews. In each of these minority cultures and others, the act of sharing personal matters with people from outside the family and culture may be seen as leading to unwanted and threatening attention from outsiders.

In some cultures personal matters are discussed indirectly, if at all. The more that is left unsaid, the better. In Spanish there is a saying, *La mejor palabra es la que no se dice* ("the best word is the one that is left unsaid"). This saying refers to the need for discretion and care before speaking out. Similarly, Ide (1995) writes, "In Japanese communication, people expect others to guess about a certain unstated part of the message. . . . In effect, it is a receiver's responsibility to be sensitive to the speaker's true message" (p. 26). In Japanese, the term *ishin denshin* describes the idea of "an immediate communication between two minds which does not need words" (Morsbach, 1987). From a Japanese perspective, an interviewer who insists on direct explicit statements may be showing a reprehensible lack of skill as a listener.

Despite these obstacles, we're often faced with the problem that we *do* need to obtain a direct explicit statement for our work. (For instance, we cannot rely on our intuition or our ability to read someone's expression if legal charges are involved.) Ways to address this dilemma are discussed below.

SILENCE

Silence is more than just a lack of words.
—EGYPTIAN PROVERB

The man who does not understand your silence will
probably not understand your words.
—ELBERT HUBBARD

Just as people from different cultures use words in various ways, they also use silence differently. In Arab countries, silence is usually considered something to be avoided, and so people repeat themselves or engage in stock phrases to avoid silence. In Japan, on the other hand, there is an expression: "Those who know do not speak and those who speak do not know." The dominant cultures in the United States, Canada, and Great Britain fall somewhere in between these two extremes.

Interviewers need to become comfortable with silence. Silence does not necessarily mean the person is about to lie or needs help coming up with an answer. If we jump in too quickly as we try to be helpful, perhaps by rephrasing a question, we may actually make it more difficult for the person to speak out.

Growing up in my family, if I did not interrupt someone I could not get a word in edgewise. This is not an uncommon experience for people who come from large families or from cultural groups that value verbal swiftness such as African Americans, Jews, Puerto Ricans, Brazilians, Greeks, and Italians. In these groups people tend to chime right in while others are still speaking, often good-naturedly interrupting each other or finishing each other's sentences, "stepping on" each other's words, and responding quickly with loud voices. These groups allow a short average length of time between utterances.

On the other hand, longer pauses between utterances are expected and preferred among other cultures, including many Native American, African, and Asian societies. Their silence is a habitual cultural pause. Among the Inuit of Arctic Quebec, mature children are expected to "control their tongues" and know when to stop talking (Crago, 1992). Traditional American Indians will not speak simply to fill a silence: "Words are considered powerful and are therefore chosen carefully" (Shusta et al., 2005, p. 264). Overly talkative interviewers may see their Native American interviewees grow increasingly silent.

The Meanings of Silence

In an interview, silence can mean many things, depending on the situation and the people involved. In any given conversation you will need to decipher the meaning of the silence and proceed accordingly.

Silence can sometimes indicate a lack of comprehension. An interviewee may simply be too befuddled to speak. In many cultures, people are reluctant to question authorities who say something they do not understand. Perhaps they are embarrassed to admit that they don't understand. Or perhaps they believe their admitted failure to comprehend a statement would imply inadequacy on the part of the interviewer. The interviewee may be confused by the words themselves (jargon, complex terms, a different dialect, lack of linguistic competence) or by the context (Why am I being asked these questions? What am I supposed to say? Who will learn my answers? What agency does this person work for? What power does this person have over me?).

If an interviewer asks a question that is embarrassing, such as one that touches on a taboo topic, the interviewee may grow silent, uncertain as to how to broach the topic or how to decline to discuss the subject at all. Silence stems from the dual fears of being embarrassed and of seeming uncooperative.

Discussing certain topics in front of certain interviewers is apt to be considered disrespectful. For instance, men may refrain from discussing sexuality in general and sexual transgressions in particular in front of a woman interviewer or interpreter, for fear of seeming disrespectful to the woman. Or, a person who has been treated unfairly by a White person may have difficulty discussing the incident with a White interviewer, for fear of offending. Similarly, someone who has been assaulted by a police officer or violated by a psychotherapist may hesitate to discuss these incidents with people from the same professional group. Rather than discussing these situations directly, the interviewee may simply grow silent in response to a pertinent question.

People from many parts of the world, including Central America, Nigeria, Asia, and Haiti, are unlikely to signal their displeasure openly to a person in a position of authority. If they dislike or disagree with a message conveyed by an authority, or even if they are uncomfortable with a certain line of questioning, they may simply grow silent. If a Nigerian woman has a reservation about a suggested course of action, for instance, she is apt to remain silent, shrug her shoulders, and perhaps even roll her eyes rather than question the professional (Ogbu, 2005). Choosing to remain silent, rather than protesting, is a method Nigerians use to avoid open conflict. A Vietnamese person may avoid responding to a delicate question with a blunt "no." Instead, to prevent disharmony, the Vietnamese interviewee will find a way to evade the question or will indirectly indicate a negative response (Novak, 2005). A quote by the revolutionary leader Ché Guevara comes to mind here: "Silence is argument carried on by other means."

Silence can also be used to emphasize the significance of a topic. For instance, if an interviewer begins to ask about a trauma, loss, sacred act, or the "heart of the matter," the interviewee may pause silently to acknowledge the weight of the subject. If a question has touched on an overpowering memory or a personal loss, the interviewee might also choke up with emotion and become silent.

Fear, too, can silence people. No response may seem to be the safest response. Interviewees could be fearful about the interview itself or the results of the interview. Do the interviewees suspect that they might be tortured, beaten, arrested, or humiliated during the interview? Do the interviewees fear that someone will seek revenge if the truth is revealed? Do the interviewees suspect that they may be deported, arrested, separated from their families, killed, disowned by their family, or forced to undergo unwelcome medical procedures *after* the interview, depending on its outcome?

Sometimes interviewees grow silent because they are tired or they believe they have been misunderstood or because they believe they have already answered the question and have nothing more to say about it. Sometimes an interviewee is thirsty or hungry, wants to use the bathroom, or needs to make a phone call and is unsure how to ask to get these needs met. Sometimes people who are being interviewed in English want to express a word or phrase in their native language and feel "stuck" when they try to find the word in English. Being unable to express themselves adequately in English causes many immigrants to feel ashamed and humiliated, and grow correspondingly silent.

People from cultures that value silence may suddenly stop speaking at certain points in an interview, simply because the silence feels just as important as speech would feel. Among Koreans, being rather silent is a sign of being humble and well educated, especially for men (Im, 2005). The Chinese believe silence is a sign of thoughtfulness, and contemplative silence in the company of another person is not considered a problem. Among Pakistanis, silence is considered a virtue that is emphasized from childhood. For Pakistanis, silence usually signals acceptance, approval, or tolerance (Hashwani, 2005).

Some cultures raise their children to be extremely verbal, whereas others cultivate the opposite demeanor:

> If a worldview endorses talking as a positive act, and people believe that talking means assertiveness and intelligence, parents and teachers will encourage their children to practice their verbal skills to foster them to be expressive and articulate. If a worldview endorses silence and listening, however, and people think that silence means thoughtfulness and being considerate, parents and teachers will discourage their children from talking too much to make them serene and attentive to others. (Kim & Markus, 2002, p. 442)

Middle-class American children from the majority cultural group in the United States are usually encouraged to speak a lot, but traditional Asian and Native American children are often taught to choose their words carefully, to pause after questions, and to avoid speaking too much, "like a fool." These habits learned in childhood may continue into adulthood. In Korea, for example, there is an expression that refers to big talkers, "The empty carriage makes a lot of noise" (from Kim & Markus, 2002).

Children raised on a Native American reservations may be shy and not accustomed to interacting with outsiders, and therefore they grow silent when among them. In Puerto Rico, children are told, *Los niños hablan cuando las gallinas mean* and *Tu hablas cuando las ranas echan pelo*, which mean, respectively, "Children speak when hens pee" and "You speak when frogs grow fur," the point being that children are to be seen and not heard.

Finally, sometimes people become silent in an interview because the interviewer has made a mistake. I have confused the name of a person's husband with that of her child, or asked questions that were self-evident or questions for which I already knew the answer, or committed other blunders that were so obvious that the interviewee just waited politely for me to realize my mistake, instead of correcting me.

In sum, we must be careful how we interpret an interviewee's silence.

WHO OWNS INFORMATION?

In some cultures, information is considered to be owned collectively rather than individually. People from these cultures would be hesitant to reveal information to an outsider without checking first with their family or group. Lipson (1994) describes her attempt to conduct an ethnographic interview with a 16-year-old Afghan girl who had said she was 18:

> I had explained that we would take a walk and that we could have a conversation about her experiences in the United States and her health, and she agreed. However, once I began asking questions, she answered the majority with, "You have to ask my father about that." . . . I subsequently learned that, to interview any woman or child (a category that includes unmarried adults), the father's consent is necessary. (pp. 344–345)

In this young woman's case, the information was considered fit to be divulged only with the father's consent.

In other instances, people will want to check with their entire family, with leaders from their cultural group, with clergy, with God through prayer, or with trusted others before they decide to confide. In some cases revealing sensitive information might indeed bring benefit to the interviewee but at the same time cause harm to another person or bring shame to the interviewee's cultural group. For instance, if a woman being battered reveals her situation, the disclosure might improve her safety but endanger her batterer, bring shame to her family, and be seen as disgracing her ethnic group. To use another example, a teen who reveals that he is using drugs might receive helpful interventions as a result of discussing this; at the same time, his revelations could stigmatize his family and call unwanted police attention to members of his ethnic group. In this kind of situation and others where revealing information could influence more than one person, many interviewees will remain silent.

AIRING SECRETS AND CONFLICTS

We must be careful not to make assumptions based on our own cultural background that it is "a good thing" for people to air their conflicts, to bring secrets out into the open, or to discuss delicate subjects with interviewers. Keeping sensitive and shameful matters private is often seen as a virtue in many cultures, because it permits everyone involved to save face and avoid public shaming. Westerners prioritize freedom of speech, but East Asians also place a high value on the freedom to remain silent. In Japanese there is a phrase, *fumon ni fusu* (Chung, 1992, cited in Shibusawa, 2005, p. 343) which means "keeping things unquestioned," or the practice of not inquiring about certain topics, which is considered a virtue. Preserving secrets on sensitive topics such as financial troubles, adoption, suicide, illness, family conflicts, drug or alcohol use, and extramarital affairs may serve an important cultural function for many interviewees. It should not be confronted antagonistically or viewed as a form of resistance.

Some cultures require a strong personal relationship before secrets are revealed, making interview situations an entirely inappropriate context for discussing the intimate details of one's life. The Maori in New Zealand are described as having a spiritual attitude toward knowledge, which assumes that knowledge should be imparted to selected individuals only after a relationship in which they prove themselves worthy of receiving that knowledge. When asked to participate in research, therefore, Maori "provide answers (if they cooperate at all), which they think the researcher wants, out of politeness and hospitality; or may even occasionally deliberately distort responses according to a Maori logic not perceived or understood by the researcher" (Stokes, 1992, p. 6). Similarly, in American Indian and Latino cultures, in particular, personal revelations are likely to occur only in the context of long-standing and deep personal friendships (Sue & Sue, 2003). The Navajo have an expression indicating that if you speak too much about yourself your ears will fall off (Steele, 2007).

People who are reticent to self-disclose because of their culture may mistakenly be seen as guarded, mistrustful, inhibited, passive, or paranoid (Sue & Sue, 2003). Some interviewees are reluctant to discuss their troubles because self-revelation around difficulties is seen by their culture as unseemly, self-centered, or even dangerous. Nigerians rarely share information about their misfortune with others because they feel that the person who receives the information will consequently perceive them negatively. Rather, they are apt to share only the information that puts them in a positive light (Ogbu, 2005). Personally, I have found this attitude especially difficult. Because of my own cultural biases, I value sharing one's troubles as a way to feel closer to someone. When speaking with Nigerians I have found myself growing frustrated, feeling as if the person was trying to manage my impression of them rather than "really" talk to me, as my culture would define "really talking." I have to reign in my own biases so I won't respond negatively.

As a struggle between two or more people, conflict brings into the open different needs, values, and levels of power. Thomas and Kilmann (1974) suggest there are five ways of handling conflict: controlling, collaborating, compromising, avoiding, or accommodating. Which of these strategies a person or group uses at any one time will depend on the cultures of the people involved, their levels of power, the perceived stakes, and how the parties weigh "winning" the conflict versus maintaining the relationship with the opponent.

TABOO TOPICS

Interviewers should keep in mind the strong cultural and religious rules against talking about certain specific topics, depending on the culture and setting. For instance, in many U.S. workplaces officemates talk about topics that seem extremely intimate, including their relationships, sex life, diets, and medical problems, but decline to reveal their salary. People rarely speak about racial issues in mixed-race groups, although they may try to discern the others' racial attitudes. In workshops, I sometimes ask participants which topics are taboo in their cultures. We generate a long list including mental illness, cancer, sexuality, sexual assault, child abuse, intimate partner violence, substance use and abuse, infidelity, poverty, homelessness, illiteracy, finances, AIDS, suicide, disabilities, disease, homosexuality, death, illegal activities, and others.

In some cultures, certain words are considered so powerful that they are not uttered. For example, Orthodox Jews will not say or write the word that's considered to be God's true name and rather use a series of euphemisms (such as "holy of holies" or "ruler of the universe"). In some communities people do not say that a person "died" but rather that he or she "passed on" or "is no longer with us." Many people use the euphemism "a long illness" instead of "cancer." Out of respect, a Lakota woman may avoid using her father-in-law's name, referring to him instead as "he" (Sutton & Broken Nose, 2005).

For traditional women from most cultures, talking about sex is considered vulgar and crude, particularly with people whom one does not know well, including medical personnel. Some children and adult women have so internalized the rules about not using "garbage can words" that they feel themselves unable to speak about something that happened "down there" and may not even know words for genitals or for sexual activity that might be acceptable to utter with strangers. A Latina woman may describe an unwanted rape as "He made love to me" because she simply has no other words to describe it, or she is reluctant to use them. If she is not a fluent speaker of English, she may fear that the English words she has learned for genitals or sexual acts are vulgar or offensive. For traditional Latina women, it is considered *muy bajo* or very crude to speak about sexual activities. In Lebanese Arabic, the word for "vagina" itself is considered extremely coarse because it is used mostly in the context of cursing. To refer to female genitals, then, most Lebanese will use a French or an English word. (Understandably, this issue caused problems in a translated Lebanese production of Eve Ensler's play *The Vagina Monologues*.)

One Puerto Rican woman I interviewed described her family's taboos around sexuality like this: "Religion is something so important in making it so that things are not discussed. And sin! Where are you going to go if not to heaven? And what if God catches you speaking—or even thinking!" (cited in Fontes, 1992, p. 90). One Mexican American woman described being told that she would be a bad girl if she even uttered the word "sex," which inhibited her from disclosing that she had been sexually assaulted. Speaking about sexual acts even in the context of an interview may seem almost as dirty as engaging in them.

A Somali interpreter recently told me how she handles discussion of taboo topics with Somali immigrants. She said she asks for a long pause when a physician wants to ask men about homosexual activity or frequenting prostitutes, for instance, because the questions themselves might be considered offensive and cause a Somali man to refuse to cooperate, as both homosexuality and visiting prostitutes are prohibited in Islam. She introduces the questions to the patients by saying something on the order of, "The doctor is going to ask you some questions now that might seem offensive, but he means no offense. To track certain diseases he is going to ask about your sexual activity. He asks all the men patients he sees about these delicate matters. Are you okay with this?" She says once the men have understood the context and given their consent to the line of inquiry, they are more open to continuing with the interview.

Sometimes interviewees are uncomfortable discussing certain topics for reasons the interviewer might not suspect. For example, people from many cultures are reluctant to describe their accomplishments because this could be seen as immodest and might attract the evil eye. Or, a child could be uncomfortable revealing the race of an alleged assailant because she has been told it is bad to talk about race. Or, a Muslim, Mormon, or Jehovah's Witness might be uncomfortable discussing a situation because it involved alcohol; and for religious reasons they believe they or the people they were with should not have been imbibing. Native American children may be afraid to discuss activities that would cast members of their clan or extended family in a bad light. Sometimes people from minority cultures are embarrassed to describe distinctive cultural activities—such as making tortillas, lighting Sabbath candles, playing mahjong, or using folk medicine. And, of course, children and adults may be uncomfortable answering questions that might imply they did something wrong. For instance, if they missed school or skipped work, they might avoid revealing this. If they viewed pornography, visited prostitutes, or cooperated in illicit or coerced sexual activity, they may feel ashamed. If they visited a neighborhood, home, or business with a bad reputation, they may want to hide it. If they have been associated with undocumented aliens they may try to conceal this, too, even if they themselves are documented. Men and women who have more than one family or who have a lover may try to hide this. If the questions involve illegal activity—even if that activity is irrelevant to the interview—the interviewees may hesitate to discuss it. People also hesitate to reveal that rules have been broken, such as when someone has been living in a home but is not on the lease, or when someone's full income has not been reported to welfare authorities.

Sometimes, hesitance to address certain topics stems not from a cultural reluctance but rather from the perception that no trustworthy person is available who could listen or help. One Mexican American woman described her feeling of frustration and isolation with the family secret that their child had been sexually assaulted:

Who were we going to go talk to about this? How many agencies do you know that welcome unauthorized Mexican immigrants with very little English fluency? And in our culture, you know, there's also this fear of being discriminated against, of being deported if you're unauthorized, of being taken out of your family because a White person thinks there's too many of us living together or something. Most people in this country don't understand Mexican culture and customs. And so yeah, there's a serious fear at the thought of sharing information outside the family. (cited in Franco, 2006, p. 49)

In this case the family's feeling of being threatened overcame their strong desire to seek help for what had happened. Their hesitancy did not reflect a cultural taboo as much as it reflected their feelings of isolation.

While a wide variety of subjects can feel especially sensitive to certain interviewees for a variety of reasons, a number deserve special attention because they appear so often and their influence is so far-reaching: the abuse of drugs and alcohol, child abuse, intimate partner violence, and sexual assault. These issues are discussed in greater depth in the next four sections.

SUBSTANCE ABUSE

Why a separate section on substance use? First, drugs and alcohol frequently figure as a backdrop for many people's life, and their influence may or may not become explicit in interviews. Second, material raised about substance use may affect the outcome of interviews in life-changing ways. Will someone receive government financial aid or subsidized housing or medical insurance? Will that person risk a prison sentence? The answers to these questions might hinge on whether evidence emerges that the person is using or has used certain substances. Third, interviewers must become knowledgeable about different cultural attitudes toward specific substances, so they can inquire about them in the most sensitive and effective ways.

People acquire attitudes toward the use and abuse of substances within specific cultural contexts (Straussner, 2001). They may choose specific substances to alter their consciousness based partly on access (including affordability), trends among their peers, culture, and generational norms. Ethnic cultures also may influence where, how, and with whom the substance will be consumed.

Some substances tend to be more stigmatized than others. For instance, those who abuse illicit drugs are more stigmatized than people who abuse legal prescription drugs or alcohol. This disparity exists despite the fact that alcohol is the most commonly abused mind-altering substance in Western industrialized nations. As we know, alcohol consumption leads to a tremendously high social cost in terms of accidents, lost productivity, poverty, family violence, and other crimes committed while under the influence. Yet alcohol is seldom stigmatized as severely as illegal drugs. I am stressing this in a book on culture because your culture may have taught you to condemn certain substances while accepting others. It is important to remember that many of these ideas are indeed cultural, and they are not necessarily based on statistics about which substances are more dangerous than others.

The influence of ethnic culture is important for you to keep in mind when asking questions about substance use. Without such knowledge, it might be easy to overlook or misinterpret problematic behaviors, or to minimize the importance of the cultural context.

In some communities, the use of alcohol and other drugs is stigmatized, whereas in others it is considered sacred. In most societies, the best way to describe prevailing attitudes toward their use is "it depends." Some substances may be used without condemnation by some people in some circumstances and up to a certain state of intoxication. For instance, it may be considered permissible for college-age men to drink themselves into a stupor on a Saturday night, but this behavior would be considered irresponsible during exams week or before driving. This tolerance for drinking in U.S. colleges is widespread despite the fact that the legal age in all states is 21 for purchasing and publicly possessing alcohol. (Some states allow younger people to consume alcohol on private property or in the presence of their parents.) College men who use substances other than alcohol may be denigrated, however, as are college women who imbibe alcohol in the same quantities as college men.

Cultural Patterns of Substance Use

To learn the patterns of acceptable substance use within a given culture, you need to become intimately familiar with that culture. (Even so, it is important to avoid stereotyping; there are always variations among individuals and families within cultures.) To outsiders, it may seem as if, "All the men drink" or "all the women are popping pills," when the actual usage pattern is distinct. Yes, the men who drink may be quite visible—standing on street corners or gathering in bars. Those who do not drink may be less visible, quietly remaining at work or at home with their families.

Cultural rituals provide support for particular kinds of drinking. For instance, drinking to excess is common at Irish wakes (Straussner, 2001) and once a year on the Jewish holiday of Purim, when celebrants are invited to "drink until you can't tell Mordechai from Haman" (two leading figures in the Purim story). Jews are generally known to be moderate drinkers of alcohol and frequently drink wine in small quantities to celebrate certain holidays and at Friday night Sabbath dinners. Of course, alcohol abuse *does* exist in some Jewish families, as it does in some number of families of all cultures. Drinking alcohol to excess is common in Poland and Russia, where alcohol is used to mark life events, seal contracts, cement friendships, and show hospitality (Gilbert & Langrod, 2001). In many European countries and among the wealthier social classes in much of the world, people drink wine or beer with dinner, whether at home or in restaurants. In Portugal, drinking wine with meals is so common that expressions exist which mock requests for a glass of water with meals, such as "drinking water creates frogs in the belly" and "water is for washing your feet."

In Japan, businessmen often feel pressured to drink with their coworkers and clients. Working relationships and hierarchies are affirmed through after-hours socializing in bars, making it politically difficult for someone who wishes to abstain (Genzberger, 1994). In rural Peru and Bolivia, indigenous people often make *chicha* (a homemade fermented alcoholic drink) and some consume it until they are in a stupor on market days and special occasions. In Great Britain, Ireland, New Zealand, and Australia men tend to gather in pubs, from adolescence into old age. Throughout the world, men frequently consume alcohol while watching sports events, whether in person or on television.

Cultures provide contexts for consuming substances other than alcohol as well. For instance, some Jamaican (and other Caribbean) people of all ages and walks of society use marijuana (*ganja*) for its purported medicinal and spiritual properties. It is smoked recreationally and in rituals and used by herbalists in potions that are taken by people in regions of the country where Western medicine may be hard to access. A basic understanding of the cultural supports for the use of *ganja* would be important when trying to interview a Jamaican about this substance (Harris-Hastick, 2001).

In some Andean countries, people chew coca leaves, in South Asia, some people chew betel, and in some African and Middle Eastern countries, people chew cola nuts or *khat* for their stimulant properties and to ward off hunger. These substances do not get their users "high" or drunk or impede their functioning. However, people can grow dependent on them and suffer withdrawal if their access to these substances is cut off. Similarly, in Argentina, Uruguay, Brazil, Paraguay, Lebanon, and Syria, people drink *maté* (a tea with stimulating properties). The consumption of *maté* is so ubiquitous in Uruguay and Argentina that people can often be seen with a thermos of hot water slung over a shoulder with a strap and a hollowed calabash gourd which is used like a cup in their hands in public places ranging from subways to parks to workplaces. This is akin to the constant consumption of tea and coffee in much of the Western world.

In many traditional cultures, on special occasions people consume mushrooms, teas, or potions with hallucinogenic properties, to initiate contact with the spirit world. These substances may be used by the entire community but more often are consumed by a restricted group, such as shamans or the men who are preparing for a hunting expedition. The most famous of these hallucinogens is probably peyote mushrooms which were popularized in the fictionalized Don Juan books by Carlos Castañeda about a Mexican shaman. An entire religion has sprung up in Brazil around the consumption of a potion made from a plant traditionally used by shamans, called *ayahuasca*. This is considered a sacred plant by its users, enabling insight into the self and the universe. In an interview, it would be important not to equate its use with the recreational use of other drugs. *Ayahuasca* has been decriminalized in the United States

Finally, contexts in mainstream culture often support the use of alcohol and other substances. For instance, undergraduate and graduate university students often consume prescription stimulants (such as Ritalin or Dexadrine) as well as illegal drugs (such as cocaine) to help them stay alert to study for tests or write papers. People who frequent dance bars sometimes inhale alkyl nitrates (poppers), which is thought to enhance sexual pleasure. And using alcohol, cocaine, and other drugs to excess almost seems compulsory among celebrities.

Discussing Substance Use and Abuse

Legal restrictions can make it especially difficult for certain people to discuss substance use and abuse. For instance, people who are not citizens in the United States may face deportation if their use of illicit substances becomes known (even if they have legal residency). People who are convicted of drug-related crimes in the United States face the likelihood of being denied federal student loans, access to public housing, and the opportunity to work in many jobs, including the role of foster parents, for the rest of their lives. We need to be cautious when our interviews touch on issues of drug use. We should let interviewees know about the rules of confidentiality and its limits.

Latter Day Saints (Mormons), certain kinds of Baptists, and Seventh Day Adventists do not permit any use of alcohol or other mind-altering drugs. A person who uses these substances may be excommunicated. In some cultures, if one family member uses drugs or alcohol, it will hurt the marriageability of all the family members. People from minority cultural groups that are already subject to stereotyping and criticism may feel they are inviting more of the same if they openly admit to using substances, or if they need to take time off work to enter treatment to kick their habit.

It can be particularly difficult for members of ethnic groups who are stereotyped as using particular substances to discuss their use of those substances with outsiders. For instance, alcoholism has frequently been described as "The Irish disease" (although of course alcohol is used and abused by individuals in many other ethnic groups). Prominent Irish writers ranging from James Joyce to Frank McCourt have written at length about how excessive drinking has blighted Irish men and their families. The pub has historically been an important social center, where men from a community gather, tell stories, celebrate, and support each other. Men are expected to buy a round for the neighbors with whom they are drinking. "In practical terms, this custom means that if five people enter a pub together, each one in turn is expected to purchase a round of drinks and therefore to consume five drinks" (O'Dwyer, 2001, p. 204). Although Irish women drink more now than they once did, drinking alcohol is still stigmatized for women, and so they are both more likely to drink in private and to deny that they are drinking, even when they are in alcohol treatment programs (Corrigan & Butler, cited in O'Dwyer, 2001). When an Irish man is interviewed, he might minimize his use of alcohol because it feels normative (just what men do), or he might be hesitant to discuss it because he fears it will confirm a stereotype about the Irish. He might also neglect to mention his use of alcohol because he believes the interviewer already assumes he is a heavy user.

We should be careful in our use of language related to substance consumption. Speaking of addicts and addiction or alcoholics and alcoholism may be perceived as extremely threatening and insulting. Some interviewers intentionally use these direct words as an intervention, but they should be aware of their impact. Terms such as "problem drinking," "frequent drinking," "regular use of drugs," or "losing himself in weed" will be better received than more general or pejorative terms. You may also choose to use the interviewee's language. If you do, at some point you would be wise to inquire as to what their terms mean. When they say "got a little high" or "put down a few" or "took the edge off" or "a sip to help me sleep," what does this mean? What substance was used? In what quantity? How intoxicated were they? What were the consequences? And how often does this happen?

To make the initial inquiry about the use of substances, it can be helpful to use "presupposing questions" (see box in Chapter 4, Types of Questions, p. 74). This would mean, for instance, saying, "Tell me about your use of alcohol" or "Tell me about your use of prescription medicine and other drugs," rather than "Do you drink?" or "Do you use drugs?" When posed sensitively, these kinds of questions can reduce the shame for interviewees asked to describe their use of substances, while still allowing those who do not imbibe to indicate this.

Treatment for Substance Abuse

We may grow impatient with the people we interview who have not taken advantage of treatment for their substance use, or who have failed to quit using. It is important to remember that the treatments available for alcohol and drugs are not equally acceptable to people from all groups. Viewing substance abuse as a disease is a strange concept for people from many cultures where substance use may be seen as a moral weakness, an indication of a lack of faith in God, a sin, a key aspect of masculinity, or an integral part of everyday life. As part of their substance abuse treatment, some people respond well to discussing their feelings. Others respond better to discussions of responsibility, or to education about the effects of substance abuse on their family or colleagues.

When recommending a treatment strategy for substance abuse, it is important to determine its "fit" with a particular interviewee. For instance, Alcoholics Anonymous groups vary greatly in their ethnic, racial, social class, and professional composition. The Tuesday evening group held in a church basement may feel right to a person, while the Wednesday morning group might be offputting. Same church, same city, but a different group of people. For people whose substance use seems closely linked to regular social events (e.g., a gathering at the pub, a card or domino game, "girls night out," "hanging with the guys," or Sunday afternoon football), it may be helpful to recommend social events that do not involve substance abuse, such as religious events, fundraising for worthy causes, mutual aid societies, continuing education of some kind, and sports teams.

A Muslim, Jew, Buddhist, Hindu, or atheist might object to an Alcoholics Anonymous meeting that ends in the Lord's Prayer. A Jew, Muslim, or Seventh Day Adventist may not be comfortable in a treatment center that serves pork. The format of sitting in a circle and revealing personal information may feel alien and upsetting to people from cultures where self-revelation in general is frowned on. This intimate sharing will be particularly difficult for some people if it is expected to occur in a mixed-gender group.

Often substance-abusing mothers cannot participate in treatment because they lack child care. Immigrant mothers, who are particularly isolated, may have difficulty finding someone to care for their children when they enter treatment. Mothers from cultures that consider the care of children the mother's sole domain face similar challenges.

CHILD ABUSE AND NEGLECT

Few areas are more stressful for caretakers to discuss than suspicions regarding any hint of child abuse or neglect. The stresses are also extreme for the interviewer, who may be under pressure to complete the process quickly and obtain all the necessary information in just one session. In situations of possible child abuse, interviewers know that their work may directly influence criminal prosecutions, family integrity, and children's safety and mental health. If the child discusses abusive incidents, the material is often painful for the interviewer as well as the child. If child abuse and neglect are revealed, the interviewer may be required to take further action with the police, child protective services, and possibly the schools and medical personnel. It is no wonder, then, that as indications of child abuse emerge, interviewers often find themselves experiencing dread and a wish that the interview would just head in another direction. When language and cultural differences enter into the mix, achieving sufficient rapport to elicit complete and accurate information may seem to be nearly impossible.

All the suggestions in this book regarding cross-cultural interviews in general can be helpful in interviews about child abuse. In addition, interviewers should keep in mind the intense shame that many children and adults feel regarding acts that they have suffered, whether involving physical abuse, sexual abuse, neglect, or emotional maltreatment, especially when these acts are perpetrated by family members (Fontes, 2007). It is not uncommon for children (or for adults who have suffered abuse as children) to want to protect their abusers, to deny the severity of what they have suffered, or to redefine what happened to them as not abuse or as their own fault. This allows them to preserve an image of their caretakers as benevolent.

Cultural taboos can increase these feelings of shame. One Mexican American woman described how she was inhibited from disclosing that she was a victim of sexual abuse because of a priest's sermon which said that thinking and talking about sex was a sin (in Franco, 2006).

Some of the most contentious cultural issues involve the line between physical abuse and discipline. What is considered acceptable punishment in one culture may be considered abuse in another. While extreme forms of violence against children are condemned as abusive in all cultures, less extreme punishments may be considered either abusive or acceptable, depending on the culture, the moment in history, the child's perceived infraction, and the adult's relationship to the child (Fontes, 2005b). For instance, in the United States children are sometimes sent to bed without supper as a punishment. Depriving children of food when they are hungry would be considered cruel and abusive in many nations. Beating children with a shoe, a wooden spoon, or a belt is acceptable in many nations, but if such a beating leaves a mark on a child, it is apt to be considered physical abuse in the United States and northern Europe.

When inquiring about possible physical abuse, it is usually best to avoid words that imply a judgment, such as "abuse." You are more apt to obtain accurate information if you ask in more neutral ways, such as "What happens when your father gets really angry at you?" or "What happened the worst time you were punished?" With caretakers, the question can be phrased, "How do you usually punish your children?" or "Tell me about a time you punished your child(ren) in an especially harsh way." Whether people respond openly or not will, of course, depend on many factors. (For further discussion of physical abuse, discipline and culture, see Fontes, 2002, 2005b).

It would be a mistake to suppose, however, that children from immigrant groups are at greater risk of maltreatment than native-born children. Indeed, research into this area in the United States and Canada shows a great deal of agreement across cultures as to what constitutes abuse and neglect (e.g., Maiter & George, 2003). The experience of immigration can prove stressful to parents, who often find themselves isolated, discriminated against, with reduced power over their own and their children's lives, and sometimes dependent on their more acculturated children. This immigration stress sometimes leads to an increase in family conflict.

When sexual abuse of children needs to be discussed, it can be extremely difficult for people who have been victimized, for victimizers, and for people who believe they should have been able to protect the child. The abuse itself involves taboo acts and violates customary relationship boundaries. The abuse is likely to be shrouded in secrecy and overt or implied threats, making it a hazardous topic to approach in conversation. Victims and their family members often fear the gossip that may emerge if knowledge of the abuse becomes known. Girls who have been abused by men may fear the abuse will hurt their marriage prospects. Boys who have been abused by men (and their families) may fear that the boy will be perceived as gay or as a potential future abuser. Where no weapons or overt physical violence were used, young people who have been abused by older teens or by adults commonly feel responsible for their abuse and may underestimate the coercive aspects of the encounters.

A full discussion of the cultural issues that emerge in discussing child sexual abuse is available in other literature (see Fontes, 1995, 2007). Remember to proceed slowly and gently, ask interviewees to explain their perspectives, and do not assume that you know the best way to resolve any particular situation unless you have studied the various cultural implications.

Questioning about child abuse of all kinds puts families at risk. In the United States, perpetrators of family violence who are not citizens may be subject to deportation, even if they are permanent residents. In many countries, families know that the adults may be subject to arrest and the children subject to removal if authorities learn about child abuse in the family. In the United States, there is overrepresentation of African American, Native American, and Latino families in the child welfare and foster care systems. Once minority families become involved in these systems, they are more likely than White families to experience adversarial interventions and to have their children permanently removed from the home (Roberts, 2002). In addition to these legal problems, families may be subject to gossip and excommunication from religious institutions. Immigrant families may fear being shunned in their ethnic community in the host country and also in their country of origin if reports of the child abuse become known. These heavy pressures cause many families to conceal information about abusive incidents.

INTIMATE PARTNER VIOLENCE

Intimate partner violence is a gender-neutral term for what was formerly called wife battering or woman battering. This broader term is designed to apply to a wider range of violent couple relationships including gay and lesbian relationships, nonmarital relationships, and the rarer but still important heterosexual relationships in which the man is victimized by his woman partner.

Cultural complications abound in discussing intimate partner violence. In some cultural contexts, wife beating may not be seen as extraordinary or problematic but, rather, as part of a woman's lot in life. In some nations, husbands may physically and sexually assault their wives with impunity. (The husband's extended family may be seen as possessing the right to castigate her physically, too.) Legal sanctions against woman battering and wife rape are relatively recent even in Western industrialized nations, and their enforcement tends to be sporadic. In every culture that I've seen, couples try to keep the violence that occurs secret, to preserve family privacy. Victims of battering often believe they can handle the violence on their own, and indeed they engage in a wide variety of strategies to escape from the relationship or reduce its lethality.

The reluctance to discuss intimate partner violence therefore makes it a particularly difficult topic to broach in an interview. Victims may not want to reveal what is happening because they've been threatened and fear for their safety if they make their plight known. They may be dubious that any benefit will result from disclosing. They may not have the financial means to support themselves (or their children) if the batterer leaves the home. They may love the batterer and believe that their love or their commitment to him precludes revealing information about the violence. They may blame themselves for their victimization. If they are immigrants, their visas or residency documents may depend on the batterer. They may fear ostracism from their communities if they speak up. They may believe that their victimization is their lot in life. Some victims also fear that their children will be removed from their custody because they will be seen as having failed to protect them from the batterer. Any combination of the above reasons, and others, make it difficult for victims of intimate partner violence to speak up.

Even where they do disclose information about the abuse, research shows that victims of intimate partner violence are apt to minimize that violence and omit information (Dunham & Senn, 2000). Women victims who consider the abuse acceptable are most likely to minimize its severity and omit details. This finding argues against a serious practice that is all too common, in which professionals discard an entire disclosure when they encounter a single discrepancy in a victim's account (see also the section "Truth, Lies, and Immigration" in Chapter 12 on common misunderstandings). For all the reasons discussed earlier, victims sometimes contradict their prior statements, which can be confusing and frustrating but should not be cause to discard disclosures in their entirety.

Victimizers are unlikely to discuss the abuse because they fear arrest or social sanctions including—in some cases—deportation. They may also believe strongly that the violence is justified and a private affair. Children hesitate to discuss the violence they witness because they have been threatened, have also been abused by the batterer, have been failed on prior occasions by official systems such as the police, or, while the violence scares them, may have come to see the violence as a normal part of life.

When inquiring about domestic violence, it is usually best to use nonstigmatizing language. Helpful questions might include, "Do you ever feel afraid? Why?" or, "Are you ever afraid of [your partner]? Why" "Are you concerned about your (or your children's) safety?" "What happens when you and [your partner] argue? Does it ever become violent?" "Does [your partner] ever push, slap, or hurt you in other ways?" People who are subject to violence at home often do not categorize this as "abuse" or "domestic violence" but may still be willing to respond affirmatively to specific questions that are less accusatory.

If a person gives indications of being victimized but seems reluctant to share details about it, you may find it helpful to inquire about the source of the concern. For instance, "You indicated that you are scared of [your partner] but you don't seem to want to discuss it. Can you let me know why that might be?" In that way, the interviewee may share with you information about threats or feared consequences that you can address. It is also possible that a person who is victimized will share information only with a person who is a part of the same ethnic community, or who is *not* from the same ethnic community, or only with a woman, or only with an advocate who is not a police officer, for instance. It is always helpful to have a list of resources for the person to turn to, if you cannot provide the needed assistance yourself or if the person is rejecting your help.

Sexual violence within marriage can be particularly shameful. Many women believe they are obligated to perform the acts requested by their husbands, even if they find those acts painful or humiliating, or they fear consequences such as pregnancy or sexually transmitted diseases such as HIV/AIDS. These issues must be approached with extreme sensitivity and care. Where applicable, it may be important to inform women about the local laws regarding sexual violence in marriage and a range of services they can choose to access, including telephone hotlines, online information, support groups, and counseling.

SEXUAL ASSAULT

Single or multiple instances of sexual assault are all too common in cultures throughout the world. These read like a catalogue of horrors. For instance, Vietnamese women refugees have been raped by pirates while fleeing in boats. College women are often raped on campus. Boys and men sometimes assault other boys or men as part of their initiation into scout troops, sports teams, fraternities, or gangs. Sexual assault of children and adult women is rampant in refugee camps. Men and women who are detained for political reasons sometimes endure sexual assaults, humiliation, or mutilation as part of their torture. Men and women are often assaulted by other inmates or guards while incarcerated. Impoverished people from all backgrounds find themselves forced to exchange sexual favors for food. In the course of war, women and children from Bosnia to Liberia to the Congo and Indonesia have been assaulted. People are sexually assaulted in their intimate relationships. And, finally, people are sometimes forced to exchange sexual favors to gain or keep their jobs or their shelter, or to gain good grades.

Depending on your responsibilities, you may need to ask about sexual assaults. These are, of course, among the most difficult subjects for interviewees to address. The interviewees may be filled with shame, and speaking about such issues may stimulate traumatic memories. The victims may feel they were responsible for their victimization because they were in the wrong place at the wrong time, were intoxicated, or in some other way put themselves at risk. They may also fear condemnation by their ethnic communities or rejection by their parents or intimate partners if these people learn about their assaults. Additionally, they may fear that the act of discussing these issues implies a desire or willingness to press charges. To speak about sexual assault is to relive it through words. For some victims, this is just too painful.

Related issues have been touched on in the foregoing sections on child abuse and intimate partner violence. Here let me advise you, once again, to avoid categorical words such as "rape" when you address these issues, and instead ask question such as "Has someone touched you sexually without your permission or in a way that made you uncomfortable?" "Many people have had sexual experiences that worry or upset them. Please tell me if this happened to you." Remember, women from many cultures simply will not discuss these issues, particularly with male interviewers. If this information is important, such as in building a case for asylum, you may need to enlist the help of a woman who is experienced in inquiring about these issues. Men who have been sexually assaulted by men may be unwilling to disclose their victimization for fear of being perceived as less masculine or gay. If this information is important, you should convey why it needs to be discussed.

If interviewees deny a history of sexual assault but you have reason to suspect they have been victimized, try to leave open the door for addressing this subject at a later date. For instance, "There may be topics that you did not want to address with me today. It can be hard to discuss certain issues. If you think of more things, this is what you should do. . . . " Try to determine if the person is currently safe from assault. If not, he or she is unlikely to disclose. And finally, make sure the person receives indicated medical attention.

INTERVIEWER STRATEGIES FOR ADDRESSING RELUCTANCE AND SILENCE

For a productive interview, you may need to invite directly an exception to a custom of silence by saying something like, "In many situations you may not speak a lot. But here, it's great if you can tell me everything you know about the questions I ask." Or, with a child, "In many situations, adults don't want children to speak a lot. Here, I really need to hear what you have to say." Of course, it would be naïve to think that a person who is shy will suddenly become talkative, or a person who has learned culturally to be quiet around authorities will drop this custom easily. Ultimately, we can only control our own side of the conversation, making sure we are as respectful, open, nonjudgmental, and engaging as possible, and making sure we give people an opportunity to be interviewed in their preferred language.

It is wise to allow some silence in an interview. Don't be too quick to fill the silence, jump in with a new question, or rephrase the previous one—this may make the interviewee feel interrupted and rushed and cause him or her to shut down. Try to gauge if the silence is comfortable or uncomfortable *for the interviewee*, and this will help you decide how to proceed. If you decide you do need to step in, you can repeat part of what the person has just told you; repeat the question; ask a new, less threatening question; or comment on the silence itself. The following comments may be helpful: "This seems to be a hard topic for you to discuss," or "Something about my last question made you grow silent. Please tell me a little about what's going on," or "What's on your mind now?"

Sometimes it can be helpful to comment in a different way on people's silence, by saying something like "It looks to me like you haven't decided yet whether you can trust me, and that's fine. What do you need to ask me that would help you make that decision?"

We often have to pursue information persistently, even if it is sensitive for cultural reasons, or even if our authority initially intimidates the interviewee into silence. For instance, if a child protective services investigator fails to pursue information adequately, children will be left vulnerable to further abuse. Or, if an investigator fails to ask for details about a crime, a case may remain unsolved. To assess a person accurately in psychological, educational, and other contexts, we sometimes need to pursue material that the interviewee would rather not address.

Interviewees may speak more openly if you give them specific information about the expectations of the encounter, such as "Please try to answer my questions as completely as possible," or "Tell me everything that happened from beginning to end, even if it doesn't seem important," or "For now I'd just like to get a general picture of what happened. Later, my colleague will be asking you more detailed questions." Make sure the interviewee is clear about the nature and purpose of the conversation.

Consider mixing in remarks with your questions that recognize the difficulty of the interview, such as "I know I'm asking a lot of questions. That can make you feel tired." Demonstrate your caring with remarks such as "How is it going for you?" You can also offer reassurance with remarks such as "We're almost done," or "You've been doing a fine job answering some really tough questions." These remarks, which focus on the process rather than information itself, will help the conversation seem more natural and humane.

We need to use all of our rapport-building skills to improve the forthrightness of the communication, including asking open-ended rather than yes-or-no questions, providing assurances about confidentiality, presenting our questions with a reassuring manner, and simply explaining why frank communication is necessary. It can be helpful to say something like "I know this is a delicate matter to discuss, but I need to hear exactly what happened."

To gain trust you may need to persuade the interviewee (and sometimes his or her family) of the good that will be accomplished by revealing the truth and the details surrounding it. This persuasion will be suspect if it is too strong-handed. It will take gentle calm and time to win this trust (Fontes, 2005a).

In some contexts, persuading others of the advantages of confiding in you poses an ethical dilemma. For instance, our desire to get the details in cases of child abuse stems from our assumption that revelation of the abuse will help improve a child's life and provide greater safety for society as a whole. But our systems lag behind our desire to help children. Once they disclose, children are left with all the problems that often follow—including seeing family members go to jail, losing the only family they have ever known, and sometimes having to participate in hostile legal proceedings. Many children tell social workers that if they had it to do again, they would never disclose (Folman, 1998).

So what does it mean to work to gain interviewees' trust while participating in a system that might harm them? This is an ethical dilemma that each professional faces alone with his or her conscience. And, of course, it varies with the systems within which we work. Potentially, the results of our interviews may range from always helpful to sometimes helpful to often destructive. Undoubtedly, we each do our work with the understanding that it ultimately is for the good, even if it does not appear that way at first or for every interviewee. If we cannot assume this, we should try to change the systems in which we work.

Offer reassurances when you need to. Assure interviewees that it is okay to talk with you about sensitive matters in this setting. If an interviewee seems to be struggling over how to say something, you can offer supportive comments, such as "It's all right," or "You can say it," or "You're doing fine." Some interviewers reassure clients with a comment such as "Nothing you tell me today will shock, anger, or upset me. You don't have to worry about that. I speak with people every day about these kinds of matters."

If you have the impression that the interviewee does not wish to talk about something but you consider it important to do so, ask the interviewee what makes the subject so difficult to discuss, and see if you can diminish these barriers in any way. For instance, the interviewee may fear the spread of gossip and need reassurances about confidentiality. Or, the interviewee may be afraid he will be judged harshly by you, the interviewer. Or, the interviewee may be afraid some particular evil will befall her if she tells (e.g., deportation, arrest, the evil eye, involuntary hospitalization), and you need to address these concerns before the interview can proceed. If you ask them, some interviewees may advise you about specific strategies that might make it easier for them to speak, such as closing their eyes, turning their back to you, speaking in their native language, dimming the lights, or covering their face with their hands. Some interviewees speak only when recording equipment has been turned off. Others prefer to tell their story alone to a tape recorder, without the interviewer in the room.

Some interviewees have been explicitly or implicitly threatened about the consequences if they reveal a secret. For instance, a sex offender's influence often shapes an interview with a child victim because the offender is in the room in spirit. He has told the child everything that will happen if the child discloses, such as: "No one will believe you. You will lose your family and your friends. I will lose my job and go to jail. Your Mom will have no money. Your mother will blame you and be mad at you."

Unfortunately, a great deal of what the offender has threatened may become reality after disclosure. This is much more complicated when the child also has to worry about someone in the family getting deported as a result of the disclosure, or possibly the only adult family member who speaks English being carted off to jail.

Threats can inhibit open discourse in other situations as well. For instance, a person may have been told he is not likely to get hired if he tells the truth about a conflict with a former boss, even if the conflict was truly not his fault. Or, a patient may have been advised by his folk healer not to tell a Western doctor about the herbs he is using because it will make him appear backward. A little boy I interviewed had been told by his mother that if he revealed what was happening in the home he would be taken into foster care and brutally assaulted every day for the rest of his life.

Living in a dictatorship or other oppressive political environment inhibits tremendously people's willingness to trust officials, or even their neighbors or coworkers, with personal information. They might grow silent, lie, make jokes, or be evasive in order to avoid revealing information to others whose motives or affiliations they are not entirely certain about. They may be hesitant to discuss trauma, tribal affiliations, torture, detention, refugee camps, political activity, and so on, because it was not safe to do so in their country of origin. They may see the interviewer as part of the government and, therefore, suspect.

I have conducted research and trainings on sensitive family issues in Chile, Portugal, Argentina, and Brazil, all of which endured brutal dictatorships with secret police at one time. In each one of these countries people reported difficulty trusting others with even the most banal information about their families, work, or politics. The default position was, "Say as little as possible," at least until you got to know someone and discovered their affiliations. These countries have moved out of their most repressive times, but unfortunately many nations still suffer from civil wars and dictatorships, which make silence the safest path by far. It may be extremely difficult or impossible to help someone open up in an interview who has been raised in such a perilous environment.

The people you interview may be facing dangers that inhibit their ability to converse with you openly—factors you may overlook if they are not part of your world. For instance, a small number of the immigrants you interview will be in your country as part of the sex trade; as virtual prisoners of abusive men; as involuntary domestic servants, factory workers, or farmworkers; or perhaps as mail-order brides who have arrived to unsafe homes. Some of the teens and adults you interview may have been, or may currently be, members of gangs. Or they may have family members who are involved in gangs, whose very life is threatened if they cooperate with you. As always in sensitive interviews, ask the people you are interviewing questions such as "Are you safe now?" "Is there anything else I should know?" "Will you be safe when you leave here today?"

The interviewee may be struggling with a concern that is unrelated to the question being asked, but that still inhibits the discussion. For instance, I accompanied Madina, a Somali refugee, to an interview that took far longer than we had anticipated. Suddenly, she grew quiet. When the interviewer gently asked what was going on, she said that her young daughter would be arriving home from school before long and there was no one to receive her. Madina had not felt she had the authority to cut the interview short. The interviewer called a premature end to the conversation to allow this mother to meet her child, and we rescheduled the second part of the interview for a more convenient time.

Sometimes it helps to offer alternative modes of communication. A person who is reluctant to describe a traumatic incident or sensitive issue verbally may be willing to write about it and then respond to questions about the written statement. The writing in and of itself can ease some of the person's fears about addressing the material. Depending on the circumstances, the written statement might also become an important legal document.

IMPROVING OUR OWN COMFORT WITH DIFFICULT TOPICS

The more comfortable you yourself feel in discussing sensitive topics, the greater your ability to put interviewees at ease. I suggest that you increase your comfort in speaking about sensitive topics through planned practice. Practice by yourself, asking questions to an empty chair in different ways, and rehearse with colleagues. Repeat the words that are especially difficult for you but necessary to speak in your work, until they no longer cause you discomfort. Practice different ways of phrasing questions, and ask colleagues for their opinions.

As interviewers, taboos in our own cultures can make us want to avoid certain topics or examine them only superficially. A psychology undergraduate student from Burundi told me sadly that she thought she would never be able to work as a professional psychologist because she was raised to be so uncomfortable talking about sex that she does not even discuss it with her American-born husband. I assured her that every professional has personal challenges of one kind or another. I congratulated her for recognizing her limitation and urged her to read a great deal, seek further training, and practice talking about sex until she could find comfortable ways to discuss it. I assured her that her own experience struggling with the difficulty of talking about sexual matters could eventually make her an especially effective psychologist in treating other people who are raised to avoid talking about sex—if she is willing to engage in the hard work of overcoming her own reluctance. These kinds of inhibitions would, of course, apply to people from a variety of cultures.

When possible, learn from your colleagues. Request permission to review the tapes of your colleagues' work, read their reports, or sit in on actual interviews. Compare techniques and question each other. This can be an eye-opening experience as you see how others approach and handle sensitive issues. While it may be most tempting to compare notes with a senior colleague, it can also be helpful to discuss interviews with junior colleagues, who may have fresh perspectives and innovative approaches. A veteran police officer told me she encourages experienced as well as rookie officers to accompany her to interviews in statutory rape cases because they have rarely been trained how to speak kindly, gently, warmly, and nonthreateningly to young women victims (A. Velázquez, personal communication, February 2006).

It can also be helpful to conduct role-play interviews with a colleague in front of a video camera and then critique each other's work. If you usually video- or audiotape your interviews, obtain supervision and peer supervision on these tapes. If you conduct interviews in front of a one-way mirror, ask a trusted colleague to observe a session and take notes exclusively for supervision purposes (obtaining proper consent first, of course). The best interviewers receive frequent feedback about their work and adjust what they do accordingly. Even experienced interviewers will find that the occasional supervision session serves as a "tune-up" to keep their skills fresh.

At one point in my life I worked full time as a psychotherapist. I had many clients, including children, teens, and adults, who had been abused sexually or who suffered from other kinds of family violence. I would ask the intake supervisor to give me different kinds of cases, and so she'd send clients my way who had no known history of sexual abuse. After gaining their trust and asking the right questions, many of them ended up disclosing an abusive history they had not revealed before. I remember the feeling in the pit of my stomach as I began to recognize the signs that the person was about to disclose. One aspect of that feeling was a certain measure of dread because I knew the case was going to become more complicated and might necessitate protective action on my part. I had to work hard in supervision and in my own psychotherapy to make sure this dread was in no way communicated to the client because the clients would have shut right down to protect me from their news. People in other fields, too, have to keep themselves "fresh" through supervision, vacations, peer support, meditation, exercise, friendships, professional development, and whatever else it takes to avoid burnout, so people can reveal what is truly important to them in our interviews.

CONCLUDING OBSERVATIONS

Through this discussion, I hope you have come to understand some of the many cultural and systemic reasons why interviewees may be reluctant to divulge information to us, may be reluctant to address particularly sensitive topics, may choose to be silent at times during an interview, and/or may be intimidated by our authority. I also hope you have learned some strategies for overcoming these areas of reluctance, so you can increase the amount of information garnered in an interview.

At the same time, I encourage you to respect interviewees' desires to remain silent at times and keep some information to themselves. In most circumstances, we should no more use coercive techniques to pry information out of reluctant people than we would forcibly open their mouth and grab their tongue with pliers to set the tongue in motion. Even if the interviewer's intentions are to "help," such helping can inflict significant damage to the recipient, including pushing interviewees to see themselves differently, to break taboos, or to put themselves at risk in other ways. When under the effects of trauma such as natural disaster, illness, war, terrorism, or other violence, interviewees may have a reduced capacity to cope or protect themselves from exploitation, fraud, and incompetence (Sommers-Flanagan, 2007). Because they are less able to use their judgment, people interviewed in crisis situations may be more likely to "cooperate" in ways they will later regret.

If we find ourselves pressing reluctant interviewees to speak, we must be sure that we understand our motivations. Do our actions comply with the ethical mandates of our professions? Are we motivated by concerns for the interviewee's or the public's welfare, or are we simply curious, titillated by the subject at hand, or fulfilling our own motivation to be helpful? Are we motivated by a personal conviction that "getting it all out" will be cathartic, while we fail to understand that for some people "getting it all out" may provoke intense shame—perhaps even leading to suicide? Are we perhaps enjoying, too much, our ability to push people into areas of discussion that make them squirm?

Under what circumstances do we have the moral or ethical right or obligation to pressure interviewees to speak with us if they'd rather not? When—if ever—do we have the right or obligation to push interviewees to address certain topics if they'd rather not? Do we ever have the right to press people to address topics that they might find distressing or retraumatizing?

The answers to the aforementioned questions fall along a spectrum. Some might assert that it is never okay to push people to respond, or only acceptable if it's a matter of life and death. Other professionals might be less adamant in this regard and believe it is all right to use a certain amount of coercion to coax answers from someone who has information that could help ensure their own or others' safety and well-being. I don't believe I can answer for you the question of when it is okay to push people to talk in your particular field at any particular moment. But I do hope you will consider this question thoughtfully, along with colleagues, and address the ethical issues involved. For some, choosing to keep certain information from us may be one of the few forms of asserting themselves that are available to them. Silence can be a healthy, soul-affirming form of resistance.

The people we interview usually have a right to privacy. The Centers for Disease Control and Prevention (1999) defines privacy as "having control over the extent, timing and circumstances of sharing one's self (behaviorally, physically, or intellectually) with others. The information belongs to the person." Does awareness of interviewees' right to privacy change the way we interact with them? Should it?

The people we are interviewing may have legitimate reasons to conceal information from us that we cannot imagine. They may have real concerns about their physical, emotional, or social safety, or they may have valid cultural reasons to hold their tongue. They may simply prefer to stay silent. If there are consequences to their refusal to divulge information, we should make sure interviewees know about these consequences. But we generally should avoid being too forceful in our attempts to gather information. Often, all that is needed is a little more time, and a few more steps to fortify the interviewing relationship.

Questions to Think about and Discuss

1. Discuss three reasons why an interviewee might grow silent during an interview. If possible, give examples of people from specific backgrounds in particular kinds of interviews.
2. Describe how cultural taboos might make it difficult for both the interviewer and the interviewee to discuss sexual matters.
3. What are some of the techniques that you have used to help people open up during interviews? Describe times when these have worked and when they have not worked.

RECOMMENDED ADDITIONAL READING

Adelman, J., & Enguídanos, G. (Eds.). (1995). *Racism in the lives of women.* New York: Harrington Park Press.

Fontes, L. (1995). *Sexual abuse in nine North American cultures: Treatment and prevention.* Newbury Park, CA: Sage.

Levesque, R. J. R. (2001). *Culture and family violence: Fostering change through human rights law.* Washington DC: American Psychological Association.

Minow, M. (1999). *Between vengeance and forgiveness.* Boston: Beacon Press.

9 Interviewing Culturally Diverse Children and Adolescents

Children are all foreigners.
—RALPH WALDO EMERSON

In a sense, all interviews with children are cross-cultural, because as adults we are so outside children's perspective. We are apt to have different status, habits, schedules, values, and worldview than younger people. This chapter focuses on interviews with children and adolescents from ethnic cultural groups that differ from the interviewer's and therefore are even less familiar.

The results of interviews with children and adolescents influence important decisions regarding academic placement, psychological diagnosis, suitability for employment, guilt or innocence, school admissions, and a host of other issues. Cultural differences, linguistic misunderstanding, and potential abuses of power figure strongly in interviews with children, as they do with adults—exacerbated further by the developmental and legal limitations inherent in childhood.

The art of interviewing children and adolescents is discussed in every chapter in this book. If you interview children, please make sure you read the other chapters. This chapter supplements but does not substitute for them. This chapter teaches ways to prepare for interviews with youth from a variety of cultures and to assess them properly. You will learn how to avoid misinterpreting their behaviors and some tips for communicating with school personnel about cultural issues. You will also learn about some of the stumbling blocks that are especially apt to creep up in interviews with adolescents from a culture that is different from your own, and ways to avoid these. This chapter will enhance your ability to interview young people from a variety of cultural groups competently and fairly.

SPECIAL ISSUES IN INTERVIEWING CHILDREN

Even in the best of circumstances, interviewing children is more complex and takes longer than interviewing adults. To begin with, interviewing a child (or adolescent) usually requires the consent and participation of at least two people—the child and a caretaker. In fact, the interview (or assessment) process often involves a crowd of people that may include parents, siblings, members of the extended family, foster parents, social workers, educators, therapists, guardians ad litem, and medical providers. Although not all these people will be present in the interview room at the same time, a number of them may need to be interviewed in person or on the phone, or asked for their consent or records. They may also need to fill out assessment instruments. Access to all these significant individuals is often difficult to obtain: Some are located in other states or countries. Some don't speak English. Some may be overworked, hospitalized, incarcerated, homeless, living without a telephone, or undocumented and trying their best to avoid official contacts. I know mental health professionals who refuse to work with children, or who severely limit the number of children in their caseloads, to avoid that burden of collateral contacts, especially because the additional time spent on this effort may be unreimbursed.

With minors, various parties may need to be consulted before permission can be obtained for the interview or assessment to take place. All too often, the interested parties will not agree with one another on the need for the interview, the nature of the problem, its significance, or the best way to proceed (Bereiter, 2007). When the child and his or her family are immigrants or come from a minority cultural group, these complexities may increase exponentially. The process may be muddled by resentments and mistrust on both sides, linguistic and cultural misunderstandings, and different philosophies about what is best for children. If the family has been betrayed in the past by professionals, or has felt less than satisfied with the results when a professional promised to "help," they may be especially hesitant to trust a professional again with something as precious as decisions about their child's future.

Because of their vulnerability, children arouse strong feelings in professionals, family members, and concerned others. This can make every contact concerning an interview with a child emotionally charged, and it can increase the likelihood that differences in perspective and opinion will flare into troublesome conflict. Caretakers and professionals, alike, are apt to have strong feelings about many topics concerning children, including discipline, diet, religion, manners, education, friendships, dating, sexuality, and daily routines.

Let us consider the following scenario:

> A 14-year-old boy in rural Appalachia, Tommy, has been mandated to seek assessment and treatment for his aggression before he can return to school after a violent episode. A mental health clinician is faced with a sullen adolescent and his furious parents, all of whom are still upset about their prior experiences with "shrinks" and are waiting to see if the new clinician will side with the family or with the school. The family seems to unite around only one issue, which is their shared mistrust of "shrinks." None can imagine a treatment relationship in which the mental health professional might be neutral or helpful.

Clearly, interviewers need to tread carefully when working with children, adolescents, and their families.

Although it is often ideal to interview children and caretakers alone and together, at separate times during the same visit, this can be difficult to accomplish if no one is available to care for a young child or siblings while the adults are interviewed. If the child has served in the past as the family interpreter, or as a cultural broker between the family and the wider world, the child may already be privy to information he or she would not otherwise have.

LIVING IN TWO WORLDS

Immigrant children often live in two distinct worlds: the home world and the wider world. Immigrant children may feel exceedingly stressed if their parents cannot help them negotiate contact with broad society, including school. Consider the following situation:

> A 6-year-old girl from a Russian family, Alina, is being bullied at school, often refuses to attend school, and soils herself during the day. As a school social worker begins meeting with the mother and child, the mother bursts into tears and describes extreme feelings of frustration, boredom, and isolation in her new country. The social worker

tries to focus the discussion on the child, who by this time has begun sucking her thumb and rocking. What should the social worker do to gather the needed information while protecting the child from a potentially disturbing interview?

Children from minority cultural groups are often caught between worlds and have trouble articulating their dilemmas. For instance, a Mexican child, Rosario, included in her prayers each night a request to her recently deceased grandmother, but she understood that the non-Mexican interviewer might view this negatively. Rosario was confused about whether she should tell the interviewer about her practice. A Pakistani boy, Omar, was told not to reveal that his uncle and aunt, with whom he spent the summer, were undocumented. He was feeling stressed and anxious because he had been hearing anti-immigrant comments at school and in the news and he was afraid to discuss this issue with anyone, including the interviewer. Graciela, from Brazil, called home from the school office and then froze with a panicked look on her face. Her grandmother who spoke only Portuguese had answered the phone, and Graciela was embarrassed to speak Portuguese in the office—she was trying to hide the fact that her family was not "regular American."

Planning Cross-Cultural Interviews with Children

Although it is not possible to devise stock answers to all the dilemmas involved in cross-cultural interviews with children, it may be helpful to think through some of the problems in advance and plan for various contingencies.

Language Fluency

Caretakers and children may have differing levels of English-language fluency. Do not create a situation in which children are responsible for interpreting for their parents, or in which children are artificially overempowered because of their greater comfort with the English language. (See Chapters 6 and 7 on language competence and the interpreted interview, respectively.) Do arrange for appropriate interpreting and for documents in the interviewees' language.

Referral Rationale

Where disempowered by lack of language competence or where harried professionals have given inadequate explanations, neither children nor their caretakers may truly understand the reason for the referral, and they may not understand which "symptoms" or behaviors were considered problematic by the referral source. Try to obtain this information directly from the referral source beforehand, as well as asking the caretaker and the child during the interview for their understanding of the problem. If the care-taker or child is coming into the interview situation with incorrect assumptions about what is going to take place, this could distort the interview or make it difficult to com-plete. See if you can determine where the idea for the interview originated, and with what goals in mind. Sometimes, it may turn out that the interview is inappropriate and should be canceled.

I am reminded of an 8-year-old boy and his mother with whom I was scheduled to hold an intake interview for possible psychotherapy. As soon as they entered the office, the mother turned to her son and said, "This is the lady who's going to figure out how f-d up you are and if they're going to put you away or what." The boy was angry, fright-ened, and completely inhibited in his conversation with me. I was grateful his mother had made those remarks in my presence, because it gave me a chance to correct their misperceptions. I began to wonder how often children might come into our interviews with misinformation of this kind, without our knowledge, and how gravely this might af-fect their demeanor and behavior. Although this was an extreme example, often the children we interview are uncooperative or overly frightened because they think we are trying to discover something crazy or evil within them or their history, with potential di-sastrous consequences if the negative elements are discovered.

Externalizing and Internalizing Symptoms

Some children do a better job reporting the ways in which they suffer (internalizing symptoms) than they do reporting their acting-out behaviors (externalizing symptoms). They may feel guilty, ashamed, and confused about their outbursts or the ways in which they hurt others, and so they keep this information to themselves. Parents, teachers, and other caretakers may view these externalizing behaviors as willful mis-conduct rather than seeing them as a product of emotional conflicts, difficult circum-stances, or mental illness. Other children, including those who are eager to maintain a tough facade, are more likely to conceal the ways they are suffering inside and speak more openly about their misbehaviors.

Child's Physical State

Children are especially affected by their physical states. Try to keep healthy snacks available for children whose caretakers may not have provided them with a meal or a snack shortly before the interview. Hunger, thirst, fatigue, and a need to use the bath-room will affect a child's memory and ability to perform on tests. (Remember, as dis-cussed in Chapter 2 on preparing to interview, that a child may not accept food or drink when first offered, because it would be impolite in some cultures to do so.)

Obtaining the Case History

With children and adolescents, it's especially important to obtain a thorough history through key documents, because the youngsters themselves may not have full infor-mation about their past. Relevant documents may need to be obtained from caretakers and multiple agencies and providers including pediatricians, therapists, classroom and special education teachers, guidance counselors, sports coaches, psychiatrists, social workers, and so forth. Regrettably, it does take time to obtain releases for this valuable information and then to obtain the information itself, particularly if the family has moved from one geographic area to another. Often, if an interview is expected to result in a clear treatment plan, the final report may need to be deferred until the essential people are contacted and necessary records are reviewed. (You may want to suggest that certain steps be taken in the meantime to protect and support the child.) At other times, when these documents are unobtainable, as often happens when the family has emigrated from another country, you may need to obtain important information about past health, school, and development through a careful interview with the family, alone.

Interventions

The process of recommending interventions can also be trickier for children than for adults. More people have to be consulted, there may be concerns about the interaction of the treatment with the child's developing brain or body, there may be concerns about how the intervention might stigmatize a child, and the adults may wonder how they are going to persuade an unwilling or reluctant child to comply. Religious or cultural mandates may make it difficult for a family to agree to share information with outsiders, give their child medication, or engage in other recommended interventions. Bereiter (2007) offers the following example of a 10-year-old whom a psychiatrist wants to treat with medication:

> The mother may agree, but the father may think that all the boy needs is more discipline; or both parents may agree but the grandparents tell the parents that the problem is their parenting; or their friends say "I'd never put my child on drugs"; or the parents agree but the child refuses; or they're worried about the addictive potential because the mother used to abuse methamphetamine; or because of reports they saw on television.
>
> Parents feel guilty about "putting their child" on medication. They may blame themselves for bad genetics or for not being good enough parents. Children and adolescents may refuse medication because they do not understand the reasons for taking it, because they do not want to be different from their peers, or because the medication is difficult to swallow.

We must figure out ways to solicit the support of the "village" that is involved in a child's care if we want the intervention we recommend to be accepted, complied with over time, and successful. This is apt to be especially true with children from more collectivist cultures, where rearing children is an activity of the extended family and community and not just the parents.

Emotional Responding

Our protective impulses, as professionals and as human beings, often come to the fore when working with children and teens. We may find ourselves becoming angry with caretakers who have been absent or abusive, furious at systems that have failed, frustrated with our own inability to make a difference, sad about the circumstances in which a young person lives or has lived, despairing about the possibility of recovery, baffled by dilemmas that seem impossible to solve, impatient with the pace of change, and so forth. Interviewing is often emotionally wrenching, and even more so when the interviewee is a vulnerable child. Be sure to maintain awareness of your feelings and allow time between interviews or at the end of the day to process them. Seek the support you need to process your own emotions related to your work. Yes, it is normal to feel such emotions, but it is important to know what to do with them. By contrast, if you ever find yourself emotionally numb to professional situations, consider the possibility that this is an early sign of burnout, and look into ways to keep yourself "fresh."

BEHAVIORAL OBSERVATIONS WITH CULTURAL MINORITY CHILDREN

Numerous cultural practices could potentially confuse an interviewer, and many have been addressed elsewhere in this volume. Their particular relevance in this chapter is that *children* may have special difficulty explaining these practices because they don't understand the rationale, they're embarrassed, or they have been told not to discuss them with outsiders. Perhaps these practices are such an integral part of the worldview of the child (and the child's culture) that the child considers them self-evident and unremarkable. Before reaching the conclusion that a particular behavior, belief, or aspect of a child's appearance is evidence of pathology, inquire about it with the child's caretaker and/or a cultural informant to see if it has a more benign, perhaps cultural explanation. Observing the parents' dress, hygiene, and behaviors may also help you determine whether the root of something that appears problematic is in the child or in the child's caretakers.

Here are some child behaviors that may appear to be evidence of psychopathology when in fact they may have a cultural explanation: Children may report hearing the voice of a loved one who has died. Or, they may report speaking with and getting advice from a deceased spiritual leader, a saint, or a god. A child may fast or avoid certain foods for reasons that don't seem to make sense to others and may appear to be indicative of an eating disorder or an obsessive personality. The child may wear amulets or engage in rituals or prayers to gain protection from the evil eye or the devil. A girl may avoid certain activities (wearing gym clothes, stripping for a medical exam, attending co-ed events, holding hands in a circle) for reasons of cultural modesty but may decline to explain why. A boy's refusal to take off his baseball cap may seem like ordinary adolescent recalcitrance, when in fact his religion requires him to cover his head, and he has chosen a baseball cap as an unobtrusive way to follow this religious precept.

We can try to be objective in our observations, and certain techniques may help us: counting the number of times a certain behavior is exhibited in a minute, for example. This approach is apt to be more objective than a simple behavioral impression. However, cultural factors can emerge even in structured observations. For example, Azar (2007) tells about training a team of graduate students to rate videotapes of mother and child interactions on a range of variables. She was surprised when a Japanese student noted vastly larger numbers of "disapproving behaviors" by a mother than did the other members of the team. It turns out, the Japanese student had been noting and recording subtle paraverbal cues such as clicks of the tongue and pursing of the lips that had gone completely unnoticed by the other observers. In this case, the cultural training in noticing subtle nonverbal expressions had rendered the Japanese observer a more finely tuned instrument for detecting maternal disapproval than the observers from other cultures. The fact that the observers were being trained as a group to increase their interrater reliability (the likelihood that they would rate observations in the same way) reduced the likelihood of cultural bias in the rating of the tapes. In many observation situations, however, professionals simply record their "impressions"; thus there is ample room for unintended bias to sneak in.

When we are not members of a given culture, it can be extremely difficult to know how to interpret what we are seeing. This is discussed in some depth in other chapters of this book, including Chapter 5 on nonverbal communication and in the section on behavioral observations in Chapter 10 on interview reports.

Correctly Interpreting the Behavior
of Children from Minority Cultural Groups

If you are interviewing a child, you may have received a report that the child displays certain negative traits. Keep in mind that such a report might fail to consider adequately the "cultural disconnects" causing those behaviors. It is easy for people to misinterpret observations of children from a cultural or linguistic group with which they are relatively unfamiliar. In this section the kind of negative interpretation of a child's behavior that often appears in educational assessments or school reports is listed along with other possibilities that should be considered. This list is meant to be suggestive, rather than exhaustive, and applies to children from immigrant families and children who are part of minority cultures in their schools. While the examples given here are mostly from schools, the issues apply equally to child care, camp, group residences, and other settings. The examples include suggestions for intervention in some cases: These may be helpful to share with teachers, therapists, and others who intervene directly with children, if you do not.

Unsociable

Children can appear aloof and unfriendly when they feel left out and unwelcome or inadequate because of their limited language ability, their accents, their newness to a community, or identity group factors that set them apart. Interventions with the individual child and with the entire student group can help the child become better integrated into the children's social fabric.

Distractible and Inattentive

Children may have trouble focusing their attention, may daydream, and may have difficulty approaching tasks systematically if they don't understand the instructions being given or are unable to complete the assignments because of linguistic or other difficulties. Children of immigrants may appear to be focused at times and not at other times, as they tire of the interview or classroom language and tune out for a while as a coping mechanism. Children who are eager to comply may not be clear about where to turn their attention. For instance, should they focus on the teacher, who is giving an assignment that they are having trouble understanding? Or, should they focus on their classmates who are beginning to execute the assignment already, and whose actions they could copy?

Impulsive and Hyperactive

Children who do not fully understand the instructions being given may appear to act out impulsively, as they try to comply with the words they thought they understood. They may be unaware of behavioral norms that are specific to the situation. They may also have cultural mandates that seem to supersede the classroom rules. For instance, if Antonia believes her best friend is being unfairly picked on by another student or by the teacher, she may jump in to defend her friend, and she may end up in trouble herself. Her intentions were honorable, as she stepped in to support someone she cared about. Although Antonia's intervention looked impulsive, it was not—it was a culturally based desire to defend her friend's honor. Finally, behaviors resulting from prior or current traumas can make children appear hyperactive (see section "Trauma Symptoms in Children").

"Overly Social"

Children who do not speak the classroom language well, or who feel separate from the other children in class because of cultural reasons, may check in regularly with people who do speak their language or with whom they do feel connected. While this may appear to the instructor to be inappropriate socializing, it may feel like a very question of survival for the child. It can be helpful to seat a child next to a person who speaks the child's language, or with whom the child feels comfortable. Also provide the child with specific information as to what kinds of communications are permissible (e.g., "You can pass notes in class about schoolwork, but not about other topics"; or, "You can ask for help after the assignment has been given, but not while the teacher is still talking"). If this arrangement is too disruptive, it may help to schedule into the day regular times when the child can socialize more easily, such as at lunch or recess. In addition, the instructor may want to speak openly with the children about guidelines for communicating that will benefit learning but will not distract other children. Margarita, who did not speak the classroom language well, asked me sadly, "What am I supposed to do? I can't understand what the teacher is saying. I can't always be raising my hand and asking. I get in trouble if I ask the kid sitting next to me to help, but then I also get in trouble if I don't do what the teacher says. What should I do?" Indeed, it is not clear what a child in Margarita's shoes *should* do; but it is clear that she should not be negatively labeled because of her attempts to get the information she needs.

During their first experience in school, young children frequently wander the halls to check on their siblings or friends from their community. They may not understand that staying with the group is a security issue. Indeed, "making sure my little brother is safe," may feel like a duty. Where possible, this caretaking impulse should be channeled rather than completely censured or repressed. Perhaps a time can be arranged each day for the two siblings to check in with each other, such as during recess or on the way in to lunch.

Undisciplined

Sometimes children from countries where the classroom demeanor is rather formal and strict (such as China, Korea, and Japan) are giddy, chatty, and a bit wild in their behavior until they find the right balance. It may appear to them that their classroom in the United States, Canada, or Europe has *no* rules because it looks rather informal in comparison. Sometimes children who come from families that use corporal punishment and/or a direct, stern demeanor with children will have trouble following the more gentle invitations to obey, so common in some classrooms (Ballenger, 1998).

Overly Serious

Children from a variety of cultural groups may decline to engage in acts that seem "silly" to them because they don't share the cultural background of the school. For instance, in many schools practicing the Responsive Classroom (Charney, 2001) model, young children engage in a variety of games to reinforce and support the values they've agreed upon. These activities may involve tossing balls, calling out names, nonsense words, and a great deal of laughter. Some children have been raised to think of schools and education as extremely serious pursuits. They do not understand how the teacher can encourage such silliness, and they prefer to opt out of these educational games.

Overly Physical

In some cultures, people tend to touch the people with whom they are speaking lightly on the arm, and they may stand closer to their speaking partners than is the classroom norm. One little girl from Puerto Rico, Marta, suffered great humiliation when she heard the teacher tell her classmates to stand a few feet away from Marta when she tried to speak with them because she touched other people "way too much" and didn't seem to want to change (M. O'Neill, personal communication, June 2007). A high schooler from

Jordan, Mahmoud, was considered "weird" by his classmates in Oklahoma because he stood close to them and often touched them when he spoke. They thought this meant he might be gay. (See Chapter 5 on nonverbal communication.)

Depressed

Children who are isolated in school or who are unable to communicate adequately in the language of the classroom sometimes appear to be depressed. Of course, this diagnosis may sometimes be accurate. But it's essential to observe the youngsters in a setting with other people with whom they feel comfortable, or who speak their language, to see if the problem is primarily internal or situational. One Mexican boy, Eduardo, said to me of his classmates who did not speak his language:

> They don't know me. They think I'm this serious, shy, goody two-shoes who is always sad. I'm not! But there's no way to show them who I really am. I want to laugh at jokes like the other kids, but I don't understand them so I don't know when to laugh. I want to say funny things but I can't. In the beginning I was smiling at all the wrong times and I looked stupid, so I stopped smiling. Why would anyone want to spend time with me, anyway, when they have their friends already, who they can speak with easily?

Eduardo certainly looked depressed in the school setting, but he brightened up with Spanish speakers including his family. He was not suffering from a mental health problem but rather from language difficulties. He was embarrassed by his accent and didn't want the children to make fun of him. He needed intensive language instruction and classroom intervention aimed at easing his adaptation—not psychopharmacological intervention. (See Chapter 6 on language competence.)

Cheating

We must be certain children have understood the expectations of a given situation before we assume they are cheating. In a classic study, Greenfield (1997) found that Mayan children consider collaborating natural and expected—*not* collaborating feels strange to them, and it feels like a failure to use the important adaptive skills of pooling knowledge. Children who may have been physically punished or verbally shamed in previous school situations may find that the internal pressure to achieve a correct answer outweighs the command to do individual work. New norms would be best taught through patient and gentle instruction, rather than through a humiliating reprimand.

Students who have been unsuccessful in school by honest means may become habitual cheaters. To break this pattern, the teacher or counselor and student will need to openly discuss the pattern and devise a plan for the future, without blame.

Slow to Begin or Complete Tasks

Children who do not easily comprehend the classroom language (or the language of testing) will not perform to the best of their abilities. They may take extra time to begin or complete tasks as they translate the instructions to themselves into their native language, and then perhaps translate back into English to compose an answer. Children who feel uncomfortable, unwelcome, or stressed in the school (or testing) environment are also apt to perform at a level that is lower than they would under more ideal circumstances. Two strategies that teachers sometimes find useful is to warn children ahead of time that they will be asked questions on a given topic, or ask the children to tell another child their response to a question, which gives them a chance to rehearse the answer before they are called upon or need to write it down (E. Fernández-O'Brien, personal communication, June 23, 2007).

Disorganized

Children who have had little formal schooling, such as refugees, may have difficulty keeping track of their school supplies or assignments. Organizing tasks that seem like second nature to some children—such as keeping specific items in separate sections of a notebook or backpack; keeping a neat cubby, desk, or locker; or recording assignments in a calendar—may prove challenging to a child with less school experience or a child who has historically owned very few possessions. The same would also be true of children who simply have not been taught the value of organization. Children who live in unstable home environments such as shelters, or who rotate among the homes of various family friends and relatives, may also exhibit disorganization both in the school setting and in a testing situation. While it is accurate to describe them as "disorganized," it may be important to note possible sources of the problem, rather than attributing it to a basic character trait. (Remember the fundamental attribution error from Chapter 3.)

Some children from chaotic environments respond extremely well to guidance about ways to organize their work, their notebooks, and their schedules. Keeping their belongings in order gives them a sense of control over their life. Sometimes they are able to transfer these skills to their home life, reducing the chaos in that environment as well.

Forgetful

Children who do not fully master the language of instruction may appear to be forgetful. It is much harder to remember an assignment, instruction, or fact if you don't understand it clearly. Additionally, children whose lives are otherwise overwhelming because of trauma or disruption may have trouble keeping schoolwork "in mind" because they are preoccupied with other urgent matters. These children will be helped by gentle advice and by concrete systems that assist them in keeping track of tasks or information.

In addition, cultures vary in what they consider important to know, attend to, or remember. Various researchers have demonstrated that East Asians pay more attention to an abstract field or context than do Westerners, who pay more attention to separate objects (Okawa, 2008). If an East Asian child is being asked to recall a separate object or the actions of individuals only, the child may appear to have a poor memory. That child might perform better than a Western child on tasks involving more contextual memory. However, contextual tasks are not usually part of school or testing activities.

Uncooperative or Defiant

Children may appear to persist in misbehaving, or they may consistently fail to live up to expectations, despite repeated admonishments and instruction. This misconduct may not be deliberate. It is important to make sure the child fully understands the expectations of the environment. Schools have many unwritten codes in addition to the written ones, and often rules are interpreted differently in various classes. For instance, expectations around speaking with classmates may be different in physical education, math, and science class. Within a given class, from one day to the next, the expectation may change if there is a different instructor or if students are asked to engage in cooperative projects. In addition, individual teachers often interpret the same rules in a different way (e.g., the procedure for leaving the class to use the bathroom, or the policy around missing homework). Children who appear to have difficulty complying with an expectation may not understand it well enough to comply. I remember a Sudanese boy, Ismael, who did not speak or write English well. He could not tell when something written on the board was a homework assignment due the next day, when it was a long-term assignment, or when it was something else. He diligently copied whatever was on the board each day, and then rather consistently was reprimanded the next day for failing to complete the assignment. He had no one to ask at home to help him understand what he had written down.

Children from cultures that are more relation based may comply better with instructions that are clearly expressed by an individual they care about, rather than with abstract rules that emerge impersonally from an unclear source. The more explicit the instruction, the more likely children are to comply.

Greedy

Sometimes children take more than their due. They may grab a handful of candy or several pencils when instructed to take only one. While children need to be taught classroom norms, teachers should avoid responding in an overly critical or punitive manner. Explanations other than greediness may clarify this behavior. For instance, the child may be collecting extra pencils or candy to bring home to a sibling as an act of love. Hoarding is also common among children who have experienced chronic neglect or deprivation.

Poor Skills in a Certain Subject

Children who possess skills in a given area may be unable or uninterested in showing them in the context of school, an interview, or testing. A wide range of ways to measure children's abilities do exist, and yet current testing approaches are usually quite limited (Sternberg & Grigorenko, 2008). For instance, a child may skillfully use math at the family grocery store, or in selling trinkets on the street, and yet fail to perform abstract math problems at school. Delpit (2002) describes creating learning situations that stimulate middle school girls' interest in math, chemistry, patterns, accounting, business, and so on, by applying them to their real-life interest in running a hairdressing shop.

School personnel would also do well to remember that at all ages, many children and teens rely on their parents for help with their homework. This important resource is simply not available to children whose parents don't speak the language of instruction well, have little formal schooling themselves, or who work long hours (or at night) and therefore are not on hand after school when their children need help with homework.

Some students do poorly on standardized math tests because they are weak readers; they may be ashamed of their inadequacy. Some children perform poorly because they have undiagnosed vision, hearing, or other medical problems which stand in their way.

USING ASSESSMENT INSTRUMENTS WITH CULTURAL MINORITY YOUTH AND FAMILIES

Although this book focuses on interviewing rather than testing, I am including a section on assessment instruments here. Often a formal assessment forms a crucial part of the interviewing process, and testing presents numerous opportunities for biases of all kinds to creep in. Testing should be fair, accurate, and impartial. We must be alert to the assumptions behind the assessment instruments, interview guides, or procedures we use in our interviews with children and their families. (For a more thorough discussion, see Suzuki & Ponterotto, 2008.)

The testing situation itself assumes that children will be able to sit still and focus on one activity at a time, be motivated to perform well for the assessor, and understand the verbal and nonverbal communication of the assessor. Where these conditions are not met, a child may not be able to perform to the best of his or her abilities, and therefore the child may be mistakenly classified as underperforming.

It is difficult to determine which instruments will best provide the information on children of a certain age and their families in a given context. This task is infinitely harder when the people who are being tested are not fluent in English, or do not hold the same concepts or even approaches to testing as the dominant culture. Often, the usual approach to assessment is inappropriate with a child or group of children from a particular culture, and we need to determine if particular parts of the assessments process are, indeed, even necessary. If they are, we should be creative in our attempts to search for alternative procedures to test similar areas. Using the wrong assessment instruments or using instruments in the wrong ways is seriously harmful and unethical professionally and yet it occurs all the time, especially with children from cultural minority groups (Suzuki & Ponterotto, 2008).

Children from minority cultural and linguistic groups benefit from an ecological assessment system (Gopaul-McNicol & Thomas-Presswood, 1998). This system offers children opportunities to demonstrate their full capacities beyond the restrictions of timed and highly restrictive tests. So, for example, children might be allowed to attempt math problems that they were initially unable to complete with the help of a pencil and paper. Using this system, children's language abilities on the playground and the lunchroom will be noted, along with their language performance in the testing situation. Children's memory might be tested using names of familiar objects, rather than just digits, as is done in standard intelligence tests.

Instruments that are purported to measure cognitive aptitude or academic achievement such as IQ tests and the SATs (Scholastic Aptitude Tests) have received the most vehement criticisms for biases against children from ethnic and cultural minority groups. However, instruments that purport to detect learning disabilities and/or psychopathology have also been subject to severe criticism (Parron, 1997; Caplan, 2004). Problems with assessments include inappropriate items (such as asking a recent immigrant from Mexico about snow or asking an inner-city child about farm equipment); inappropriate tasks (timed tasks such as puzzles for children who have no exposure to puzzles), poor-quality translations (e.g., translating assessments into a form of Spanish that is not understood by children from particular countries), tests that have not been normed on the group to which they are being administered, tests given under inappropriate conditions or in inadequate settings (such as when a child is hungry or in a noisy hallway), tests that are administered, scored, or interpreted by inadequately trained personnel, tests that are poorly explained to the children who take them, and so on.

Children who are not thoroughly fluent in reading and writing the language of the test will not be able to demonstrate the top range of their abilities. Important decisions regarding school placement, diagnosis, and treatment are often made based on scores on these tests. Consider the following:

> Ruben was a 14-year-old boy from Puerto Rico, who had emigrated to New York at the age of 9. At 11 he was given a battery of cognitive tests in English and placed in a class for moderately retarded students. Three years later when he was retested, this time bilingually, he performed much better. Unfortunately, he had already taken on some of the habits and mannerisms of his more severely disabled classmates. (M. O'Neill, personal communication, June 2007)

Some of the formats used in Western testing will be unfamiliar to young people from other cultures, including multiple choice, true–false, graduated rating scales, sentence completions, and the use of puzzles, blocks, or other objects that the child is asked to manipulate. Different levels of familiarity with the test materials or format can render the results of tests invalid. In one test, children in Zambia and England were asked to reproduce patterns using wire, pencil and paper, or clay. The English children were best with pencil and paper, the Zambian children performed best with wire, a material with which they were more experienced, and the two groups performed equally well with clay (Neisser et al., 1996, cited in

Gopaul-McNicol & Thomas-Presswood, 1998). We can see how children who are not from Western industrialized nations would be penalized in assessments that rely solely on pencil and paper or verbal achievement.

Tests where points are given for speedy answers favor children from Western cultures, which typically value speedy performance. Children from Eastern cultures typically have been taught to value careful thought and reflection rather than speed.

Even the tests used to screen children's motor performance may contain cultural biases. For instance, Asian children are typically unfamiliar with skipping and may have trouble differentiating between hopping (one foot) and jumping (two feet) (E. Fernández O'Brien, personal communication, June 23, 2007).

Increasingly, computers are used to administer cognitive, achievement, vocational and psychological assessments. There are certain advantages to using computer-based assessment. Apparently, some people are more willing to reveal sensitive information to a computer as compared to being interviewed by a real person face to face. When used appropriately, computers can improve the ability of people with learning or physical disabilities to demonstrate their capabilities (for instance, a person with a hearing impairment can use a talking computer, and a person who has difficulty writing with a pen may have greater ease with a keyboard). Additionally, computer-based testing also reduces opportunities for bias in the testing situation—the computer is not scoring based on the race of the test takers. (Bias is not completely eliminated, however, because there is usually some human contact in the testing endeavor. For instance, uncomfortable encounters with a receptionist or discriminatory readings by an interpreter can still skew results.)

Interviewers would be wise to exercise caution in their use of computerized testing with culturally and economically diverse populations (Ahluwalia, 2008). It is important to determine the degree of familiarity with computers among the people being tested. In addition, you must determine if the people being tested are fluent readers of the test language. If the people being tested are not familiar or comfortable with computers, or if they cannot read the testing language well, their performance might be hindered in unexpected ways.

Assessments that involve asking a child to copy a figure or put together a puzzle or identify how two pictures differ may seem straightforward, but they may be all but impossible for children from certain backgrounds. I remember a Somali child who at the age of 5, and after being in the United States for 6 months, still had never held a drawing or a writing implement. I was shocked because I had given his family paper, crayons, pencils, and pens months earlier. His family had simply stored away these valuable items for adult use. They said the children would rip the paper if it was given to them, and it was too precious to waste. The boy's lack of familiarity with writing and drawing implements did not indicate any cognitive difficulties, but it might have appeared this way to an uninformed observer or tester.

Projective tests may seem more neutral in terms of culture, but they are not. The idea of seeing things in inkblots, or putting pictures together into stories, or free associating from images is very foreign and all but impossible for some people. In addition, without cultural information it may be difficult for the interpreter to properly interpret the child's response. For instance, "red indicates happiness and prosperity in Chinese culture but danger, aggression, and sexual impulse in American culture" (Uba, 1994, p. 168). This could affect the responses of Chinese children to inkblots and how these responses should be interpreted. Another example, José from Puerto Rico, was referred to family therapy because he had not included a chimney in his drawing of a house, which was seen by the test administrator as indicating a lack of warmth in the home (rather than an indication that the child had grown up with houses that did not have chimneys, because they were in a warm climate).

There are no perfect or easy answers as to how to choose assessment instruments for children and families from minority cultures. Only a thorough multimodal assessment will allow people with diverse cultural experiences to show their true capabilities and personalities. In many areas, adequate tests do not exist—thus increasing the importance of the personal interview.

ASSESSING DEVELOPMENT IN CHILDREN

When interviewing children, we often want to determine whether the child is "developing normally." While the need to answer this question is obvious in medical, mental health, and educational settings, it can also be important in legal and criminal justice settings where we may need to determine whether a child has special vulnerabilities or will be a credible witness. The enormous potential for bias in conducting developmental assessments with children who belong to a different cultural group than the assessor will not be fully addressed here. Rather, this section orients readers to some of the issues involved and provides references for further consultation.

We should remember that bilingual children may know differing words in each of their two languages. For instance, children may know "school words" such as ruler, blackboard, cafeteria, and recess in English, while knowing "home words" such as sofa, closet, and the names of family relationships in their first language. For this reason, bilingual children who are assessed in just one language may not be able to express their full vocabulary or full conceptual knowledge. Therefore, they may appear less advanced academically or developmentally than they really are.

Children who are not native speakers of English may have even more difficulty than other children with complex verb forms like would have, should have, may have, might have once wanted, and so on, to say nothing of constructions such as: "Where were you when you first told someone that something had happened to you in the alley behind your aunt's building?" Interviewers should keep their questions short and direct, using no embedded clauses. Every so often, interviewers should ask if the child understands the questions. If the interviewer has the sense that the child does not understand, the interviewer should pause and try to ascertain what is happening. Interviews with young children and with children who are non-native speakers of the test language can move slowly, requiring a great deal of time and patience.

To assess development we often try to gather information about a child's early milestones to determine if the child is growing well and developing age-appropriate skills. Psychiatrist Carolyn King, who practices in both Detroit and nearby suburbs, comments that children often have subtle symptoms that they can mask for short periods of time. To achieve an accurate assessment, King recommends that clinicians observe children closely "and get a complete history, starting from birth and straight through every single developmental milestone" (Carey, 2006). While this is the ideal backdrop to any child assessment, it is often hard to achieve.

Questions about milestones can be frustrating for parents and professionals alike, particularly when working with people from a different cultural background. Questions such as "When did your child roll over?" or "How old was your child when she said her first sentence?" may seem bizarre to some parents. For some Native American families, for instance, these events simply are not a milestone, whereas the child's first laugh might be one (Joe & Malach, 2004).

In some cultures, such as Filipino, Lebanese, and Mexican, children will achieve certain developmental milestones such as self-feeding, weaning, self-soothing, and sleeping by themselves at a much later age than in Western industrialized nations. These children are more dependent on their caretakers because they are typically held and carried constantly and consoled immediately if they are distressed. Also, children often sleep with their mother at night, either in the same bed or in the same room (Santos & Chan, 2004; Sharifzadeh, 2004; Zuniga, 2004). In these cultures, young children are often indulged and may experience little in the way of expectations for discipline or achievement until they enter school. For instance, young children may be allowed to drink from a baby bottle, and their mothers may cut their food and tie their shoes for them until a much later age than would be expected in the United States, Canada, or Northern Europe.

Children whose parents come from many parts of the world such as

Somalia, the Sudan, and parts of India will not be comfortable using silverware, because they are used to eating with their hands. (Conversely, children from Western industrialized nations often lag behind their peers from developing countries in their ability to use kitchen knives, work with fire, complete household chores, and care for younger siblings [Rogoff, 2003]. However, *these* tasks do not form part of typical developmental assessments.) These developmental differences are not a question of one culture making its children more advanced than another. Rather, different skills and qualities are emphasized to shape children to be the kinds of adults who will fit in with the values and gender roles of their culture. If the methods we use to assess children rely solely on one set of skills, such as reading and writing, they will be inadequate to measure development in other areas.

The way these developmental questions are phrased in assessments may create a situation in which children who are not from the culture on which the test was based will appear delayed. For instance, the test question may be phrased as, "Does the child _____" rather than "can the child _____"? The answer to "Does the child feed herself" will be "no" if the child is usually lovingly handfed food by her grandmother, although the child may be capable of this.

Conducting Developmental Assessments with Children and Their Families from Diverse Cultures

- When selecting instruments, choose only those that are appropriate for the child's and the family's language and culture.
- Use an interpreter, as necessary, for people with limited English proficiency (see Chapter 7 on the interpreted interview). Remember, however, that most standardized assessment instruments will not be valid if they are not conducted in the original language in which they are validated. We cannot simply have an interpreter spontaneously translate and administer an instrument and then expect the results to mean the same as if the assessment was conducted in the original language.
- Make sure all important family members with caretaking responsibilities are included, where appropriate and possible. This may include the father, grandmother, godparent, or even an older sibling. Remember, many families emigrate in waves. The most important caretakers in the child's early life (e.g., a grandmother or aunt) may have remained behind in the country of origin.
- Conduct the assessment in a place that is comfortable for the child and family.
- Gather only the necessary data. Limit the number of forms, questionnaires, and other types of paperwork, as these can be especially cumbersome and offputting for people who come from cultures where paperwork is less common.
- Do not overwhelm the family with multiple professionals, especially in the beginning.

- Tend first to the issues that concern the family most.
- Explain every step of the assessment to the family as many times as necessary.
- Incorporate cultural rituals such as handshakes, bowing the head, warm greetings, and/or serving tea, as appropriate (see Chapter 5 on nonverbal communication).
- Be sure that input from the entire family is solicited and encouraged, individually and collectively. Some family members may not be comfortable speaking in a large group but may wish to contribute their insight and opinions in a more private setting.
- Allow time for the family to question *you*. Some families are too embarrassed to ask questions in the context of a formal interview. Be prepared to discuss the kinds of issues that have been raised by other families from similar cultures in the past.
- It is also important not to draw conclusions too quickly as to what it might mean if a child is quieter than other children. (See Chapter 8 on reluctance.)

Note. Partially adapted from Lynch and Hanson (2004, pp. 459–461).

Using Alternative Media with Children

Where children are reluctant to talk, sometimes you can make it easier by letting them make a drawing or diagram of what happened, explaining what they are doing as they create it. It is important, however, not to cut off people who are about to speak by thrusting a piece of paper and crayons at them. Generally, the verbal explanation is preferable first. The drawing may be used to demonstrate the interviewee's knowledge of the details of a place or person, or may help the interviewer understand exactly what happened and where the people described were placed in relation to each other.

Numerous studies suggest that children provide more details about events when given an opportunity to make a drawing about the events (Faller, 2007). Drawings may be used in interviews with children to improve rapport, to decrease anxiety, and as a way to collect information related to the event in question. However, research does *not* prove that drawings are accurate tools that in and of themselves prove the existence of particular conditions or histories (Faller, 2007).

Sometimes children prefer to use dolls or puppets to recount an incident. We must be careful here if we are working in a forensic context or if our interview may later be challenged in court. Some jurisdictions disqualify interviews in which dolls or puppets have been used because they are thought to make a child prone to engage in imaginative play. Research has shown, however, that when used properly, dolls can help children show interviewers what happened and provide additional details (Faller, 2007; American Professional Society on the Abuse of Children, 1995, 2002). Dolls, like drawings, if they are used at all, should be used after and as a supplement to verbal inquiry, not to substitute for it.

Trauma Symptoms in Children

Trauma symptoms can complicate a developmental assessment. For instance, a child who has been traumatized may suffer from any combination of separation anxiety, school phobia, bedwetting, encopresis, depression, compulsive behaviors, anxiety, poor concentration, mood disorders, anger, substance abuse, suicidality, and/or nightmares, all of which might obscure an accurate developmental picture (Greenwald, 2005). A child who has been traumatized may be afraid of loud noises, sirens, yelling, airplanes, and fire alarms and may startle easily. Conversely, another child who is traumatized may seem to seek out frightening situations, appear to be afraid of nothing, and respond violently to minor incidents. A traumatized child may have to be coaxed into eating or may bolt down food quickly and sloppily, looking as if this is his or her last meal.

Trauma symptoms can easily be misinterpreted as indications of an organic difficulty, poor parenting, or oppositional behavior. Refugee children commonly face traumas prior to migration, during the migration process, and after migration. These damaging traumas may include the "disappearance" of family members, hunger, thirst, homelessness, sexual assaults, seeing dead bodies, being wounded, physical threats and beatings, confinement, torture, rape, seeing relatives killed, witnessing atrocities, being forced to violate their own moral code, and living for prolonged periods in fear for their lives (Delgado, Jones, & Rohani, 2005). Life in the refugee camps is often tenuous and traumatic, including violence, illness, inadequate food and shelter, and overcrowding. Undocumented immigrants and people who have come from countries with repressive governments, even if they are not official refugees, may also have experienced trauma in their countries of origin and/or during an arduous voyage to their new lands. But life in the new country may not be safe or secure for the immigrant child, who may observe his or her parents unable to communicate, uncertain of how to proceed, and subject to the vagaries of bosses, landlords, social service providers, and others. It is also traumatic for a child to live as an undocumented alien, or to have loved ones who are undocumented and risk deportation on a daily basis. Sometimes immigrant children are isolated, humiliated, mocked, and even beaten by peers in their new countries.

Sometimes we assume that a child who was very young during traumatic experiences was somehow shielded from them. However, some mental health experts believe that when children have experienced trauma before they developed language skills, they actually have a more difficult time healing than older children who transformed their experiences into words as they occurred (Pynoos, Steinberg, & Goenjian, 1996).

When assessing a child who may have been traumatized, it is important to take a full trauma history and inquire about the child's behavioral changes over time (Greenwald, 2005). This assessment will help you determine the origin of the child's symptoms and the best course of action. When working with children who were adopted, or who come from extremely chaotic environments, such a thorough history may unfortunately not be possible.

The process of immigration itself has been found to be traumatizing for many children and families, as are chronic experiences of racism, discrimination, and exclusion (Bryant-Davis & Ocampo, 2005). Consider the ongoing trauma of a child who is thrust into an unfamiliar school filled with people who speak another language, and who have different sets of behavioral norms. The child is apt to feel isolated, confused, and perhaps invisible for hours every day, without end. One child who spent 3 months in a school where he did not speak the language told me he felt like a ghost at school—everyone was moving around him and occasionally looked in his direction, but because he could not communicate he felt as if they couldn't see him. Children whose caretakers are unable to serve as a bridge to the school system are apt to be particularly lost without a guide in their new environment. Because they have a limited set of experiences to draw on, children may not understand that they *will* adjust to their new environment, the disorientation is *temporary*, they will learn the new language and make friends. The despair that they feel initially will seem like eternal damnation. It is especially important for school personnel to reach out to children who are new in school, and particularly to those who come from a radically different culture. These outreach efforts must be sustained for at least the first 2 years of the child's entrance into the new environment, and more if the child appears to continue to struggle academically or socially.

Where professionals perceive a child's symptoms as resulting from trauma, family members will often have another explanation. For example, Webb (2004) described a Chinese high school student who attended school near the World Trade Center and suffered nightmares, poor concentration, and declining grades after witnessing the September 11, 2001, attacks. The student's parents rejected the school counselor's recommendation of counseling and rejected the notion that the student's difficulties stemmed from trauma. Instead, the mother reported being ashamed of her son's performance and suggested he meet with his uncle, a significant family figure. She rejected talk of posttraumatic stress disorder (PTSD). She did not want her son stigmatized as having a mental health disorder.

The actual symptoms of people who have suffered trauma also appear to vary by culture. For instance, in a UNICEF (United Nations International Children's Emergency Fund) study of more than 3,000 Rwandan children, fewer than 20% reported difficulty sleeping, more trouble feeling happiness or love than before the slaughter, difficulty concentrating, strong waves of feelings about the event, and startling or being nervous. However, despite the consistent lack of these common PTSD symptoms, these children did report high rates of avoidance and intrusive thoughts that are typical of children with PTSD (Dyregrov, Gupta, Gjestad, & Mokanoheli, 2000). In other words, although the trauma manifests differently across cultures, these children suffered from the trauma to which they had been exposed.

SPECIAL ISSUES IN INTERVIEWING ADOLESCENTS

Adolescence is not recognized as a distinct phase of life in many cultures. Instead, children in those cultures pass directly from childhood to a state where they are judged and treated as adults. Sometimes the transition from childhood to adulthood is marked by a coming-of-age ritual such as a confirmation or bar/bat mitzvah, an initiation ceremony that might include painful circumcision and/or joyous dancing, a Sweet Sixteen, or a Quinceañera party. Sometimes this transition is marked by a practical rather than symbolic change in circumstances, such as getting married, giving birth, joining adults in traditional labors, going off to college, or getting a job.

In contrast, in many Western industrialized nations the adolescent phase is a long, prolonged one, ranging from when a young person leaves elementary school (at 12 years old or so) to when he or she assumes full adult responsibilities, which may not occur well past the college years, for those who go to college. For the purposes of this discussion, however, I use the term "teenager" or "adolescent" in its traditional sense, to describe the years from 13 to 19. We should recognize that this is a somewhat arbitrary demarcation. These years vary greatly for young people, depending on their circumstances. For some, these years may be filled with fun, sports, summer camp, school, and parties. For others, they may be filled with substance abuse, homelessness, giving birth to and taking care of one or more young children, working, or any combination of these activities and more. These are years when the values of a teen's family and culture, which often predominate in childhood, may be challenged by the values of their peers.

In Western industrialized nations, adolescence is often considered a period of exploration, self-involvement, and risk taking. In other cultures, however, adolescence may be viewed quite differently. It may be seen as a time of increasing responsibilities toward the family (e.g., caring for younger siblings, cousins, or older relatives; getting married; or helping in the family business), and toward the community (e.g., praying, hunting, farming, or selling items at the market). In traditional cultures, adolescence is often a time when increasing restrictions are placed on girls' movement and modesty. Orthodox Muslims and Jews often require their daughters to cover themselves or isolate themselves from boys and men, as the girls reach puberty. A young Muslim girl who is permitted to play in a teeshirt and jeans with the boys next door may be restricted from such play and required to cover her head, arms, neck and legs, as she matures. She may be forbidden from participating in mixed-gender activities such as sports, afterschool clubs, and theater. If her classmates include non-Muslims, she may resent the restrictions and look back longingly on her young childhood of relative freedom. All these pressures need to be considered when interviewing adolescents and their families, who are from cultures with which we may be less familiar.

In part because the teenage years are lived so distinctly in different nations, immigrant parents are often puzzled and angry about the behavior of their more acculturated offspring. Some of the questions they may ask about their teen children include: Why do they suddenly think they are so grown up? Why do they want to stay out with their friends until all hours of the night? Why are their friends so disrespectful of their parents? Should I be treating them like children or adults? If they are adults, why do they still go to school instead of working hard the way we do? Being a parent of one or more teenagers is bewildering enough for people who are very familiar with the society in which they live—it can be overwhelmingly disorienting for people who come from other cultures.

An interview or assessment may be confounded by the dissonance between the visions of this life stage held by youngsters and their immigrant caretakers. The teen and the adult often hold different definitions of both the problem and the solution. The strong feelings that may be experienced on both sides need to be handled with care.

Adolescents and Cultural Identity

Identity is a process of negotiation through social
relationships and power and culture.
—DAVID MURA

In the United States and other Western industrialized nations with majority White populations, most young White youth spend most of their time with people from the same race. This is usually seen as natural and expected. When young people of color "hang out" together, whether in the school lunchroom, or in neighborhood parks or street corners, this social behavior is often interpreted by others as unfriendly, standoffish, or indicating that the youth are part of a gang.

Being a teenager in Western industrialized nations is often difficult—

including negotiating rapid hormonal changes, new role expectation, decisions about school, employment, dating, and substance use. A teenager who is caught between two cultural worlds faces additional challenges. Add to that a special situation such as a sexual assault, school failure, mental or physical illness or disability, a special talent, or a teenager realizing that he or she might be gay or lesbian—the teen years can be minefields, indeed.

As they struggle with questions of their own individual identity, adolescents often examine their peers for signs of nonconformity to group norms concerning gender, sexual orientation, race, social class, and culture. They can be merciless in their teasing of those who do not fit neatly into identity boxes either because of factors beyond their control (e.g., having parents of different races) or because of choices in their lifestyle, apparel, manner of speech, or behaviors. In many contexts, teenagers also have especially rigid and narrow ideas about what it means to "act like" a member of a given cultural, racial, or social class group. Young people from minority cultural or racial groups who strive for academic success, or who speak Standard English or who have many White friends, may be accused of being "White on the inside" while superficially belonging to a minority group. Some of the terms used are:

- "Twinkie" or "banana" (for Asians, meaning yellow on the outside and White inside) or "Chonky" (an Asian person who "acts White");
- "Apple" (for Native Americans, meaning red on the outside and White inside);
- "Oreo" (for Black people, meaning Black on the outside and White inside);
- "Coconut" (for Latinos, Blacks, or Filipinos, meaning Black on the outside but White inside); and
- *Pocha* (which in Spanish can mean faded or overripe)—used pejoratively by Latinos to describe other Latinos who are considered *over*assimilated.

Minority youth often feel caught between societal norms that tend to privilege those who conform to the dominant styles of dress, language, and lifestyles, and their peers, who may promulgate a contrasting set of values.

Growing up in Trinidad, Joanne Kilgour Dowdy spoke such proper English that she was asked to represent her grade school in choral speaking competitions and storytelling festivals:

My mother always reminded us that we needed to learn to "curse in White." By this she meant, or I believed that she meant, that we should always be aware that we had to play to a White audience. We could protest, we could show anger, but we had to remember that there was a White way, and that was the right way. (Dowdy, 2002, p. 5)

Dowdy was teased by her peers, however, for her use of Queen's English, the language of the colonizer. She describes being caught between speaking the way her mother, grandmother, and teachers wanted her to speak and speaking the language of her peers—the rich mixed English patois that reflects the many cultures that make up Trinidad. Dilemmas of this kind are typical for youth who participate in more than one culture, and who need to choose many times a day which one to favor at any given moment.

Adolescents often have little tolerance for their peers who are seen as posing as something they are not. In general, they may be called *wannabees*. Some specific terms that are often used disparagingly include:

- "ABCD" or "CBCD" (American Born or Canadian Born Confused Desi) (a person of South Asian heritage who is confused about his or her cultural identity);
- "Chinig" (an Asian person who is trying to "act Black");
- "Pretendian" (someone with little or no Indian background who claims this heritage);
- "Wexican" (a White person who tries to act Mexican);
- "White chocolate" (Whites who try to act like Blacks);
- "Wigger" (meaning White nigger, and used to describe White people who "act Black," or Black people who "act White," or people of mixed White/Black racial background); and
- "Wink" (a White person who hangs out with Asians or tries to "act Chinese").

Adolescents sometimes display harsh attitudes toward their peers who date outside their race or culture. This may be seen as yet another attempt to enforce conformity to a narrow cultural identity. Some terms that are used include:

- "Chocolate dipper" (someone of a different race who dates a Black man or woman);
- "Race traitor" (someone who dates or has children with a person of a different race); and
- "Rice king" (a non-Asian man who dates Asian women).

Children of mixed racial or ethnic background are often special targets of other youth, who appear distressed by the difficulty of placing them into easy categories. A short list of the many terms used to describe these young people of mixed heritage include:

- "Blaxican" or "Mexicoon" (Black and Mexican heritage);
- "Blew" or "jigger" (Black and Jewish heritage);
- "Bumblebee" (Black and Asian heritage);
- "Halfrican" (half African, half another heritage);
- "Jewarican" or "Portajew" (Jewish and Puerto Rican heritage);
- "Zebra" or "milano" (White and Black heritage, in reference to the cookie);
- "Pakoniggy" (Pakistani and Black heritage);
- "Pinto" (mixed White and Native American heritage after White and brown horses);
- "Sortarican" (Puerto Rican and any other heritage); and
- "Spink" (Hispanic and Asian heritage).

I include such a long list of terms, and there are many more, to convey some of the difficulties adolescents of mixed background may face in constructing their identity. Where this is the case, simple questions about cultural background and race may be extremely delicate.

Interviewing Adolescents without Their Parents

In some situations, such as police interviews, it is important for parents to be present or to give their consent for an interview with a minor. This gives the adult opportunities to help protect the minor's rights. However, in other situations, such as social work, health, or mental health interviews, the interview is apt to be more effective if the adult is *not* present. Legally, a caretaker's consent may need to be obtained for the interview to take place, however.

Many adolescents are hesitant to reveal sensitive information about a long list of issues in their parents' presence. Of course, this list includes dating, sexuality, and substance use but is not limited to these. Some teens do not want to discuss their schoolwork in front of their parents, either because they are struggling or because they are pursuing an independent path that they believe will disappoint or anger their parents. Some teens do not want to discuss their friends, especially if their parents want to restrict their friendships to people from specific ethnic or religious groups, or exclude people from specific groups, or exclude friends whom they consider a bad influence. Some teens are keeping secret from their parents the fact that they have paid employment, have suicidal feelings, have sought counseling, or play on a sports team. Some teens lie to their parents regularly about their whereabouts, if they consider their parents overly strict. Some teens will not tell their parents that they are applying to college. Consider María Luísa, from Puerto Rico:

> "No one in my family ever finished high school, much less college. I couldn't tell them I applied because they would have made fun of me, or told me that I wasn't good enough, or that they couldn't afford it. I was even worried they might send me back to live with my grandparents in Puerto Rico to stop me from going. I was worried that they would think I would get too far away from them if I kept studying. I forged their names on the applications and the forms from the guidance office. Then when I got the acceptances and told my parents, they were actually really happy for me. They didn't want me to move out, but they were so glad that I was going to get to keep on studying, they cried. If I had told them beforehand, I still think maybe they would have tried to stop me."

Immigrant parents may be hesitant to allow their teen children to be interviewed alone, demonstrating an attitude of "my daughter (or son) tells me everything!" In their parents' presence, of course, youth often deny that they need to keep information private from their parents. However, interviewers who aim for a complete picture of the teen's life may need to insist on an interview with the teen alone, explaining to the parents that this is standard practice. At the same time, it would be important to explain the limits on confidentiality to both the teenager and the parents.

Generational Status for Immigrant Youth

The concerns of youth vary greatly, depending on whether they are the first generation (born outside the country where they currently live), second generation (born in their current country of residence, but with at least one parent foreign born), or third generation or greater (youth and both of their parents born in their current country of residence).

For youth who have immigrated themselves, the age when they immigrated partly determines their level of acculturation and their ability to speak the language of the new country. Consider the following Somali family:

> Timira and her three children arrived in the United States with little more than the clothes they wore and their settlement papers as refugees. The children were ages 2, 4, and 13 when they arrived. Three years later, Timira gave birth to another son, Isaac. The eldest child, Abshir, had suffered from malaria for a prolonged period as a child and was generally in ill health. He entered the fourth grade, although he was more than 2 years older than his peers there. The school district hoped the extra years in elementary school would give Abshir a chance

to learn English and learn to read and write. However, he was not given adequate instruction in English as a second language, nor the special attention that would have enabled him to catch up to his peers. From his first day at school he experienced mostly failure, frustration, and loneliness. He had no one to help him with his schoolwork at home. He couldn't wait to drop out and avoid the misery and isolation that he suffered in school. Isaac, on the other hand, attended a Headstart Preschool Center from the age of 18 months, where he quickly learned English and made friends with children from a variety of backgrounds. At home he spoke Somali with his mother and mostly English with his siblings. As he got older, he was able to ask his siblings for help with his schoolwork. He was the same age as his peers in school and not only kept up with the schoolwork but also excelled in both math and sports. How different Isaac's teen years were from those of his brother Abshir! Isaac enjoyed friends from a variety of cultural groups, mastered the English language, and looked forward to school. He was largely comfortable with U.S. norms around dress and dating. Within the same family, Abshir is a first-generation immigrant and his brother Isaac is a second-generation immigrant, and their needs and issues are quite different.

CONCLUDING OBSERVATIONS

Whether they comply or rebel, children know that they are largely subject to the will of adults. Young children may not comprehend the implications of an interview, and they may view it as a simple conversation or an opportunity to draw and play. Older children are apt to understand that an interview is yet another situation in which an adult will assess them, pass judgment on them, and make decisions about their future.

When we interview a child or adolescent we are taking on an enormous responsibility. We need to be aware of ethical issues that may be complex and difficult. When the interview involves a child from a culture different from our own, we need to be even more cautious and conscientious than usual.

Questions to Think about and Discuss

1. How might a person's understanding of his or her own culture change with age? How would it be different for a preschooler as compared to a third-grader as compared to a high school senior?
2. Describe an interview you conducted with a child from a different culture. What cultural issues emerged?

3. Imagine a 10-year-old child from a particular ethnic group in your area. What are some of the cultural issues that might emerge in assessing the child's development?
4. A 14-year-old girl has been crying frequently at school and stealing from her classmates. She sits alone at lunch and stands in a corner of the gym during physical education, without interacting with the other children. How does your evaluation of her behavior change when you learn she is a recent immigrant from Croatia or Liberia, or that she recently saw her brother shot on the street of her neighborhood?

RECOMMENDED ADDITIONAL READING

Canino, I. A., & Spurlock, J. (2000). *Culturally diverse children and adolescents: Assessment, diagnosis and treatment* (2nd ed.). New York: Guilford Press.

Delgado, M., Jones, K., & Rohani, M. (2005). *Social work practice with refugee and immigrant youth in the United States.* New York: Pearson.

Gopaul-McNicol, S., & Thomas-Presswood, T. (1998). *Working with linguistically and culturally different children.* New York: Allyn & Bacon.

Rogoff, B. (2003). *The cultural nature of human development.* New York: Oxford University Press.

Suzuki, L. A., & Ponterotto, J. G. (Eds.). (2007). *Handbook of multicultural assessment: Clinical, psychological, and educational applications* (3rd ed.). New York: Jossey-Bass.

10 Interview Reports and Documents

In Chapter 3 on boundaries and biases I discussed the relationship between observing in interviews and taking notes as parallel to the relationship between seeing and drawing. Let's add another layer here. Observing, taking notes, and writing reports is like seeing, drawing, and producing a finished work of art. The first two steps are essential preludes to the third, but most people have contact only with the finished work of art, or—in our case—the final report.

The report, which is the tangible "output" of the interview, should reflect the same skill and sensitivity that were used in the interview itself. Unfortunately, however, report writing is too often accomplished either as an afterthought or in a rush. After all, who has this kind of time or energy to dedicate to their paperwork? Few of us entered our respective professional fields with the intention of focusing on our paperwork. Most people view report writing as a tedious and unglamorous part of their jobs. Unfortunately for those who abhor, delay, or resist paperwork, an interview is often only as valuable as the report that stems from it. Recall that the written report exists in perpetuity, representing your and your agency's work. Some people suggest writing reports with the mental image of a vigorous attorney on one shoulder and a professional from your own discipline on the other shoulder (W. Moore, personal communication, June 2007). We should be that careful.

Better interviews lead to better reports. The stronger the relationship between the interviewer and interviewee and the more thorough the interview, the more accurate the information gathered is likely to be. However, the effectiveness of an interview report also hinges on what happens *after* the interview has concluded—the organizational skills and the writing or presenting skills of the person making the report. This chapter discusses some of the difficulties you may encounter in writing unbiased reports after an interview with someone from a cultural group that differs from your own, and ways to overcome these challenges.

The finished product typically reflects a triad of global components: objective data, history, and "presentation." Objective data are arguably the more quantitative aspect of a broad assessment, which might include a drug screen, legal record, and educational or psychological test data. History, which is often considered the best predictor of future behavior, most likely involves broad and disparate information such as family composition, psychiatric hospitalizations or suicide attempts, educational achievement, medications taken, and work record. Presentation is the most subjective domain of these three elements and results from observing the interviewee and noticing his or her reactions to the interviewer's prompts.

RECORDING BEHAVIORAL OBSERVATIONS OR PRESENTATION

You may be expected to write about the interviewee's behavior during the interview. Without a videotape, a person who reads your report relies entirely on what you write to understand what transpired. If the interviewee cries, sighs, moans, or laughs; responds sarcastically, sweetly, or angrily; sits rigidly, slumps, or rocks wildly; wears rags or a suit or a uniform; has needle marks, scars, or bruises or other unusual physical characteristics which might be relevant—all this will be lost in your report unless you find an effective way to record more than just the interviewee's words. The behavior displayed in the interview is assumed to be in some way representative of the interviewee's behavior in other situations.

Our perceptions of people we interview cannot be entirely pure or neutral. As discussed in Chapter 3, we bring our biases into the interview room. We see people through our own eyes, and we hear them through our own ears. Exactly what we see and hear depends on which factors stand out enough for us to notice them. Our biases and expectations filter our perceptions and memory in ways that may escape our awareness. For example, people have much greater difficulty remembering and distinguishing faces of people from a different race than their own (Anthony, Cooper, & Mullen, 1992).

Beyond what we actually perceive, our expectations and biases also help determine what we consider worth recording and what we leave out. Think about a recent event that you shared with others—maybe a meeting, a meal, or a holiday celebration. Picture two other people who attended the event. If they were to write about it, do you think they would record the same things as you, and the same as each other? Or, would certain statements and certain happenings seem more salient and worth recording to some people than to others?

Your profession and the goals of the interview will also determine what you notice and what you record. Interviewing the same woman, a physician may be likely to notice her flushed skin whereas a social worker observes her halting speech. A college admissions officer might note her comfortable use of a large vocabulary, whereas a detective might focus on the fact that she checks her watch and cell phone throughout the interview but denies that she is in a hurry.

When writing about an observation that is largely speculative, be sure to state it as such. For example, an odor of alcohol might also be attributable to other sources, and unless you have your interviewee use a breathalyzer, conclusions about alcohol use can only be described as speculations. (Police officers who believe they smell alcohol on the breath of a person who is operating a vehicle can take the driver out of the car and perform a roadside sobriety test, but an assumption of intoxication is not made unless the person also fails that test.) Similarly, if you see scar tissue on the underside of a person's forearm, the origin of the scar could include self-mutilation, suicidal gestures, cooking burns, or injuries sustained in a work environment. Record the observation of the scar, without a description of its source, unless you are certain of it

REPORTING THE INTERVIEWEE'S ATTITUDE, DEMEANOR, AND AFFECT

Depending on your setting, you may be asked to report on interviewees' general demeanor and attitude toward you. This is commonly included in a mental status exam, for instance. Some dimensions that are commonly discussed include cooperative/uncooperative, open/closed, and friendly/hostile.

Correctly Interpreting and Writing
about Interviewees' Presentation

Let's examine several ways culture can complicate your assessment of an interviewee's attitude, focusing on some negatively tinged words that are commonly used:

Impatient

An interviewee who sits on the edge of her seat, tapping her fingers or feet, checking her watch, or verbally expressing that she's in a hurry may be described as "impatient." This word comes across as a criticism implying a resistance to the interview process if it is used without context to describe possible reasons for the apparent impatience. We must be careful before we use this word to find out the reason behind the behavior—perhaps it is legitimate in this particular situation and not an indication of an objection to the interview process itself. Perhaps this is not the first interview of this kind that the person has endured, and the others did not produce results. Or perhaps she has to be at work in 20 minutes, or use the bathroom, or pick up her children, and is uncomfortable saying so. Perhaps the decision based on the interview is much more important to her than we can imagine, and her anxiety about the interview appears to us like impatience.

Indifferent or Passive

Sometimes reports indicate that the interviewee did not seem to care about the outcome and was indifferent or passive. I heard this expressed once regarding a father who chewed gum while attending a custody hearing about his son (Azar, 2006). The social worker interpreted his gum chewing as lack of concern, but in fact the father was very tense. He was chewing gum because smoking was prohibited and he didn't want to step out to smoke, concerned that he might miss part of the proceedings.

I have also seen situations in which Cambodian refugees responded in a way that appeared disturbingly passive to their social workers in the United States, and their behavior was interpreted as indifference toward their children. In fact, the parents were upset and terrified, but they were afraid to express their opposition to what was happening because of previous horrific experiences when they opposed authorities in Cambodia.

One final example: I was speaking with a Somali refugee once through an interpreter, trying to elicit her opinion about educational decisions regarding her elementary school-age children. She brushed off my questions and kept asking me to make the decision myself. Finally, she reminded me that she had never attended school a day in her life and barely knew what happened inside a school, although we had visited the school together. She said she did not know enough to make the decisions and would like me to do so on her behalf because she trusted my judgment and considered me a second mother. Far from being indifferent, in fact, Yasmin cared too much about her children's schooling to make an uninformed decision.

Manipulative

Interviewees are sometimes described as manipulative if they try to get people to meet their needs without stating their needs directly. It is important to remember, however, that making direct requests is considered bad form in many cultures. People from cultures that rely on indirect communication are more likely to suggest and imply rather than ask directly, and they depend on others to infer what they mean from what they are saying (or not saying). Cultures with indirect communication tend to be more collectivist and to emphasize harmony: Speaking obliquely is a way to avoid conflict. So, for instance, picture this dialogue between a Portuguese patient and his doctor:

DOCTOR: (*looking at the chart*) Is your knee still bothering you?

PATIENT: (*Laughs and rubs knee.*) A little.

DOCTOR: (*writing in the chart*) Okay, so it's better.

The doctor interpreted the patient's comment literally, to mean that he was experiencing only a little pain, while the patient was trying to describe continued suffering without seeming weak or like a "complainer." If the patient dares to return to the issue at all, it may be through indirect means, such as by describing how often he has to push heavy machinery and climb stairs at work, hoping that the doctor will understand that he needs some kind of intervention so he can use his knees. Accustomed to more direct communication, the doctor may entirely miss the patient's hints, or might experience the patient as trying to manipulate him into prescribing painkillers or recommending time off work. The patient expects the doctor to tune into his subdued expressions of distress and find a solution. Clearly, there are many opportunities for miscommunication when direct communicators and indirect communicators interact.

Ingratiating or Overly Eager to Please

Interviewees are sometimes described as ingratiating if they seem overly eager to obtain the interviewer's approval, seem to curry favor, or seem to work too hard to present themselves in a positive light. Pleasing an authority, demonstrating respect, and presenting oneself as positively as possible may be expected in the interviewee's culture (see Chapter 8 on reluctance). In addition, the interviewee may overestimate your power, or may assume that behaving obsequiously is appropriate, given the circumstances.

Hostile or Aggressive

Interviewees are sometimes described as hostile or aggressive if they speak loudly or in a harsh tone, or if their nonverbal behavior seems to communicate contempt or anger (see Chapters 4 and 5 on setting the right tone and nonverbal communication, respectively). Remember that you may be misinterpreting their tone of voice and manner of speaking. Police officers sometimes misinterpret East African men as hostile because they are apt to get out of their cars and approach the police vehicle if stopped for a traffic violation and are apt to stand quite close to the officer, as is customary in their part of the world.

The interviewee may be misinterpreting the nature of the interview or what you are saying and therefore respond in a hostile way to a perceived insult or threat. While such behavior may be worth noting, it's important to clarify the misunderstanding rather than simply using a charged word such as "hostile" in an interview report. For example, I knew a graduate professor who habitually asked applicants to her doctoral program if they had concerns about paying for their education. She asked this question of all applicants. However, people from certain groups may perceive this as an insult, thinking, "Why does she think I can't pay for college? Does she assume I'm poor because I'm Black?" While candidates are unlikely to ask this question aloud, they may bristle from the perceived insult and be mistakenly described, thereafter, as hostile.

Numerous examples of misunderstandings of this kind are provided in this book. Here I will add just one more. While speaking with a mother, Eva, a first-grade teacher mentioned that 6-year-old Ramón sometimes acted "very silly" with his friends. Eva, who was Colombian, had been living in the United States for several years but was not entirely familiar with the word "silly." She knew it meant something like ridiculous or clownish and took offense at the teacher's description of her son. She became angry, and gave only curt replies during the rest of the conversation. While it might be technically accurate to describe the mother's behavior as hostile after the misunderstanding, to do so without exploring the motivation is to convey a false sense of her as *a hostile person*, rather than as a person who was affronted by a perceived insult to her child. This is an example of the fundamental attribution error, described in Chapter 3— mistakenly attributing a behavior to an enduring characteristic rather than the situation.

Uncooperative, Closed, Standoffish, or Guarded

In Chapter 8 on reluctance, we reviewed many reasons why interviewees may hesitate to cooperate, are reticent to speak, or are wary of discussing particular topics. If some of these reasons apply, general descriptors such as "uncooperative" will not help the reader understand the interviewee.

Resistant

This term is apt to be used by people in the mental health field, particularly those with some psychoanalytic training. Clients are "resistant" when they decline to agree with a professional's assessment of a situation or do not follow a recommendation. This word implies that the professional knows best. While this is often the case, sometimes people behave in ways that looks resistant because the professional is mistaken in his or her assessment and the conclusions or recommendations do not fit the situation. For example, a school counselor recommends to Pakistani parents that they encourage their son to take a wide variety of courses in high school and that they support his desire to join after-school clubs and activities. The parents nod. But when it comes time to signing their son's course registration, they insist that he take an academic overload and avoid all courses in the arts, and they refuse to let him participate in after-school activities. It would be natural for the school counselor to see the parents as resistant. Further exploration of the problem would reveal motivations that are far more complex, however: The parents left their elegant home in Karachi so their sons could attend high school in the United States. The parents were both physicians in Pakistan. Now, the mother works at a department store and the father maintains his practice in Karachi, visiting with his family only once a year. Not only has the family made tremendous sacrifices for this son's education, but his help is also needed after school to care for his grandmother so the mother can be free to work the afternoon and evening shift at the store. "Persistent" might be a more apt term than "resistant" to describe these parents. Should the guidance counselor therefore abandon her assessment of what would be best for the student? Not necessarily. But she may need to explore with the parents the advantages of a varied curriculum and after-school activities, both for the boy's development and for his college admissions profile.

Defensive

Reports sometimes describe an interviewee as "defensive," meaning that the person rejects a criticism or perceived criticism without considering it sufficiently. Cultural differences could create a situation in which the interviewer perceives a deficiency in an interviewee and communicates this judgment, but the interviewer is mistaken in his or her appraisal, or the interviewee sees the situation differently. For example, Cecilia, an African American mother of three, arrived 20 minutes late for her intake interview at a mental health clinic. As the meeting began, the interviewer told Cecilia that she must "feel worried about this appointment" and "not really want things to change." Cecilia's face grew flushed and she gritted her teeth as the interviewer spoke, mumbling, "You really don't know what's going on with me." The interviewer described this response as defensive. Had she been asked, Cecilia might have described the interviewer as ignorant and mean, because she failed to ask Cecilia about the source of her tardiness.

Seductive

Reports sometimes describe interviewees as seductive. While interviewees from a variety of cultures might indeed intentionally behave seductively, it is also important to note that norms around flirting vary widely by culture. The line between friendliness and seduction, when to flirt, how much to flirt, the intention behind the flirting, and even what constitutes flirting can vary by culture. In addition, a host of nonverbal behaviors including eye contact, touch, interpersonal distance, posture, and clothing choice can easily be misinterpreted among people from different cultures as seductive when the intention is far more mundane. What is considered an acceptable amount of cleavage to show in San Juan, Rio de Janeiro, or Buenos Aires would be nearly scandalous in professional contexts in much of the United States and Canada and might provoke an arrest in some countries of the Muslim world. Finally, before making assumptions that someone is trying deliberately to behave in a seductive way, it would be important for the interviewer to identify what it is, exactly, about the interviewee that merits this label. If the interviewer simply finds the interviewee attractive but the interviewee is not behaving or dressing in any particular way to invite the attention, it is probably inaccurate to use the term "seductive." Feeling attracted to an interviewee does not necessarily mean the root of the issue is in the interviewee—we must be careful not to assign responsibility to interviewees for what we ourselves are feeling (countertransference). Keep in mind that the use of the term "seductive" can be a minefield if you are asked to testify in court: This term can be portrayed as sexually biased and discriminatory.

Shy, Withdrawn, or Timid

Cultures cultivate different personalities and ways of being. For example, in traditional Japanese culture an ideal person behaves as inconspicuously and undemonstratively as possible (Ellsworth, 1994). There is even a saying, "The nail that sticks up gets hammered down." In the United States, on the other hand, an inconspicuous and undemonstrative person is apt to be seen as pathologically shy and in need of intervention. When you are recording your observations, therefore, try to limit yourself to describing rather than interpreting. For example, "Mr. Fukayama spoke only in response to direct questions" is a neutral statement, whereas "Mr. Fukayama showed extreme shyness and an inhibited ability to express himself" is judgmental.

At this point you may be wondering how you can possibly describe your interviewee's demeanor or attitude toward you, as it might seem that almost anything can be "explained away" by culture. I am not suggesting that you ignore or disregard what you see. Rather, I advocate for describing as much as possible rather than drawing conclusions or using overly general summarizing words. So, for instance, you might write, "Mr. Luong asked many questions before he signed the form" rather than that he was "uncooperative" or "suspicious." Further, if you think his reluctance stemmed from his difficulty understanding the form, you could ask him about this and make a note of it in your report. If Ms. Rollán asks you a number of questions about why you are taking notes and where the notes are going, you can describe exactly this if you need to, rather than using a summarizing word such as "suspicious" or "paranoid." (If her questions about the notes are accompanied by scanning the room repeatedly, glancing out the window, and asking about hidden cameras and microphones, then you might want to describe each of these behaviors and summarize them with a phrase such as "presenting a pattern of suspicion." Wouldn't it be ironic, however, if you later discovered that she is being stalked by her ex-husband who has hidden microphones and video cameras in her home and workplace? Her "suspicion" would then be seen as warranted and situational, rather than a reflection of her character.)

Mental health workers are frequently expected to comment on an interviewee's "affect" (the expression of feelings). Words that are used commonly include "labile" for someone who seems to fluctuate rapidly between emotions such as from happy to sad and back again; "flat," for someone who does not show much emotional expression; and "inappropriate to content," for someone whose expression of emotion does not match the content of what he or she is saying. These kinds of conclusions need to be drawn with caution in cross-cultural interviews because of the varied norms concerning emotional expression across cultures (see Chapter 5 on nonverbal behavior).

It is misleading to comment on whether a person is responding "appropriately" to an event without knowing what that event means to the person involved. For instance, some Christians may respond to a loved one's death with rejoicing because they see heaven as a glorious, welcoming place. Similarly, some Hindus and Sikhs will respond to the death of a loved one with equanimity because they believe the soul remains alive and immortal even when the body dies (Zachariah, 2005). A Lebanese father may seem overly despairing or angry when he finds out that his young daughter has engaged in sex play with a similar-age neighbor's child because—in his community—she and the entire family will be seen as disgraced if the word gets out. If a family's emotional, verbal, or behavioral response to an event seems unusual to you, be sure to ask what the event means to the family.

How was the eye contact? (You can note this, even if you are not entirely sure what it means at first.) At what point in the interview did you note nonverbal changes such as hesitating, blushing, sweating, or averting the eyes? Did the interviewee display any unusual mannerisms or other nonverbal behavior? Remember that many aspects of what you note in the interview itself may be culturally based, including what you consider unusual. (Review Chapter 5 on nonverbal communication and consider consulting someone from the interviewee's culture before you decide what any particular nonverbal behavior means.)

TAKING NOTES

Better note taking during interviews facilitates better reports. A careful record of the interview can help you guard against a tendency to confuse this interview with a prior one with someone else who—in some way—reminds you of this interviewee. Some interviews are recorded with video or audio, but most often the only record will be your notes. Even if you believe an interview is being recorded mechanically, you may still want to write notes as the interview progresses. I'm sure I am not the only interviewer with disaster stories caused by mechanical glitches. In one case, the batteries failed in my handheld tape recorder in the middle of an interview and I did not realize it until the interview was over. In another instance, I interviewed a woman in her home on an extremely hot day. The noise from the fan operating in the living room made our audiotape completely unintelligible. If you rely entirely on mechanical recording, you risk regret. It's great to have your notes as a backup because you will not be able to remember everything about an interview even 10 minutes later, let alone hours or days later, without written notes. Keep in mind that a variety of laws might ensure that the interviewee can obtain a copy of your notes. Personal shorthand facilitates the note-taking process; however, be prepared to explain this method if asked.

Usually, you'll want to take notes in a way that would help other people read and understand them easily. This poses certain challenges for people who are conducting interviews in a language other than English. Which language should you use for taking notes? Many bilingual people who are conducting interviews in a language other than English end up taking notes in both languages—recording notes to themselves in English, perhaps, and then quoting what the interviewee says in his or her native language. For interviews that are conducted in a language other than English in an English-speaking country, the advantage of taking notes in the original language is that it may help keep you "in the moment" by not obligating you to work with two languages at once. Also, any quotes in the interviewee's own language are more likely to be precisely accurate.

In our notes, we must be careful not to use shorthand stereotypes. For instance, José Lopez, Assistant Police Chief of Hartford, Connecticut, told me that his office uses "John Doe" and "Jane Doe" to protect the anonymity of child victims of sexual abuse. At one point officers began a trend. They would write, "Juan Doe" and "Juanita Doe" for Latino victims and "Tyrone Doe" and "Oprah Doe" for African American victims, trying to outdo each other in how outrageous and creative they could be in signaling the ethnicity of the victim through their naming. Lopez said he put a stop to this practice, considering it disrespectful and mocking (J. Lopez, personal communication, January 2007).

THE AUDIENCE FOR YOUR REPORT

Think about the goals of your report. What is it meant to achieve? Who is the intended audience or reader? These answers will partially shape both the content of the report and the manner in which it is written. The report could be intended to serve more than one purpose. For instance, the report on a mental health intake interview could be intended to guide the ongoing clinician who will work with the client, and also to document the intake interview for insurance purposes. In all cases, be alert to the use of jargon and gear the language of the report to the intended recipient. If you are writing a psychological report for a court proceeding, for instance, you'll want to either avoid psychological jargon or explain its use. If you are writing an educational assessment which will be read by a parent, be sure to explain all the technical terms you use.

It is also important to remember that your report may have an extended shelf life and become available to secondary audiences, whether or not this is your intention. For instance, although it's not common, a judge could subpoena a mental health intake interview report for a custody or competency hearing or a criminal trial. The report may be reviewed as part of a quality assurance assessment for the agency, or in a lawsuit filed by the client, by the client's family, or perhaps by someone hurt by the client who was interviewed. For instance, a colleague was appalled to see excerpts of a mental health exam that he had conducted in a high-profile trial printed in a prurient tabloid—someone had apparently stolen the confidential report from the interviewee's hospital file.

While an educational assessment is most often used to develop an education plan for a child in school, it could also be examined down the road as part of a disability or insurance claim, or in a class action lawsuit against the school. So while we craft our reports to the audience who will soon make decisions based on the interview, or the entity that commissioned the interview, it's a good idea to have our eye on the horizon and ask ourselves, "In my worst nightmare, who could end up with this report in their hands?" We should write our reports so they will withstand examination at this later point as well.

NOTATIONAL BIAS

Bias can manifest in reports much as it does in other phases of the interview process. Notational bias, mentioned in Chapter 3, refers to ways in which the instruments we use for measuring, our terms, our categories, and even our forms can bias our findings. This bias is introduced when the available notation used to describe something influences our ability to describe and approach it. For instance, if there are a limited number of categories for race included in a form, a person who thinks of himself as "Black and Filipino" may be forced to describe him- or herself as "other" or "biracial," which clearly omits important information.

Notational bias is also introduced when we use shorthand ways of identifying problems, which may have limited validity. For instance, in a study we may use "receives special education services" as a shorthand way to identify children in the sample who have learning disabilities. However, of course, there are many factors influencing whether children receive special education services including their parents' attitudes toward such services, the availability of screening programs in schools, and so on. Thus when we have only two categories for learning disabilities—stating that someone receives or doesn't receive special education services—we may be missing the categories of those who once received such services but no longer do, those who should receive such services but do not, those who will receive such services in the future, those who have been identified as needing such services but whose parents refuse to permit it, and so on.

Our forms often do not allow the reporting of shades of gray. We must record the father as either living in the home or not—there is nowhere to record his sporadic presence. We may have to check one box only to describe a person's profession, although that person engages in a number of different jobs. We may be forced to give a person a diagnosis who doesn't fit neatly into a category. The forms and categories used in our report may themselves introduce unintentional errors. We can guard against this by working to improve our forms, and noting the complex reality in the narrative portions of our reports.

WORD CHOICE

We inevitably make choices about which elements of an interview to highlight or play down and the order for presenting the information. For example, notice the words available to describe an interviewee who taps his feet and fingers as he speaks: agitated, restless, impatient, jittery, fidgety, hyper, high strung, anxious, and nervous. Each of these words conveys a tone that would influence the readers' perception of the interviewee. The most accurate description and the one with least bias, of course, would be to record simply, "The interviewee tapped his fingers and feet throughout our conversation." The slight valences of meaning contained in our word choices can influence the conclusions readers reach about the person described in the report. We need to make sure words are chosen without prejudice.

Our choice of words can evidence multicultural understanding or ethnocentrism and can contribute to just or unfair outcomes. It is important to eliminate biased word choice from our reports. This is hard to do, as much of the language we use on a daily basis contains biases that we may not even be aware of. For example, the word "gyp," meaning to cheat or swindle someone, comes from the word "gypsy," and thus it is an unacceptable ethnic slur.

In another example, sometimes people use the term "inner city" to describe a school or neighborhood that is rundown and inhabited mostly by people with a low income. In the United States it usually carries the implication of being populated by Blacks and Latinos. Within the city of New York, for example, there are top-notch schools that rank among the best in the nation as well as schools that are run down, dangerous, and low achieving—but only the latter would receive the designation "inner city." "Inner city" is essentially a modern reinvention of the word "ghetto." I recommend using more specific terms. For instance, if you want to describe a school, use specific terms such as "overcrowded," "underfunded," "in a decaying building," "brightly decorated," "dedicated school staff," or whichever terms are most appropriate and exact to the situation at hand rather than the coded term "inner city"—which seems to say a lot but may be misinterpreted.

The same would be true for describing a neighborhood. Use specific terms, giving the name of the area where an interviewee lives if it is apt to be known by the consumer of the report or specific details such as "a neighborhood of high-rise subsidized apartments that police say has the highest level of crime in the city," rather than more general terms.

We especially need to be cautious in describing people. When referring to their clothing, write that "Jean wore all black clothes, ripped lacy stockings, black eye liner, and black lipstick," rather than that she was "dressed like a Goth." Or write that James wore "baggy pants that he had to hitch up several times during the interview, a baseball cap on backward, a thick gold chain, and several large rings on his fingers," rather than that he was "dressed in gangsta style."

Sometimes individuals or their caretakers who are not very sophisticated, or who are not comfortable with English, may provide inaccurate or confusing information about their own or their child's condition. They may not be able to articulate, for instance, the type of "disability" a child suffers from, confusing a learning disability with mental retardation or a lack of motivation. You may want to use the individual's own terms ("John's mother reported he obtained extra time for formal testing in school") even as you seek more complete and accurate information from other sources. If you use the interviewee's terms, be sure to put these in quotation marks and make clear who said them.

REFERRING TO RACE, ETHNICITY, AND OTHER IDENTITY GROUPS

You may wonder how you should refer to the interviewee's race, ethnicity, or other identity group characteristics. In some situations you will have no choice—there will be a box for you to check with a limited number of categories. For instance, the face sheets or cover sheets that usually accompany the narrative in police reports often contain demographic boxes, as do the demographic questionnaires that are usually part of the intake process in health and mental health care settings. These determinations are important. Data on birth and death certificates, population studies, and health research have all too frequently been found to be inaccurate because of misclassifications—for instance, misclassifying people as White who, when questioned directly, identify themselves as Native American, Asian or Pacific Islander, multiracial, or "other" (Wilson & Williams, 1998).

In general, it is best not to guess about a person's race or ethnicity. You may be interviewing a child who appears White and whose mother is White, but actually the child is biracial. How do you categorize someone whose family is of Japanese origin but who grew up in Brazil? You may see that someone's name is Roberto Sanchez and therefore you assume the person is Latino—but he might come from the Philippines instead. Your workplace may have specific guidelines about how to ask these questions. If it doesn't, I recommend that you proceed as sensitively as possible without making assumptions. I like to ask, "How would you like me to identify your race or ethnicity?" If this process would not work in your circumstances, you may read the categories to interviewees and ask how they identify themselves. Bi- or multiracial people often object to having to choose "other"—it can make them feel "other than" human. Many demographers and activists are advocating for the inclusion of the category "multiracial," for people whose parents come from more than one of the four official racial groups (Wilson & Williams, 1998).

We all have ideas about race and ethnicity that may be outside our immediate awareness but can shape the way we respond to an interviewee and write up the interview. The more we can become aware of these ideas and responses, the less apt we are to inject bias into our interviews or our reports.

In general we should try to avoid writing in a way that could cause offense. When possible, we should use the terms that are chosen by the interviewee to describe him- or herself. If we are concerned that this term is not professional, we can put it in quotes to say, for instance, "When asked how she identifies herself, Josefina said she is a 'queer spic.' When asked to elaborate further, she said that she is a Mexican American who likes both men and women." Clearly, this would be appropriate in some contexts but not in others.

The *Publication Manual of the American Psychological Association* (2001) recommends that we avoid labels that might be stigmatizing—for instance, by referring to a person in a clinical study as a "patient" rather than a "case." It recommends that we avoid equating people with their conditions. For example, rather than writing "Jim is a schizophrenic" we should write "Jim was diagnosed with schizophrenia." It also recommends that we avoid contrasting people with an imaginary group called "normal" people, for example, writing that "Sam is more self-absorbed than normal children." In general, we should use terms that *put the person first*, such as " 'person with _____,' 'person living with _____,' and 'person who has _____,' " rather than using nouns such as a cripple, a stroke victim, or an AIDS patient (American Psychological Association, 2001, p. 69).

In regard to race, the American Psychological Association manual recommends that we respect current usage, which changes periodically. At the time this book is being written, in the United States *Black* and *African American* are both considered acceptable although not identical terms, while *Negro* and *Afro-American* are not considered acceptable. The terms "Black" and "White" should be capitalized when they are used as adjectives or proper nouns to describe or refer to a person or a group. Color words such as yellow, brown, or red should not be used to describe other groups.

The terms "Hispanic" and "Latino" are preferred by different people who fall into these largely equivalent categories. Because the word "Latino" is a Spanish word, whereas the term "Hispanic" was invented in English by the U.S. census, the word "Latino" is gaining popularity. Whenever possible it is best to use more precise geographical references to say that "Ramón is Cuban American" and "Wong is from Hong Kong," for instance, rather than using less specific terms such as Latino or Asian.

Most Native Americans in the United States would rather be referred to by their tribe, as Navajo or Ojibwa, for instance, rather than by the catchall terms "Native American" or "American Indian." The terms "Native American" and "American Indian" are both considered acceptable to refer to the indigenous peoples of North America. "Native American" is a slightly broader term encompassing the native peoples of Hawaii and Samoa. The term "First Nations" is currently gaining use to refer to the original people of Canada.

The term "Asian" is preferred over "oriental," which is considered overly exoticizing. The terms "White" or "European American" are preferred over "Caucasian" because the latter term is rooted in biological models of race that we now know are largely inaccurate.

As with race and ethnicity, we allow interviewees to describe their religion. "Latter Day Saints" usually prefer this term over "Mormon"; Jews strongly prefer to be called "Jewish" rather than "Hebrew," and so on. When in doubt and when it is relevant, ask. We should be careful not to confuse the term "Muslims" (describing people who practice the religion, Islam) with the term "Arabs," which broadly describes an ethnic group. It is also important to remember that simply knowing a person's religion without knowing how observant the person might be in regard to practicing that religion, or which branch of that religion the person practices, will probably not reveal much about how the person lives.

In referring to age, the manual recommends that we avoid the term "elderly" and use "older person" instead. "Boy" and "girl" are considered acceptable when referring to people of high school age and younger, although many teenagers would rather be referred to as *teens* or *youth* or *adolescents*. For persons 18 and older, use "men" and "women." Rather than "young man" or "young woman" we should specify the person's age or approximate age.

The American Psychological Association manual recommends using the terms "gay men" and "lesbian" (for women) to describe specific people or groups. The term "homosexual" is considered dated and has had negative connotations in the past and, therefore, should be avoided. Not all people who have sex with people of the same gender consider themselves gay, lesbian, or bisexual. For instance, some men are married to women and live their lives as heterosexuals but occasionally engage in sexual activity with other men. If asked for their sexual orientation, they will probably describe themselves as heterosexual. But if asked about sexual activities with other men, they may admit to these.

It is also important to avoid using the term "homosexual" to refer to sexual exploitation or same-sex sexual assaults of children. That is, it is more accurate to write that "Stewart reports that his choir director, Tomas Jones, asked him to stay after practice and then touched his genitals" than to use more general and inaccurate terms such as *homosexual assault* or "homosexual rape" or "gay abuse." (Adult men who sexually abuse boys should not be confused with gay men—adult men who have consensual sex with other adult men.)

Nations other than the United States have their own terms to refer to their majority and minority populations. A comprehensive discussion of every term is beyond the scope of this book. When in doubt, choose the term preferred by the interviewee, and/or consult with recent central texts in your field for further guidance.

In most reports it is necessary to identify the race or ethnicity of the subject of your report, but not ancillary people. For example, if a physician is interviewed about a patient, that physician's race is apt not to be important and therefore should not be included.

GIVING YOUR OPINION

Some reports are intended to present the facts without conclusions or judgments, whereas others expect a certain amount of opinion or synthesis and recommendations. For instance, a police report on a crime scene is intended to be a mental photograph of what was seen, smelled, heard, and experienced. The exact details are extremely important—entire cases may hinge on details that did not at first appear central. In their reports, officers are instructed not to editorialize, add personal opinions, conjecture, or predict outcomes. The reports are expected to be truthful, complete, unbiased, and professionally written. Police reports provide primary and secondary witness testimony (both what the officer witnessed and what witnesses recount). Police reports are meant to stand on their own in case the officer cannot testify in court (A. Velasquez, personal communication, June 26, 2007). Police reports, are, therefore, on the objective end of the spectrum. Police reports present the facts, and the decision making is expected to lie with the judge or jury that reads the report and considers other evidence.

Even police reports can be biased, however. One officer told me how his colleagues knew exactly which facts to include or omit, depending on whether they wanted the case to hold up in court. This officer said he had often witnessed racial prejudice at work in this regard, where a fellow officer would be more likely to include sufficient information for a conviction when investigating a crime perpetrated by a Black man, but leave out those kinds of details when investigating a crime perpetrated by a White man. When intentional, this selective reporting of facts constitutes unethical and possibly illegal behavior.

Other reports need to integrate material from the interview and a variety of other sources and then present a recommendation. Some reports require synthesizing and analyzing vast quantities of information and therefore necessarily include the interviewer's perspective. For instance, diagnostic interviews by psychologists and psychiatrists often include a "case formulation." This case formulation may be written in a variety of ways. One format includes a brief restatement of the case history, a differential diagnosis (a list of the possible disorders), a best or most likely diagnosis, contributing factors and strengths, additional information that is still needed, a treatment plan, and prognosis (Morrison & Anders, 1999).

Some interview reports are intended as little more than vehicles for the interviewer's conclusion. Those conclusions range from psychological diagnoses to educational, employment, custody, mental health, social work, or admissions recommendations.

Clearly, there is extensive room for personal opinion and judgments in many reports. Care must be taken to be fair at all times, reporting strengths in addition to weakness, and avoiding a tendency to assign certain diagnoses or treatment plans to people from particular ethnic groups, for instance, based on their group membership. Unfortunately, the interviewee's ethnic or racial identity has been found to unduly influence legal, medical, mental health, and educational decision making (DelBello, 2002).

YOUR VOICE AND CHOICES AROUND IT

Make sure you preserve a feeling of the humanity of your interviewee, even if this person has been involved in objectionable activity (e.g., sexual offending) or is suffering from an ailment that might make him or her seem "less than" others (e.g., mental retardation). The person is not simply a case, a patient, a client, a problem, a depressive, a victim, or a suspect: The person is a human being with many facets. When in doubt, err on the side of professionalism and respect. Ask yourself, "How would I want to be referred to if I was in this person's shoes?" Or, "How would I want my mother (or my daughter) described if she was in this position?"

CULTURAL FORMULATION

The *Diagnostic and Statistical Manual of Mental Disorders* (DSM-IV-TR; American Psychiatric Association, 2000), which is the diagnostic bible of the mental health professions, recommends including a "cultural formulation" to provide sufficient information about an individual's background. In practice, however, unfortunately these elements are absent from most mental health reports. I recommend including a cultural formulation in a wide variety of interview reports. Here, I am adapting the DSM recommendations to make them more broadly applicable to a variety of interviewing situations. In the report, include the following sections, where it would improve the report's ability to convey the interviewee's situation.

A. The individual's cultural identity: including cultural reference groups, language abilities, use and preferences and—for immigrants and member of other cultural minority groups—their degree of involvement in their minority and the dominant culture. For example, "Sam identifies as a Black Dominican. He speaks Spanish and lives in a Dominican enclave in Washington Heights."

B. Cultural explanations of the individual's condition. Find out how the person or the person's family explains his or her condition. For example:

1. How are symptoms expressed (through *nervios* or nerves, somatic complaints, crying spells, etc.)?

2. The meaning and perceived severity of the person's condition according to the cultural reference group (e.g., slight signs of spirit possession or exhibition of total takeover by such a spirit).

3. Any local condition category used by the person's community (e.g., *calores* used by Salvadorans to explain somatic symptoms that appear to result from trauma or extreme stress).[1]

---

[1]DSM-IV-TR includes a list of culture-bound symptoms and idioms of distress. See also Bartholomew (1995) who discusses culture-bound syndromes as a form of deception.

4. The perceived causes or explanations of the person's condition.
5. Current and past experiences with professional and traditional sources of care. For example:

> Laura reports being troubled by nightmares since her father died. She says he is angry for her for not having been able to visit him as he was ill in her native Cuba. She had an exorcism with an *espiritista* which seemed to help for a while, but the nightmares have returned. She reports that this is the first time she has sought the help of a psychotherapist, which she did reluctantly, at her daughter's urging.

C. Cultural factors related to the person's psychosocial environment and functioning. Note culturally relevant interpretations of social stressors and culturally specific supports, including religious and extended family networks.
D. Cultural factors influencing the relationship between the interviewer and the interviewee. Indicate cultural and social status differences between the interviewer and the interviewee and the difficulties these might have posed in the interview situation. For example, note language or communication difficulties and culturally based difficulties in establishing rapport.
E. Overall cultural assessment for diagnosis and care. In this section, indicate the importance of cultural factors in realizing the reports' recommendations.

CONTRIBUTING FACTORS

If you are writing a mental health, social work, or educational report, you will probably include a section on contributing factors, where you identify various factors that may have contributed to the interviewee's situation. Here, be sure to mention cultural, linguistic, socioeconomic, and religious factors or environmental changes that may be important. It would be reasonable to write, for instance, that "Jane's mother said Jane isn't doing well in kindergarten because she had nothing to play with when she was younger and 'spent all day every day watching TV.' " In this case, you are not drawing inferences but rather reporting what the mother has stated. In referring to the same situation it would also be reasonable to write, "Jane's mother reported that Jane did not have many toys at home and spent 10 or more hours daily watching television. Perhaps this lack of direct stimulation at home has inhibited Jane's ability to participate in classroom activities." It would be wrong, though, to write, "Jane doesn't know how to participate in classroom activities because she comes from a poor family."

RECOMMENDATIONS AND PROGNOSES

For many interview reports, you will need to conclude with a recommendation or a set of recommendations. This could concern a decision with only two options, such as to hire or not hire someone, to award visitation to a father or to deny it, and so on. Frequently the recommendations you make will be more textured and subtle than the two just listed. For instance, you might be expected to develop a treatment plan, an educational plan, or a custody agreement.

If your data are incomplete and insufficient to make a decision, you can often recommend gathering more information. While this may not be the ideal outcome, it is far better than making a decision based on inadequate information. Your interview and the report undoubtedly will still have helped complete the picture, and you have identified the gaps that need to be filled before recommendations can be rendered. Cross-cultural interviews often *are* incomplete because of difficulties building rapport or linguistic misunderstandings, among other causes.

Your recommendations should take into account all the relevant data as well as practicalities and legal obligations. Before developing recommendations, consider the following:

1. The accuracy of the interview findings.
2. The strengths and deficits of the interviewee.
3. The strength and deficits of the system that is receiving your recommendations.
4. Additional resources that might be usefully added to the recommendations.
5. The clarity and precision of your writing.
6. The inclusion of sufficient detail in the recommendations, including which individuals or organizations will implement which parts of it.
7. The need for additional assessments or evaluations.
8. The need for follow-up—when and by whom. (adapted from Sattler, 1998, p. 236)

Your suggestions should be based on the individual and not a formulaic or cookie-cutter response. Unless your agency protocol specifies otherwise, your suggestions should be written in order of priority, with the most urgent issues mentioned first. The recommendations should be practical and concrete and based on the ethics and best practices of your profession.

Be careful about employing code words such as "high risk," or negative, gloomy predictions. Many pathways can lead to the same outcome, and a single event might have many outcomes down the road. You can indicate how the interviewee is doing now and give some kind of indication about the future based on the past, but you should be extremely careful in conveying too much certitude about your predictions, especially those concerning the distant future. Make sure you state clearly your degree of confidence in any claims you make about the future. Use information from your observations and interview to help the reader understand the basis of your recommendations and prognoses.

For example, in a psychological report it would be inaccurate and inappropriate to write about an 8-year-old: "Ramón was sexually assaulted by his stepfather and will suffer for years as a result. He can be expected to show continued behavioral problems and should be carefully watched for further sexual acting out." However, it would be accurate and appropriate to write:

> "In conclusion, Ramón has been evidencing encopresis, frequent public masturbation, and angry outbursts at both school and home since September 2006, when his mother's boyfriend moved into the home. As reported, the symptoms have steadily worsened over time in terms of both frequency and severity. Ramón's behavior, the medical findings, Ramón's verbal statements during our interview, and the police report are all consistent with the finding of possible sexual abuse by the stepfather. Until now, his mother has refused to acknowledge that the abuse occurred and has blamed Ramón for the problems. It is important to secure safety for Ramón and support for his family to prevent a continued worsening of his symptoms, and to assure a healthy outcome. The following strategy is recommended. . . . "

If you make a presentation to the interviewee that includes recommendations, try to address practical and cultural barriers which might impede the person from following the recommendations. You may be able to anticipate some of these, such as child care and transportation, and provide solutions. If you are familiar with the culture or have the opportunity to consult with a person who is, you may be able to identify other possible barriers to carrying out the recommendations and identify ways to overcome them. For instance, a Somali woman with whom I worked suffered from disabling monthly cramps. Her gynecologist recommended that she use birth control pills to limit the pain. It was important to explain to the doctor and the interpreter that they should communicate to the woman that although these pills can be used for birth control, they were being recommended in her case for other purposes. This was a sensitive subject. This woman was unmarried and had two children as a result of sexual assaults in refugee camps. She was rejected by other Somalis for having born children out of wedlock. It was important to reassure her that the doctor was not impugning her morals by recommending birth control pills.

It is always helpful to ask people if the recommendations seem like something they could or will carry out and what might get in the way. For immigrants, lack of services in a person's country of origin, or lack of enforcement of certain laws, or lack of legal protections, can lead to differential use of services in their new country. For instance, it is difficult to obtain a divorce in Japan if one partner refuses. Yoshihama (2001) suggests this contributes to the finding that battered Japanese women in the United States do not think divorce is an option if their husbands indicate that they are unwilling to consent.

Finally, to increase the likelihood that a recommendation will be carried out, identify ways the intervention can be immediately helpful, if this is the case. Many immigrant and low-income families are unfamiliar with the services that many agencies offer or do not expect that our interventions will help. Pointing out something concrete that agencies can do which is helpful, such as translating a letter from a landlord, making a call to a teacher, arranging for day care or fuel vouchers, enrolling a parent in English lessons, contacting a soup kitchen, or putting the family in contact with a medical provider can make for the beginning of a trusting relationship. Low-income families and immigrants who are less acculturated in particular need support of all kinds. The abstract, more long-term "help" that we often promise may be less readily understood or valued than something a family can put their hands on or eat that very night. Once the family trusts that the agency or individual means well and can deliver, they are likely to be immensely loyal.

If the data are inconsistent, be extremely careful in drawing conclusions. Inconsistent data suggest avenues for further exploration (Sattler, 1998).

MAKING ORAL REPORTS

Oral reports can range from informal telephone or hallway conversations to official and ritualized court hearings. People usually feel little anxiety about the former and a great deal more about the latter. However, it is important to be professional at all times, and not to fall unfairly into gossip or stereotyping about interviewees simply because a situation lacks formality.

Reviewing Your Completed Report

Once you have written your report, examine it with a cold eye. Check for the following:

- Have you recorded the person's name correctly?
- Have you recorded the interviewee's demographic information correctly and respectfully, such as age, race, profession, and country of origin?
- Is the report well organized?
- Is it complete?
- Have you avoided shorthand and jargon?
- Are you respecting the person's privacy in that you include only the information that is pertinent and appropriate? Is there anything in the report that could jeopardize the person's confidentiality?
- Have you described the person or people in a respectful way?
- Have you included necessary cultural and linguistic information to help the reader understand the findings?
- If a foreign language interpreter was used, have you recorded the interpreter's name and contact information?
- If you have questions about the findings due to possible cultural misunderstandings, have you resolved these?
- Have you avoided stereotyping by recording what you truly encountered rather than what you may have expected to encounter?
- Would you feel comfortable sharing the report with the person interviewed?
- Would you be comfortable sharing the report with your supervisor?
- Would you be comfortable sharing the report with your state ethics board?
- Is the report written with enough integrity that if it ended up printed in the newspaper, somehow, you could stand by what you wrote?
- Have you provided illustrative examples?
- Have you included quotes from the interviewee in his or her own words, where appropriate?
- Have you included specific rather than general information?
- Have you avoided overstating your case?
- Have you assessed and reported on strengths as well as deficits?
- Does the report indicate which information came from which source?
- Do the recommendations follow logically from the findings?
- Have you limited yourself to conclusions, recommendations, or prognoses that are based on facts and not inferences?
- Are the recommendations realistic and attainable, considering the context?
- Is the report written in a professional style, and have you proofread the report for content, grammar, and spelling errors? (If your skills are not strong in this area, is there a confidential person at work who can edit reports for you?)
- Have you reduced to a minimum the likelihood that your report might be misunderstood by readers?

Some interviewers present their reports in a public setting, such as in court; in an education forum with parents, teachers, administrators, and possibly others present; or in a case review. Look upon giving a report in such a situation as an opportunity to demonstrate the values of the agency you represent. Your report should be accurate; and the way you present it should increase the public's confidence in you and your agency, and therefore further your agency's mission. Be sure to know how to pronounce the interviewee's name. In addition to listening for the content of your report, in many cases the audience will also be listening to hear what kind of person you are.

In taking the witness stand, which is perhaps the most stressful way to make a report, your natural ability, general preparation, experience, and understanding of your role and of the specific case at hand are keys to your success (Stern & Meyers, 2002). Be sure to convey professionalism and respect for the interviewee in your manner, tone, and facial expression.

Be sure also to convey respect for the process. If you don't take this report seriously, no one else is apt to, either. Although you may have a position in terms of the outcome of the case, you are more apt to be taken seriously if you come across as factual, objective, and accurate rather than as advocating for a particular arrangement (unless, of course, it is your role to advocate a particular outcome).

CONCLUDING OBSERVATIONS

The interview report may be oral or written, and often is presented in both formats, formally and informally. Interview reports may range from informal conversations by the water cooler or a single paragraph to extensive legal documents that need to be defended in court, perhaps with life-changing consequences. Without minimizing the importance of the interview interaction itself, I want to underline the importance of the interview report as the public representation of the interview. The report may live on for many months, years, or decades, influencing crucial future decisions.

If "objective measures" such as the results of standardized tests are available, be sure to include these in your report. However, it is important to remember that many of these instruments have not been normed on people from minority ethnic groups, or on people who are not active speakers of English, and so the accuracy of these measures may be questionable with certain populations (see Chapter 9 on interviewing children). In many professional fields, we are known by our words as much as our deeds. It is important to make every word count and every word fair and unbiased in our cross-cultural interview reports.

Questions to Think about and Discuss

1. Discuss concerns to keep in mind when describing someone's race or ethnicity in a report.
2. Describe ways in which the forms you are required to use limit what you are able to say in your reports.
3. Imagine yourself as the interviewee who is being written about in a report like the ones you write. What would be important to say? What would you worry that the interviewer might "get wrong" in the report?

RECOMMENDED ADDITIONAL READING

Biggs, M. (2004). *Just the facts* (2nd ed.). Upper Saddle River, NJ: Pearson/Prentice Hall.
Sattler, J. M. (1998). *Clinical and forensic interviewing of children and families*. San Diego: Sattler.

11 Authority and Trust Issues for Specific Professions

Some people grow up feeling that "the system" is on their side. They are apt to trust professionals who interview them and believe that interviewers are willing and able to help them. Others grow up feeling that "the system" is against them. They are apt to keep their distance from professionals of all kinds. If they're forced to interact with representatives of "the system" they remain guarded and are ready to have their worst fears confirmed.

More than three-quarters of the world's population lives in non-Western cultures. If they emigrate to the West they bring with them their mindset and expectations about contact with officials, retaining all the complex emotions their previous contacts have entailed. People from non-Western countries may be unfamiliar with the concept of a "professional friendship"—a relationship that is friendly but is nevertheless different from a personal friendship. Or they may not understand or expect confidentiality. They may assume that all people in positions of authority share information with each other, and with all agencies of government, and perhaps even with a secret and threatening police force. They may assume that they will not be treated fairly because they are not wealthy or do not have family or political connections. They may see the interview as a test or an interrogation and not understand its well-meaning purpose and possible benefits. People who have low levels of formal education may also harbor mistaken

253

beliefs about interviews and interviewers. Some may overestimate our power, and some may underestimate it. Some may not understand unwritten codes concerning the various behaviors or answers that might help them achieve their desired outcome.

These issues concerning trust and authority affect all of us in our interview work, but the flavor varies considerably for different professional fields. The bulk of this chapter is dedicated to examining cultural competence issues for specific professions. These specific sections are designed to complement the more widely applicable advice of the rest of the book, and in no way do they substitute for it.

SOCIAL WORK

Upper-middle-class people often believe that social workers are a valuable help to families with problems. Their contact with social workers is apt to be limited to the ones employed in school and medical settings, where they usually serve as purveyors of helpful services rather than social enforcers.

On the other hand, lower-income people, and particularly low-income people from ethnic minority or immigrant groups, usually have greater contact with social workers in less favorable circumstances. Fear of child protective service social workers is rampant in many communities, and social workers may be perceived as "kid snatchers" who take away poor people's children and place them in dangerous foster homes (Folman, 1998; Roberts, 2002). Because of the real risks posed by poverty and because of bias in the child maltreatment system at every phase, people in low-income neighborhoods are far more likely than people with a higher income to be acquainted with families that have been torn asunder by the child welfare system. Therefore, they actively fear social workers (Roberts, 2002).

Low-income families are also more likely to encounter social workers in other settings, such as welfare, housing, and public health agencies, where the social workers serve as gatekeepers to services and fulfill the unwelcome task of demanding documentation, asking intrusive questions, and checking for compliance—tasks that do not endear them to their clients.

Lee (2005) describes a social worker's efforts to help a Korean-born teen who had been adopted at birth by a United States family:

> "You're afraid to face your feelings of being different," said the social worker (the self-righteous one for whom I decided that "MSW" standed for Minority Savior Woman). "And then you lash out at those around you, making quite a mess for everybody." (p. 53)

Although fictional, the foregoing paragraph signals the ambivalent feelings of many clients toward social workers who try to help. The clients may feel they are being condescended to. Or they may be suspicious of the "help" that is offered to them, however sincere the efforts of the social worker. The foregoing quote also symbolizes the extra difficulty that can emerge when the social worker comes from the majority group and is reaching out to members of a cultural minority group.

To cite another example from literature, in her novel *Push*, the poet Sapphire writes in the voice of a semiliterate African American teen who has been impregnated by her own father. She vividly describes her mistrust of social workers:

> You know she jus' another social worker scratching on a pad. I know she writing reports on me. Reports go in file. File say what I could get, where I could go—if I could get cut off, kicked out. (p. 115)

This quote illustrates a common resentment of the power social workers have over the lives of low-income people. Of course, many social workers do establish strong working relationships with their low-income clients and may even be perceived as saviors because of the services they are able to provide. However, even when a specific social worker has been helpful, this positive relationship may not change the client's attitude toward social workers in general.

Emigrants from certain countries will be unfamiliar with social workers as a group and fail to understand their professional role. They may discount the social worker's authority and ask to speak to "a real doctor" or "someone in charge." They mean no offense. Social workers should take extra care to explain their function and purpose in this particular instance. This may seem basic and self-evident, but it is crucially important. Such an explanation could look like this, for example:

> "My name is _____. I am a social worker and I work for _____ [agency]. Have you known any other social workers? [Pause for response. If they respond positively, inquire about that prior contact with a social worker.] Social workers do many kinds of different jobs. In this case, my role is to _____. We are going to be having a conversation today about _____. As a result of this conversation, _____ will happen."

Particularly when working with people who are not fully familiar with the systems in which we work, such an explanation can be extremely important, and aspects of it may need to be repeated.

Tips for Conducting Cross-Cultural Interviews in Social Work Settings

- Reduce language barriers by having care provided by bilingual personnel, using interpreters as needed, and seeing that written materials are available in the languages of your clients (see Chapters 6 and 7 on working with a different native language and using interpreters, respectively).
- Carefully explain your role and allow clients an opportunity to ask you questions about it.
- Explain confidentiality and its limits.
- Be sure to convey respect as you gather information, remembering that issues that seem routine to you may be extremely sensitive to your clients.
- If you will be working over time with one or more families from a given culture, learn as much as you can about people from that group. Read, attend social events, make friends with people from the culture, and enlist the help of a cultural guide, where necessary. All these steps will help you work better with your clients.
- If your clients are currently facing a major difficulty (e.g., illness, homelessness, or the trauma of immigration) try to assess the family's functioning prior to the current difficulty. Remember, the picture you see of their functioning today may be a far cry from how they look when in better control of their lives.
- When you are going into people's homes, be sure to find out what is expected of you in terms of accepting food or drink, taking off your shoes, and so on (see the section "In People's Homes," Chapter 2).

MEDICINE, NURSING, AND ALLIED PROFESSIONS

Every culture is familiar with doctors and healers. People of all income levels and ethnic and racial groups regard some medical professionals as helpful and skilled—whether these are Western health providers or traditional healers. However, real-life experiences with practitioners of Western medicine may vary a great deal by social class. People with access to private clinics are apt to establish an ongoing caring relationship with a particular doctor or nurse, whom they see when they are sick and also for checkups when they are well. In these circumstances, they learn to think of health care professionals as kindly, caring, and wise.

People with a lower income are more apt to seek medical care only when they are ill, and often they delay seeking medical care because it is expensive and inconvenient. They are more apt to be seen in an emergency room or urgent care setting by a provider whom they have not met previously. When you are poor, seeking medical care often involves long delays in unpleasant and overcrowded waiting rooms. When the harried providers finally appear, they are often pressed for time and cannot listen attentively.

Low-income people may also worry that their medical providers will report them to child protective services or other authorities, and this worry inhibits trust.[1] For people on the economic margins, medical providers—like social workers—often serve as gatekeepers to employment or needed social services, such as disability benefits, worker's compensation, health and life insurance, and so on. This creates a dependency that might cause the patient to resent and fear the provider.

Some people from ethnic minority groups view health providers with suspicion as authority figures who may not have their best interests at heart. Native Americans often view health workers as agents of a government that aims to disempower them as a people—perhaps dating from pioneer times when disease-infested blankets were deliberately given to Native American peoples to promote weakness, illness, and death among them. Some groups of Native Americans and Alaska Natives have refused to participate in DNA sampling, concerned that information on their genetic origins could be used to deny them their land rights, that information on heritable diseases could be used against them, or that researchers will be profiting financially from their genetic information without sharing the proceeds with those who provided it (Bowekaty & Davis, 2003).

Some immigrants are cautious with medical providers, offering no more information than that which is necessary. Let's look at Antonio's situation:

Antonio spent the first 20 years of his life in Guatemala, as the oldest son in a family of peasant farmers. During one of Guatemala's many dictatorships he was stripped of his land and forced to flee to the United States, where he eventually obtained status as a legal resident. He goes to his neighborhood *botánica* (purveyor of traditional products) and asks for various herbs and salves when he feels ill—avoiding Western doctors whenever possible. When a particularly troubling ailment does not respond to the cures supplied in the *botánica*, he may

---

[1] A variety of studies have documented overreporting by medical personnel of low-income and Black, Hispanic, and Native American children in the United States for suspicion of child abuse. In one emergency room study where the injury was later independently deemed accidental and nonabusive, Black and Hispanic children ages 12 months to 3 years were five times more likely to have a skeletal survey (series of X-rays of all the bones of the body, designed to detect previous fractures) than were their White counterparts. They were also more than three times as likely to be reported to child welfare services (Lane, Rubin, Monteith, & Christian, 2002). The over- and underreporting of certain families lead to twin harms. Those families from groups that are overreported are more likely to be scrutinized and possibly torn apart unnecessarily by social services, while children from groups that underreported are more likely to remain at risk without professional intervention.

visit a Western doctor with a mix of hope and mistrust. He is governed by the following unstated rules:

1. *One problem at a time.* This rule has two parts. The first: Don't burden the doctor with too much at the same time. Even if Antonio has various symptoms and—in fact—these symptoms may be linked in ways he does not understand, he is not apt to bring these all up at once. He doesn't want to appear weak, like a whiner or a complainer. The second: If the doctor recommends two or more medications, Antonio is likely to start with one at a time because he wants to test its effect before beginning another. He may also decide to conserve his resources by seeing if one medication helps "enough" so he won't have to pay money for another. This may be true even if the medications are prescribed for different conditions—Antonio is simply mistrustful of having too many chemicals in his body at the same time.

2. *Don't tell the doctor everything.* Antonio feels ambivalent about medical providers, as he does about all people in positions of authority. He is wary of revealing too much about his work or living situation, his family, his immigration status, his habits, or his physical condition. His years of living under a dictatorship have also taught him that authorities are not to be trusted, informants are everywhere, and it's better to keep to oneself all but the most essential information.

3. *Consider the doctor's recommendations carefully before following them.* While Antonio is grateful when the doctor makes recommendations that help him feel better, for example, if he has a stomach ache or a fever, he is hesitant to follow recommendations regarding health concerns that are less tangible and familiar, such as those that might concern cholesterol, blood sugar, and preventive medicine. If a given recommendation does not fit into his worldview and if its purpose has not been carefully explained, he is unlikely to follow it.

4. *Don't discuss issues that the doctor might frown upon.* Antonio is unlikely to tell the doctor about his use of healing teas or potions, health recommendations that he failed to follow, taboo sexual activities, or his use of substances. Antonio is not apt to tell his doctor that he has personal weaknesses or limitations. For instance, he will hesitate to make known that he is hard of hearing, cannot read, or didn't remember the instructions he'd received about how to take his medicine. He is unlikely to tell the doctor that his dizzy spells began when his wife left him, or that he cannot afford fuel for the up-

coming cold winter, or that he cannot follow through with recommended physical therapy because the copayment is too steep and he cannot afford time off from work. He won't tell the doctor that he stopped taking the antidepressant because he heard on a radio program that depression is caused by a lack of religious faith. Rather, Antonio will keep these potentially shameful or embarrassing issues to himself.

5. *Life is hard and physical deterioration is inevitable.* Antonio assumes that most of his physical problems are due to natural causes such as aging, hard work, drafts of air, worries, or inherited characteristics. He believes he got his "bad legs" from his father, his "sour stomach" from his mother, and his "nerves" from the fright he endured when imprisoned and tortured in Guatemala. Because all these ailments have an explanation or a historical precedent, he doesn't consider them worth reporting and does not expect that they will be alleviated through medical intervention. He believes suffering through ailments is just what a person has to do, and medical treatments may or may not be able to make a difference.

6. *A nurse is more trustworthy than a doctor* because nurses are closer in social status. On the other hand, Antonio may consider a doctor's word as more authoritative.

Whew! Antonio clearly represents a challenge to his medical providers. What can they do to improve the quality of Antonio's medical care? They must recognize, first of all, that the interpersonal relationship here is paramount and requires special attention. The person conducting the medical interview with Antonio must convey the utmost respect and demonstrate interest in Antonio and his beliefs and habits. The professional should establish as nonhierarchical a relationship as possible, avoiding condescension or lecturing. The provider should welcome Antonio like a long-time neighbor, behaving like a person who truly cares about Antonio's well-being. The interviewer should ask repeatedly about additional symptoms or complaints, "What else is bothering you? Anything else I can help with?" If treatments are recommended, the provider should make sure Antonio understands the purpose and protocol of each one. If relief will not occur immediately, this should be explained carefully to Antonio so he does not give up the treatment prematurely because of a perceived lack of benefit.

The provider should schedule a follow-up visit, if possible, or a phone call, to check in as to how Antonio is doing with both his condition and the prescribed treatment. If Antonio is not following the recommendations that were given to him, the provider should inquire in a nonaccusatory way about why Antonio has made the decisions he made. Antonio may have misunderstood the original recommendations. He may have feared or experienced side effects. He may have decided to delay treatment until a later date for some reason. Or he may simply not have "felt like" doing what was recommended. Although this kind of attitude can be frustrating to a medical provider, ultimately Antonio has the right to self-determination in his own care.

It is also important to remember that practical problems can interfere with medical compliance. These might include lack of foreign language interpretation, not knowing where or how to fill prescriptions, losing prescriptions, lack of health insurance, lack of knowledge of health benefits, lack of transportation, or inability to read the instructions on a medicine bottle.

People from groups with ambivalent feelings at best toward health care workers may take an extremely passive position in regard to their health care, or they may resist the regimen prescribed. They are seen as noncompliant and are therefore dismissed, ignored, or resented.

Studies have found that physicians vary a great deal in their ability to communicate with patients who have limited English proficiency without interpreters (Erzinger, 1999). Also, medical interpreters—who are meant to serve as a bridge—sometimes present an unexpected barrier between medical providers and patients. In evaluation studies, medical interpreters have been found to delete sections of conversation, direct the conversations, define problems, shape messages, and make patients feel rushed (Davidson, 2000) (see Chapter 7 on interpreted interviews).

Recent laws in some parts of the United States that restrict free care in hospitals to those who can prove legal residency have also created a serious loss of trust. These laws sometimes intimidate and drive away immigrant patients, including many who *are* legal residents but who fear having to prove it or who do not have the documents to prove it.

Gender can play a role in the problem of establishing trust between medical providers and their patients. Women from many cultures do not want to be examined by male physicians or nurses.[2] For women from some cultures, even an inquiry by a male provider into gynecological or obstetric

---

[2] We should ask individual women about their views with regard to working with male professionals, rather than making negative assumptions. For instance, a male nurse midwife in London became extremely popular among pregnant Bengali women, one of whom said with her limited English, "Nice boy midwife better than bad girl midwife" (L. Ahmet, private communication, June 16, 2006). In this case, the skills and familiarity of a particular male midwife won him popularity among a Muslim population that ordinarily would have been hesitant to have a man conduct obstetric exams or be present during childbirth.

issues is considered inappropriate and invasive. I have known traditional Chinese women who refused to permit obstetrical or gynecological exams to be performed by men, and I have known Somali women who refused to take the diaper off an infant girl when a male interpreter was in the room. A community activist described her own shock and distress when, as a recent Muslim immigrant from Iran, she was surprised to see a male physician enter the room to perform a gynecological exam. Because of language and cultural difference, she did not know this was going to occur and did not know how to object. She submitted to the exam but then avoided reproductive health care for years after (Family Planning Advocates of New York State, 2006).

Where possible, requests for female providers should be respected. We need to remember that many women have experienced sexual trauma and assault; their requests may not be "simply" about culture or modesty but may also be an attempt to prevent the exam from restimulating traumatic memories. Some Muslims permit a woman to be examined by a male medical provider if he wears rubber gloves, or if there is a woman assistant or nurse observing. When in doubt, inquire. If no female providers are available, offer an alternative such as being examined in another facility or at another time when a woman provider is available. If a woman consents to being examined by a man, do what you can to ensure her comfort. This might include having a woman nurse or aide in the room during the exam or allowing a woman of the patient's choice to be present with her during the exam (while protecting the patient's modesty, of course).

Tips for Conducting Cross-Cultural Interviews in Health Care Settings

- Reduce language barriers by having bilingual personnel provide care, using interpreters as needed, and seeing that written materials are available in the languages of your patients (see Chapters 6 and 7 on working with a different native language and using interpreters, respectively).
- Consider and discuss cultural issues that might affect care. For instance, discuss how people's usual diet or religious fasting might affect the way they follow your recommendations.
- Ask your patients what they believe caused their condition, and what they believe might make it better. Keep in mind that different interpretations of illness (such as an imbalance of Yin and Yang) is apt to result in different cures. If your recommendation goes against traditional beliefs, your patients are less apt to follow it. If you are aware of the patient's belief system you will have a better chance of presenting your recommendations n a way that they are most likely to be followed.
- Ask about what steps patients have taken prior to seeing you, including alternative

medical practices that your patients may be following. Ask about pills, vitamins, potions, or other "cures" they might be using.

- After you have made your recommendations, ask your patients if there are any barriers to following through on what you recommended. Keep in mind the possible barriers of finances, fasting, traveling abroad, and incomplete understanding of the recommendations.
- Make friends with colleagues who are from the ethnic cultures of your patients. Ask these colleagues for cultural consultations, where necessary.
- If the patient seems dissatisfied, confused, or upset, ask about this.
- Be sure to explain the reasoning behind procedures that might be unfamiliar to your patients. Procedures that may seem quite ordinary in Western industrialized nations may be puzzling to people from cultures with distinct philosophies of wellness.
- If you are working consistently with people from particular cultural and linguistic groups, see if you can make language and cultural competence training a regular expectation of your workplace.
- Use a variety of approaches for public health campaigns, including outreach to community and religious groups; distributing information at fairs and community events; radio, television and print media campaigns in a variety of languages; a telephone helpline; posting information in local ethnic shops; educating trusted community members; and making fliers available within ethnic communities.
- Consider using a cultural broker to help bridge the cultural gap between your agency and the client's culture. (For more information on cultural brokers, see Georgetown University's National Center on Cultural Competence.)

MENTAL HEALTH CLINICIANS

People who belong to cultures that traditionally rely more heavily on mental health professionals, such as Jews, or families with a higher level of formal education, may consider the sharing of the most intimate aspects of their life in a psychotherapy or counseling situation to be perfectly normal, acceptable, and beneficial. They may be "psychologically minded," which means they are already familiar with some of the basic mental health concepts that guide therapy, such as the belief that what happened in our childhood influences who we are today, or that we can be motivated by impulses that are outside our awareness, or even that talking about problems is useful.

On the other hand, in many cultures and for many people with lower levels of formal education, a distrust of mental health clinicians is the norm. In many cultures, a person who seeks help from a mental health professional is considered "crazy." Families don't understand what services can be provided by clinicians and how they might be helpful. Families will respond to a clinician with a great deal of hesitation or downright fear, because of concerns that their responses could stigmatize them and cause them to be locked away or labeled "crazy." The portrayal of mental health professionals in the popular media undoubtedly contributes to this mistrust. In movies, clinicians are often shown as incompetent (e.g., *Nuts* and *What about Bob?*), unethical (e.g., *The Prince of Tides*), or evil (e.g., *The Silence of the Lambs, One Flew Over the Cuckoo's Nest,* and *The Legend of Simon Conjurer*).

Finally, people who are less familiar with the mental health system may be concerned about who has access to their information. Could they lose their job if they confess to depression, anxiety, or alcoholism? Could they lose custody of their children if they admit to feelings of anger? Could they lose their health insurance if they describe being victims of battering, or suffering from an eating disorder? Clearly, greater effort is necessary to establish rapport with someone who feels less positively disposed toward mental health clinicians.

Mental health clinicians face great challenges when trying to diagnose conditions across cultures. Research in the United States has shown bias in this regard. For example, African Americans are likely to be diagnosed mistakenly as suffering from schizophrenia while being underdiagnosed and undertreated for mood disorders (DelBello, 2002). These mistaken diagnoses can lead a patient to extremely negative outcomes including side effects from the wrong medication, stigma, and needless suffering. African American children are less likely than White children to be prescribed medication for attention-deficit/hyperactivity disorder, which may contribute to a greater likelihood of school failure. These differences in diagnosis and medication occur despite similar rates of illness and symptom presentation in the population (DelBello, 2002). Mental health clinicians are strongly encouraged to seek further training in interviewing, diagnosing, and intervention with people from a variety of cultural groups.

Talking in order to "feel better" is a cultural construction that not everyone shares. Not all cultures believe that talking about one's problems will in and of itself be beneficial or will lead to helpful interventions. Many people simply don't know how to talk about themselves and their feelings and intimate concerns. They may feel great shame over bringing their private concerns to another person. They may feel they're being judged concerning the content of their problems (see the section in Chapter 8 on reluctance). They may feel embarrassed over being in the humble position of someone who is asking for help or who is mandated to receive help by the courts or other agents of social control. They may feel that talking about their issues is a debilitating sign of weakness.

Ideas for mental health clinicians include introducing your role, the purpose of the interview, and the possible outcomes in some detail. It can also be extremely helpful to do something concrete early on, such as setting people up with needed services or helping them smooth relations with a school system. In some cases, it may be helpful to use a simple metaphor. For instance:

> All of us have problems in our lives. At times, they become so difficult that they get in our way, almost like an overly full suitcase that we trip on every time we try to walk past it. In counseling, you take items out of that suitcase, examine them, and then either refold them and stick them back in or throw them away. In that way, bit by bit the suitcase becomes less bulky and becomes less of a problem. Eventually you can lift it and move it to the side where you'll forget about it a lot of the time. But if you never deal with it, it will stay in your way.

Helpful volumes have been written about cross-cultural therapy and counseling, several are cited at the end of various chapters of this book.

Tips for Conducting Cross-Cultural Interviews in Mental Health Settings

- Reduce language barriers by having bilingual personnel provide care, using interpreters as needed, and seeing that written materials are available in the languages of your clients (see Chapters 6 and 7 on working with a different native language and using interpreters, respectively).
- Explain confidentiality and its limits.
- Inquire as to people's explanations for the difficulties they are having.
- Inquire as to how people think their current difficulties can be solved.
- Try to present the interventions that you are recommending in the least stigmatizing way. For instance, many people respond more positively to the word "counseling" than they do to "psychotherapy" and more positively to "medicine" than "drugs."
- Provide as much information as possible about your role, the purpose of the interview, and possible next steps.
- If you are explaining mental health concepts that might be unfamiliar, be sure to provide as much background information as you can about them.
- Access for people from minority cultural and racial groups is improved if agencies are decentralized and accessible by public transportation. Locate services within community organizations, social service agencies, community action agencies, health centers, places of worship, schools, and neighborhoods.
- Ensure that agencies are able to serve all members of immigrant groups regardless of immigration status. Even people who *are* documented are sometimes intimidated by documentation requirements.
- Consider using a cultural broker, to help bridge the cultural gap between your clinic and the client's culture. (For more information on cultural brokers, see Georgetown University's National Center on Cultural Competence.)

LAW ENFORCEMENT

People who grow up in middle- and upper-middle-class White neighborhoods in Western industrialized nations usually believe that the police are kind, respond when they are called, lock away "bad guys," and keep order. Parents from these kinds of neighborhoods are apt to tell their children to contact police for help if they are lost, for instance. Adults may call the police if they see "suspicious behavior," which is often simply the presence of a person from outside the neighborhood or someone of a different race. People in wealthier areas usually have limited direct contact with the police, perhaps encountering them during traffic incidents or during the rare need to report a crime. When police are present in schools in these kinds of neighborhoods, they're usually experienced as helpful and friendly.

People who grow up in less advantaged neighborhoods are likely to hold a radically different view of the police. Parents are apt to tell their children to avoid the police because they represent a threat. One African American police officer told me that the attitude in the low-income neighborhood where he grew up was, "You don't tell the police anything. You avoid them if you can, but if they ask you something you just tell them you don't know. They are trouble."

In low-income neighborhoods where many people of color live, residents may believe the police will not respond promptly to their calls and may even aggravate conflicts. One study found that children who were being removed from their homes by police because of suspected child maltreatment saw themselves as targets whom the police were threatening, not as victims whom the police were rescuing (Folman, 1998).

In the United States, incidents of police harassing African American and Latino boys, disrespecting women, and beating up men draw more public attention than the more frequent occasions where the police have quietly done their jobs to help people—adding to the perception among many groups that police are a menace to be avoided whenever possible. One study found that 7 in 10 Latino New Yorkers worry about becoming crime victims and 6 in 10 also fear becoming victims of police brutality (Lombardi, 2000). School-based officers in lower-income neighborhoods often have difficulty gaining trust, and they may find themselves busy in the schools investigating crimes rather than simply building connections with youth. This, of course, leads them to be perceived less favorably by many students and their families, contributing to the cycle of mistrust.

Over the course of U.S. history, police officers have been called on to enforce various anti-immigrant and racist government policies. For example, police were called on to force people of Japanese ancestry into concentration camps during World War II, to remove American Indian children from their homes and place them forcibly in boarding schools, to enforce racial segregation, to arrest people guilty of miscegenation (or "race mixing") in a variety of states, to interrogate people of Middle Eastern background after the September 11, 2001, attacks in New York City, and so on. Similar processes have occurred and continue to occur throughout the world, where the police are the enforcers of government policies that target members of indigenous, minority, or immigrant groups. Because of the nature of their job, because of a few high- profile incidents that tarnish the entire profession, and because of racism throughout the judicial system, people in law enforcement often face suspicion and mistrust in low-income, ethnic minority, indigenous, and immigrant communities.

In the United States and other countries where indigenous peoples have been granted some law enforcement authority in their own territories, jurisdictional issues are particularly complicated and vary tremendously. Native peoples often live in what may be described as a parallel environment, with structures, systems, laws, customs, values, and traditions that are different from the larger society in which they are embedded. (They often move between these two worlds, with all the confusion and stress this can imply.) Also, Native people often live in frontier situations where formal resources are scarce, and where two or more cultures butt up against each other regularly. In these situations, interviewers must be prepared to observe, listen, and ask for guidance. We must be sure to follow appropriate protocol and observe both federal and tribal laws and regulations, where applicable. Exactly which laws apply where and when may vary depending on the tribal identity of the person who is being interviewed, the location of the interview, the incident under investigation, and so on. When protocols are not followed, all the material gathered in the interview may be inadmissible in court.

Some of the misgivings about police described previously may be even more extreme for people who come from war zones, where—indeed—police, guards, and the military often pose an immediate danger. For instance, many refugees from regions as diverse as Bosnia, Cambodia, El Salvador, Somalia, Mozambique, the Congo, Indonesia, the Sudan, and Liberia have experienced sexual assault or the threat of sexual assault by the military, armed guards, "peacekeepers," and police. Women from these regions are likely to fear any man who appears to work in a law enforcement profession, such as the police and security officers.

Some groups may not believe that an officer in plain clothes is truly an officer, or that a woman can be a police officer, because these concepts are unfamiliar to them. Officers in plain clothes and women officers may need to show their badges to gain credibility.

What can police officers do, then, to win the trust of interviewees who may be predisposed to fearing, mistrusting, or even hating them? I hope this entire book is helpful in that regard. In addition, when you work with people who are not suspects but who are, rather, members of the community, witnesses, or victims of crime, do everything you can to avoid intimidating.

Tips for Conducting Cross-Cultural Interviews in Law Enforcement Settings

- Partner with community members and community leaders. Learn about the ethnic and cultural communities in which you work and try to make friends with people from those communities.
- See if you can sit or stand in a way that makes you less physically intimidating (unless you are trying to be intimidating).
- Explain as precisely as you can the nature of your inquiry (e.g., that the interviewee is *not* a suspect).
- Conduct interviews in the person's native language or use an interpreter, whenever possible.
- Demonstrate empathy and respect.
- Interview people in places where they are more apt to feel safe from bodily harm, whether it is from you or from people who might seek retribution if they are known to be cooperating with you.
- Enlist the help of colleagues or advocates who have expertise working with community members from certain backgrounds or with specific issues such as sexual assault. Don't hesitate to step aside when need be, so the job can get accomplished as well as possible; this requires willingness to admit that some situations are better handled by others.
- Be part of an effort to recruit and retain a more culturally diverse police force, which will improve relations between the police and diverse members of your community.

EDUCATORS

Upper-income children are apt to go to school in pleasant circumstances with easy access to books, games, and other learning materials. With a smaller student–teacher ratio, upper-income children are more apt to establish positive bonds with their teachers. They are more likely to have opportunities to participate in specialized school activities that they enjoy, such as art, music, dance, physical education, and outdoor recess. Upper-income children are, therefore, more likely to feel that they belong in a school environment and are successful there; thus they perceive schools and educators more positively.

On the other hand, many lower-income children attend schools that are overcrowded, where they have reduced access to resources including time with their teachers. Teachers frequently hold low expectations for student achievement, and they may control student behavior through threats and other forms of coercion rather than sincere praise and rewards (Boykin, 2001). Art, music, and physical education programs are likely to be severely limited, if they exist at all. And neighborhoods may be too dangerous or facilities too inadequate to permit outdoor recess. Certainly some schools in low-income neighborhoods are successful in helping their students achieve, but on the whole, schools that are overcrowded and underfunded are apt to alienate rather than inspire their students.

The new emphasis on high-stakes standardized testing also can put additional pressure on children that makes them fear failure and may actually cause them to experience failure, beginning at a young age. The Civil Rights Project at Harvard has recently released a series of reports documenting the resegregation of U.S. schools, with levels of segregation in 2003 the same as in 1969, reversing decades of progress (e.g., Orfield & Lee, 2006). In many cities, the shoddy low-income schools are apt to be filled almost entirely with Black and Latino students while the faculty is more likely to be White. Children in these schools may feel that educators are part of a force aimed at containing them. Similar class and ethnic tensions are reported in Western Europe, Canada, and Australia.

Some children's first experience of school is one of learning that the way they and their families speak is wrong. Delpit (2002) describes a continual battle by U.S. teachers to pressure their low-income Black students to "talk right" and the children's attempts to hold onto their language as a form of identity. She suggests that when adults respond negatively to children's home language, the children end up rejecting the school's language and everything associated with the school. She asks what it means to a child who encounters an adult who aims to "speak out against Ebonics." (Ebonics refers to African American Vernacular English, formerly called Black English):

> It can only represent the desire to speak out against those who are speakers of Ebonics—to stamp out not only the child, but those from whom the child first received nurturance, from whom she first felt love, for whom she first smiled. There is a reason our first language is called our mother tongue. To speak out against the language that children bring to school means that we are speaking out against their mothers. . . . Ironically, the more determined we are to rid the school of children's home language, the more determined they must be to preserve it. (p. 47)

Delpit recommends that educators teach children standard English while simultaneously celebrating the variety of languages and dialects that children speak at home.

One Puerto Rican psychotherapist with experience working as a school psychologist in a district with a large Latino population discussed the racism she has seen among some educators. She attributed this racism to teachers' contact with people from minority groups in the most difficult circumstances:

> Teachers are sometimes racist because of their own backgrounds. And teachers sometimes become racist, or exacerbate their racist attitudes because of the situations they have to deal with in the school system. They have thirty-five children in the classroom, the majority of which don't have the basic skills they should when they reach that classroom. They do not have supportive families because these are families that are dealing with so many issues that what's happening in school cannot become one of the priorities. . . . [The families] can't look to the future because they don't have their present problems resolved. . . . So the teachers are alone in their struggle with these kids. And because [the teachers] don't have a lot of support from the school system, their anger has to go somewhere, and it goes to the kids. And the kids are victimized again. So the chances of a child feeling trust in a teacher under those circumstances—to which there are exceptions—are not very high. (cited in Fontes, 1992, p. 70)

Although overcrowded and underfunded schools and biased teachers can ruin educators' reputations among some low-income people, and therefore complicate educational interviews and assessments, it would be wrong to suggest that all or even most low-income people, immigrants, and members of minority groups are suspicious of educators. On the contrary, many people from these groups believe that education is the hopeful key to their own and their children's advancement. It would be equally wrong to imply in any way that educators working in low-income minority neighborhoods are necessarily discriminatory. Some of the most dedicated and highly qualified educators I know choose to work in low-income minority neighborhoods where they feel they are most needed.

Many Native American children have heard stories in their families about the abuses perpetrated by educators in boarding schools where their parents and grandparents were forced to live away from their families, punished if they spoke in their native tongue, and systematically stripped of their culture. Teachers who work with native children will need to show that they are different, in part by demonstrating respectful interest in the children's diverse backgrounds.

In Puerto Rico there is a saying, *La maestra es la segunda madre* (the teacher is the second mother). Teachers of some kind exist in all societies. Adults with less education often hold great respect for educators, or even awe. If they are hesitant to attend events or meetings at school and fail to speak up during interviews, it is probably due to a lack of familiarity with the school setting or lack of English-language competence, rather than a dislike of educators.

Tips for Conducting Cross-Cultural Interviews in Educational Settings

Wonderful volumes have been written for educators about multicultural classrooms and working with culturally diverse students and their families (Ballenger, 1998; Nieto & Bode, 2007). Here are a few pointers to keep in mind when conducting cross-cultural interviews in educational settings:

- Exercise extreme caution and respect when inquiring about adults' levels of education and employment. These are deeply sensitive areas. (I am reminded of my grandfather, an immigrant from Poland who wrote and spoke several languages but who never learned to write without errors in English and was painfully ashamed of his spelling and grammatical mistakes.)
- Issue personalized invitations to parents who are unfamiliar with the schools or who are uncomfortable in them to encourage them to attend interviews or events. If the parents are not very literate, you may need to make a phone call or a home visit, or encourage the child to write and read a message to the parents.
- Communicate your respect for the caretakers and for their culture in every way possible, without appearing condescending.
- Convey what you *like* about children and what they are doing well, along with the problems.
- If you have concerns about speaking in the parents' native language, make sure to ask if they want an interpreter.
- Finally, be sure to communicate what you hope the parent will do as a follow-up to the interview. For example:

> "The information you gave me today really helps me understand your child better. We are going to be giving your child a great deal of support so he can perform better in school. It would be helpful if you could ask him to show you his homework every day and make sure he gets nine hours of sleep each night as well."

Educators have the potential to serve as a helpful bridge between children from minority cultures and the wider society. Often, schools can help entire families in their adjustment to a new land, through work with the children and through outreach programs such as family literacy.

ATTORNEYS

Wealthy and middle-class people may have attorneys among their friends and neighbors; they have probably worked with attorneys and courts in purchasing houses, closing business deals, writing wills, settling estates, and so on.

However, attorneys are relatively unfamiliar figures to many immigrants and low-income people. In some states attorneys hawk their services on local television stations and on the backs of telephone books with pitches that would make a used car salesman blush. Increasingly, attorneys are being portrayed in crime shows and court dramas as clever, dramatic courtroom orators or as underhanded, conniving scoundrels who will sell their soul to the highest bidder. People from lower-income backgrounds have often experienced less positive direct contact with attorneys and the courts, perhaps limited to unpleasant issues such as child protective services, evictions, unpaid traffic fines, and criminal trials. People who have enjoyed fewer positive experiences with attorneys and the courts may believe that these professionals are geared to serving the interests of the powerful; they may mistrust the motives of guardians ad litem and court-appointed attorneys. They may feel extremely guarded and vulnerable in interviews or depositions with attorneys—even attorneys who are working to represent their interests.

Each nation's legal system has its own culture. Except in the case of religious and other traditional law, these legal systems are designed to be logical, orderly, linear, and confrontational. Information is segmented into discrete bits that are expected to be ordered into a sequential whole. Only solid facts are considered. Hearsay and opinions not supported by provable facts are considered irrelevant. The formal set of principles that guide the mainstream legal system simply do not jibe with the values and habits of many ethnic cultures.

First Nations Justice (which refers to the legal systems of the Native peoples of the United States and Canada) is more concerned with balance among the family, clan, and the natural world and bringing together the various parties (e.g., accused, victim, and their supporters) to talk things out and restore harmony and balance. The goal of this system is healing and peacemaking, and the approach incorporates spirituality (Mirsky, 2007).

The complexities of the law are difficult for any nonattorney to understand, but even more so for those with lower levels of education or for those who deeply mistrust the law's representatives. Native Americans, in particular, are apt to mistrust attorneys and the courts. The history of Native Americans is replete with broken treaties and unfair and even genocidal court decisions. "Just sign here," are neutral words for many of us, but they are words with horrendous historical echoes for many Native Americans.

Because depositions may take place over a period of months, attorneys have ample opportunities to build rapport or intimidate, explore cultural complexities, or fall back on stereotypes. The course they choose to pursue usually depends on their motives.

Tips for Conducting Cross-Cultural Interviews in Legal Settings

- If you are using a foreign language interpreter, take time before the session to create a list of the particular words that will be used to translate important terms. Give the interpreter an opportunity to discuss the various possibilities and the advantages and disadvantages of each. Often, a number of different terms could be used, but if the terms are used inconsistently, this could be confusing.
- Cultures have different approaches to conflict and different understandings of how conflict should be resolved. Many people will not be comfortable with the adversarial nature of most legal systems. Where possible, help people resolve conflicts in ways that feel more natural to them. The economic and social costs of an adversarial approach may be too high. If a more adversarial approach is apt to benefit them, explain why and how to proceed.
- Explain your role carefully along with the purpose of the interview.
- Explain whom you are representing and who is paying your bill.
- If working with an immigrant, you may need to explain briefly the basic workings of the legal system as well because this varies greatly among nations.
- Allow interviewees to ask you questions. Offer answers to the kinds of questions you think the interviewees might have in the back of their mind if they seem hesitant to make inquiries themselves. A short list includes: What are my rights here? Can I back out of this case or change my mind about how to proceed? Can I trust you with the truth, even if it is harmful to my case? What are the implications of lying? Can I be sure this information will be kept confidential?

RESEARCHERS

Researchers are viewed with suspicion in many ethnic communities. In her wonderful book on cultural conflict in classrooms, Lisa Delpit (1995) describes this attitude: "People of color are, in general skeptical of research as a determiner of our fates. Academic research has, after all, found us genetically inferior, culturally deprived, and verbally deficient" (p. 31).

The ethical guidelines of most professions that conduct research are designed to protect the rights of individual research participants, rather than the rights of a participant's cultural community (Fontes, 1998). Also, these guidelines often fail to take into account cultural differences in terms of who owns information, what it means to speak to "an outsider" (however that is defined), cultural difference in interpreting the meaning of constructs, the value of research to different groups, and so on. All too often the lack of cultural competency in research not only limits the scientific value of that research but also renders it unethical (Fontes, 2004; Gunaratnam, 2003b).

The history of research is riddled with abuse concerning people who are disabled or incarcerated, have a low income, and/or belong to a variety of minority racial and ethnic groups. African Americans remember the Tuskegee experiments in which African American men were left with untreated syphilis for decades, unbeknownst to them, and not only became extremely ill themselves but also served as vectors for illness in their communities. One third of Puerto Rican women were sterilized by 1965, most without their consent (Presser, 1980). Some would argue that the ethical history of social science research in minority communities is not much better than the medical research—with much of it serving to reinforce societal power imbalances and confirm problems and pathologies, rather than to document strengths or uncover solutions (Fontes, 1998).

Research involving people and not just archival data *always* involves a relationship:

> This relationship is most obvious in the intimate setting of an in-depth interview; but even anonymous telephone or written surveys emerge from— and create—a relationship. Researchers must ask themselves, "What kind of relationship do I have with the participants? What kind of relationship do I want to construct with them through the research?" (Fontes, 1998, p. 54)

In the research setting the researcher is always more powerful than the person who is being researched, no matter how collaborative the methods. If the researcher comes from a group that is socially more powerful (wealthier, more educated, from a more privileged race or ethnic group) the situation is even more imbalanced.

Without a thorough understanding of the group(s) being studied, it is easy for a well-meaning researcher to make mistakes. For instance, I conducted a study in a Chilean shantytown where the participants objected to the anonymity I had painstakingly assured them through the design of my study—they wanted individual credit for what they said. All too often in the past, they said, they had labored without recognition. My best efforts to assure them anonymity backfired because they valued credit for their words more than anonymity. If I had worked more closely with members of the community in designing the research before submitting it to an internal review board, maybe I would not have made such a blunder.

Other researchers have found that people from the Middle East sometimes object to being asked to sign a consent form, trusting this formality less than they would trust giving one's word orally with a handshake. Other groups of people who might shy away from written consent forms include undocumented immigrants, people who are illiterate and embarrassed to admit it, members of stigmatized groups who don't want their names associated with the research, and people who fear retribution from family members, political groups, or criminal elements if their participation is made public.

Tips for Researchers Conducting Cross-Cultural Interviews

- Make sure you have thought carefully, and consulted with others, about cultural issues in all phases of the research, including study design, data gathering, data analysis, and dissemination of the findings.
- Incorporate members of the community into key decision-making positions regarding all those research phases—not just as "covers" to gain credibility with the community.
- Investigate questions that have been identified as "of interest" to the communities you are investigating and not only questions of interest just to outsiders.
- Do not simply translate instruments or apply them to groups on which they were not initially normed and assume the findings are relevant.
- Be sure to choose study methods and instruments that make sense within the participants' cultural context. (See Fontes, 1997, 1998, & 2004, for more information.)

Without thorough integration of people from the culture in question into research teams, it is easy to fail to ask the more important questions:

"A colleague was developing a questionnaire for immigrant women about barriers to using contraception. She consulted the scant literature that existed and was putting the final touches on her questionnaire when she spoke with someone who was familiar with the culture of immigrant women although from a different field. The cultural informant replied that the women usually did whatever their boyfriends and husbands told them to do concerning contraception. My colleague added a question about this to the survey. As it turned out, this was the single most often selected item in the study."

This example points to the inadequacy of instruments that are developed without sufficient input from members of the target community. We cannot simply take an interview guide that we have developed with one group in mind and assume that it will fit another group of people, even if the instruments have been translated.

Yoshihama (2001) illustrates how easy it is to miss important elements in cross-cultural interviews with examples from her research on intimate partner violence in Japan and among Japanese Americans in the United States. There are entire categories of violence that are particularly relevant in Japan that would be missed in a standard U.S. survey. For example, in Japan abusive men are prone to overturning dining room tables. Yoshihama (2001) suggests this happens because "the dining table represents the locus of family activities and, by extension, is a symbol of women's legitimate role and place in the Japanese home" (p. 310). Additionally, abusive Japanese men sometimes throw liquid at their partner. This is seen to stem from the practice of throwing water to purify objects that are considered dirty or impure in Japan, so throwing water at a partner is a harsh insult. Yoshihama (2001) emphasizes that these practices are "socio-culturally rooted" (p. 310), reflecting sociocultural values in Japanese society, but are not unique to Japan. These acts might not show up at all using "standard" interviewing instruments, and their impact might be underestimated by an interviewer who is less familiar with Japanese culture.

These examples point to the absolute imperative that we incorporate people from the culture into key decision-making roles when we design research instruments, interview guides, or questionnaires that will be used with people from a given culture (see Fontes, 1997). To do anything less is to virtually guarantee that our questions will miss the mark.

A thorough discussion of ways to make research more fair and just for people from minority cultural groups, and to increase the likelihood that they will participate forthrightly in research, is beyond the scope of this section.

POTENTIAL EMPLOYERS IN THE HELPING PROFESSIONS

Among the upper middle class in the United States, "tooting your own horn" and highlighting your own virtues are not only seen as acceptable in job interviews but are expected. People from the more educated and economically stable classes learn to describe their experiences in the most favorable light, perhaps a somewhat exaggerated light, when communicating with potential employers. They probably have received the kinds of training that reinforce their strengths and inspire self-confidence. They probably have learned how to hold their body, shake hands, maintain eye contact, and assume a vague air of privilege that conveys their suitability for the position. They have learned how to dress to impress *professionally*, knowing this requires a different sort of clothing from what they would wear to impress in a social situation. They have learned to talk in a professional way, using a different vocabulary and style of speaking from the way they would speak with their friends. Although educated and wealthier individuals might sometimes feel nervous or intimidated during job interviews, they are still likely to convey a certain self-assurance and entitlement that helps them make a favorable impression.

On the other hand, people from a lower-income background, people with less education, and immigrants from the working classes in many developing countries may feel inadequate and intimidated in job interviews and less able to highlight their strengths. They may lack confidence in their ability to write, read, or speak English properly. Or they may just not know how to "show off" their skills.

Extreme job mobility is increasingly the norm, rather than the exception, in the United States, and U.S. residents thus become accustomed to the process of applying for a new job. Even in U.S. communities where jobs are scarce, people increasingly move from employer to employer and position to position throughout their working life. Many countries do not offer similar opportunities for part-time, temporary, and full-time openings. In many other nations, even jobs as waiters, store clerks, and factory workers are apt to be full time and long-lasting. In those societies the job interview is correspondingly more serious, and the job interviewer seems more intimidating.

Many cultures value a demeanor of humility, which might be misperceived by a job interviewer as low self-esteem or a lack of qualifications. Many cultures do not prioritize being liked and making a good impression as highly as these qualities are valued in the United States. In Australia, the U.S. attitude is described as the "obsession with making a 'good' impression" (Renwick, 1980, as cited in Wierzbicka, 1994). Scandinavian humility has been described as an admonishment to not believe you are somebody and to stay in your place (Erickson, 2005). South Asian cultures also value "a modest, self-effacing personality; the more accomplished one is, the more humbly one is expected to behave" (Lee, 1997, p. 86). Latin cultures, including the Portuguese, also value a humble demeanor. In Spanish there is a saying, *Nadie diga de sí nada, que sus obras lo dirán*, which means essentially that people should not speak for themselves but rather let their deeds speak for them. Clearly, people who tend to be more humble culturally, and more intimidated by the interviewer, are less apt to speak up on their own behalf in an interview.

One interview question that especially bothers job seekers is, "How much salary do you want?" While this is a stressful question for many applicants, experienced middle-class job seekers (especially males) will often come to an interview prepared for such a question, and they are not afraid to request an unrealistically high salary as a bargaining ploy. Women and immigrants often end up being paid less than they deserve because they fail to ask for enough money. Job interviewers should keep this discrepancy in mind because an underpaid employee will not remain satisfied for long.

Questions such as "What is it like to work with you?" or "What are your best attributes as a colleague?" or "Describe your personality" may be quite foreign and almost incomprehensible to people from many cultures. If the answers are stumbling or incomplete, the employer should not assume that the person is hiding something. Rather, it may be more productive to elicit this information from other sources.

People conducting job interviews would do well to follow the many recommendations contained in this book in terms of demonstrating respect, putting interviewees at ease through nonverbal communication, and using interpreters with nonnative speakers of English. Applicants for all jobs should be treated with dignity. In addition, when conducting a job interview you may want to remember that performing less well in an interview may not necessarily mean that a person will perform less well on the job; the skill sets may be different. It may be helpful to explain the purpose of the interview to the applicant with as much detail as possible. Knowing that people may not present themselves in the best light, the interviewer may want to ask for details about the person's job experience. For example, if you see that the person has worked as a secretary at a medical clinic, inquire as to the exact duties. It could turn out that the interviewee had managed the office, supervised several administrative employees, trained patients in self-care, written handouts for patients, and developed a complex filing system for tracking records. Sometimes immigrants will only include in applications the jobs they have held in their new country. With inquiry, a potential employer may discover that the woman who has been a clerk at a department store since arriving in her new country holds a master's degree in chemistry and managed a medical laboratory before immigrating.

Sometimes it can be hard to evaluate the personal characteristics of people who come from a vastly different background from your own. In many jobs, these interpersonal characteristics such as diligence, ability to get along well with others, and pride in one's work may ultimately be more important than prior experience. Training a new employee in the specifics of a job may require some investment early on but may well be worth the payoff later.

WOMEN'S CRISIS WORKERS

Most developing countries do not have shelters for battered women, rape crisis centers, or other agencies geared to helping women in crisis. (Even in areas where these services exist, they rarely have sufficient capacity to meet the demand.) Staff from these agencies, therefore, represent an unknown concept to most people from the developing world. Even in countries where these agencies do exist, they are little known by most of the populace.

People who work in women's crisis centers—if they are considered at all—are often stereotyped as "antimale" or "antifamily." Many people believe that a woman who meets with a crisis worker may find herself pressured to abandon her husband or family. Sometimes a woman is unable to continue meeting with a professional in a women's crisis agency unless she gets permission from her husband, boyfriend, mother, or mother-in-law—or unless she keeps them in the dark about these meetings.

People who work in women's shelters or women's crisis centers may therefore need to demonstrate their ability to understand and work with, rather than against, a woman's cultural values. These values are apt to include intense and irrefutable bonds to family. As with all the professions described previously, women's crisis centers can demonstrate their multicultural awareness and competence most effectively if they employ a diverse staff that includes members of all the major cultures in their service area. (See sections of Chapter 8 on intimate partner violence and sexual assault for more information.)

CONCLUDING OBSERVATIONS

Those of us who are in a position of authority because of our professional roles may have to cross a wide gulf to gain the trust of interviewees who have learned to avoid and fear people like us. Our rapport-building skills assume special significance when we consider the many reasons why people may be predisposed *not* to trust us. With this in mind, it is especially important for us to prepare carefully for an interview, set the right tone with an appropriate demeanor, use nonverbal communication wisely, and take full advantage of interpreters.

We are preceded by the reputation of others from our field each time we have a contact in the course of our work. Similarly, we leave interviewees with an impression of people in our field at the close of each interview session. That impression will have echoes in the interviewees, their family, and perhaps their community, long after we have closed the case file.

Questions to Think about and Discuss

1. Describe three challenges that people from your profession face in gaining trust in interviews. What can you do to overcome these challenges?
2. Describe some of the consequences of an interviewee refusing to discuss particular problematic topics in your field.
3. Describe a way people in your profession could be trained to become better at establishing rapport and interviewing people from two specific cultural groups.

RECOMMENDED ADDITIONAL READING

Lipson, J. G., & Dibble, S. L. (2005). *Culture and clinical care*. San Francisco: University of California, San Francisco, School of Nursing Press.

Ponterotto, J. G., Casas, J. M, Suzuki, L. A., & Alexander, C. M. (Eds.). (2001). *Handbook of multicultural counseling*. Thousand Oaks, CA: Sage.

Shusta, R. M., Levine, D. R., Wong, H. Z., & Harris, P. R. (2005). *Multicultural law enforcement* (3rd ed.). Upper Saddle River, NJ: Pearson Prentice Hall.

12 Common Dilemmas and Misunderstandings in Cross-Cultural Interviews

Cultural competence may be seen as a journey with a clear direction but no distinct destination. We never arrive at a place of perfect cultural competence. Rather, as we acquire greater knowledge of various cultures, deepened self-understanding, and greater insight into how to adapt our work to people from different cultural groups, we also become aware of how far we still have to go.

At the beginning of this journey toward cultural competence we are typically unaware of the importance of culture in our life and in the lives of others. We are apt to see what we do as "natural" and we may be unaware that others hold contrasting viewpoints, beliefs, and customs. In our professional work, therefore, we are apt to use our own values and behaviors as our yardstick for measuring everyone else's. This is called ethnocentrism. At this stage of our development as culturally competent professionals, we may profess to be "culture blind" or "color blind" (indifferent to race) and aim to treat all people "the same," without understanding that "the same" may not be fair to people from minority cultural groups. The mistakes we make at this stage of the journey are apt to be based on assumptions that all others share our values (or should share them!) and that "normal" is the norms from our own cultural background.

As we progress and begin to learn about the importance of culture in our work, we may see cultural differences principally as nuisances and potential obstacles to doing what we usually do. We may believe we have to understand other people's cultures just enough to persuade them to accept our services so we can influence them in the direction of becoming "more mainstream" or more similar to the dominant culture. At this point in our own development we may want to know how to adapt our services minimally to achieve some kind of "fit" between what we do and the culture of particular groups of our clients or interviewees.

As we step into still greater knowledge, we come to see cultures as dynamic and changing, flexible rather than rigid, evolving rather than fixed. Instead of simply finding out about habits of a large all-encompassing cultural group (such as African Americans, Latinos, or Asians), we come to understand each person as an individual who shares certain characteristics with some members of the same group but differs on many others. We notice that general cultural norms are adapted and changed by individuals and local cultural communities. While we may continue to find general information about "traditional beliefs" or "cultural norms" interesting, we know it does not tell the whole story about who our interviewees are, who we are, or how we can best relate.

No matter how far along the road toward cultural competence we travel, we will continue to make mistakes in our interviews. As long as we are interacting with people from cultural groups that are less familiar to us, small and large cultural misunderstandings are bound to occur.

Common Mistakes in Cross-Cultural Interviews

You will make mistakes in cross-cultural interviews—everyone does. Try to see such mistakes as learning opportunities and be gentle with yourself. Here is a list of some of the many possible errors you may make, even if you believe you should "know better."

- Interrupting interviewees because you believe they are done speaking when they are just trying to collect their thoughts.
- Viewing a given behavior or statement as evidence of a problem (pathological) when it actually is just an example of a cultural difference.
- Using a word in English or another language in a way that inadvertently offends the person you're interviewing.
- Thinking you understand what the interviewee is saying and acting on that belief, which turns out to be erroneous.
- Failing to accommodate the interviewee's culture in ways that damage rapport (e.g., scheduling an interview during a religious holiday).

- Believing a given behavior is cultural when, in fact, it is due to individual or systemic factors.
- Touching people who you should not touch because of differing cultural beliefs about what that touch means.

Although all of these errors are unfortunate, none is apt to be fatal. When you make a mistake, apologize, explain, use your sense of humor, and do what you can to avoid committing the same mistake the next time. This may require becoming more familiar with the culture of the people you're interviewing or reviewing this book or another multicultural resource.

This chapter discusses common dilemmas that have not been discussed elsewhere in this book, with the goal of helping you avoid some of the more frequent misunderstandings. I want to acknowledge, however, that it is impossible to avoid making mistakes. I know that each reader brings a set of background knowledge to this chapter, and so some elements will seem obvious, whereas others will be surprising. In balance, I hope you find information that will be new and helpful to you in your cross-cultural interviews.

GATHERING BASIC DEMOGRAPHIC INFORMATION

Gathering basic demographic information can be complicated, especially when the interviewer and interviewee come from different cultural backgrounds. Issues include atypical family configurations, information that has been lost or changed in the process of immigration, and lying.

Family Relationships and Living Arrangements

In recent decades most of us have become aware that the nuclear family of Mom, Dad, and the kids is just one of many possible family forms. Extended family members and grown siblings may live in the same apartment or down the hall. Close family friends may be called aunts and uncles and live with the family for a time, although they are not related by blood or marriage. Grown siblings, aunts, uncles, grandparents, and godparents may serve as children's caretakers and wield as much influence over children as the parents. Children may float among various households within their extended families, going to grandma's after school, eating dinner at their aunt's, and sometimes sleeping at their godparents' home. Inconsistencies in addresses may not indicate lying but may rather point to either the extreme mobility of many low-income families or the way children participate in a number of households simultaneously. Social workers can be confused if they are checking the food supply in Mom's refrigerator and find it is empty—but perhaps her children actually take their meals in another household.[1]

A situation in which extended family members raise children either instead of or along with the children's parents should not be seen—a priori—as less favorable than a situation in which children are raised by their own parents exclusively. Koul (2002) describes growing up in her grandparents' household:

> I was satisfied with the arrangement, happy to have everyone's attention to myself. In any event, we had only a vague idea that in our extended family life we had our own nuclear family. It was not something that was given much prominence; the larger tribe was crucial. Even when my mother and father were present, my grandparents were the de facto parents and heads of the household. . . . [At my grandparents'] I was a full-fledged member of the household, and far from feeling that I was not in my own home, luxuriated in being the only grandchild present. I have never felt so at home anywhere else. (p. 67)

Clearly in this case, being raised by grandparents was safe and comfortable for this young woman in Kashmir, as it is for children in many families throughout the world.

We need to ask questions in ways that allow the respondents to acknowledge the complexity of their lives, including multiple caretakers, informal adoptions, children conceived outside marriage, common-law spouses, gay and lesbian partners, and "fictive kin." "Fictive kin" is a term used to describe all those many ways in which people come to be considered or feel like family to each other, without necessarily having ties of blood, marriage, or legal sanction. In Spanish the phrase *padres de crianza* means the parents who do the raising, a term that is lacking in English.

Informal adoptions are common among African Americans (Boyd-Franklin, 2003), as family and friends help each other out by welcoming another person's child to live in their household. The circumstances that inspire this arrangement include when older relatives raise the child of a teen mother so she can pursue her education; when a family in a good school

---

[1]In many countries, people do not stock up on food in the supermarket once a week but, rather, go to the market each day to purchase the foods needed for that day's meals. A trip to the market is often a social event and an opportunity to purchase the freshest food. A social worker who finds an empty cupboard should not assume the children have inadequate access to food. Rather, he or she should inquire about shopping habits and where the family eats.

district invites a youngster to live with them to attend a better school; and when a mother is going through a hard time economically, has lost her housing, or is working odd shifts and other relatives take in a child until the mother has improved circumstances. Sometimes mothers are forced to "lend" their children to relatives to pursue their own education or attend medical or substance abuse treatment. This flexibility of households often works well as an unofficial support system for families on the economic edge, but it can also be confusing in an interview. Recently, I heard this practice referred to as "illegal adoption." I think we should avoid this term because it implies malicious or criminal intent. "Informal adoption" would be a more acceptable term.

Refugees and immigrants often engage in informal adoptions. A couple in a refugee camp who is granted refugee status to emigrate with their children may take some of their nieces and nephews with them as well, pretending they are their own children, in the hopes of saving them from war or starvation and assuring them a better life. This can confuse the interviewer who is trying to ascertain family relationships.

We should remember that the words "Daddy," "Papi," "Papa," or even "Father" might be used to describe a biological father, a stepfather, a grandfather, the mother's boyfriend, or another important male in the child's life. The child may say he lives with Mama, but he knows Mama is the grandmother and he visits Mommy on weekends. In families from India, Pakistan, and Bangladesh, as well as among many traditional Native American families, any older female friend of the family is apt to be "Auntie." A professional might also be called Aunt or Uncle as a sign of respect and affection.

Because of China's one-child policy, some Chinese youngsters describe children their own age as brothers and sisters when, in fact, they are cousins or neighbors. In Chinese and Native American families, people may be called cousins because they come from the same ancestral village or tribe. In Spanish the term for first cousin is *primo hermano*, which translates literally as "cousin brother."

People may use names for relatives that are new to you: For example, Navajo may speak of their "brother cousins." Blackfeet Indians have a specific term in their Piegan language that an older brother uses to call his younger brother, and vice versa. These terms should not be seen simply as *referring* to something—the existence of the terms themselves highlights the importance of birth order in Blackfeet culture (Ivanova, 2002). Speakers of Croatian, Bosnian, and Turkish have specific names for relatives for which there is no English equivalent, such as mother's brother and father's brother—two distinct names which in English are collapsed into "uncle."

Recently I was speaking with Habibo, a Somali Bantu woman who has limited English skills. I was trying to discern her family constellation, which was tricky because so few names are used in Somalia that she has multiple Mohameds, Ishas, and Hassans in her family. At one point she said, "My father is my uncle." I laughed to myself, thinking how a few months earlier I might have assumed that her statement was an error based on her language competence. But knowing a little about Somali culture, I now know that it is common for men to marry their brother's widows as a way of protecting the brothers' family, leading to a situation in which yes, indeed, Habibo's father is her uncle. In other words, the man who acts as her father is the brother of her biological father, who was killed in the refugee camp. As a result, Habibo has large numbers of siblings, half-siblings, and step-siblings—some of whom are also her cousins. I saw a man who was with her the other day whom I vaguely recognized. "Is this your brother?" I asked Habibo. She smiled, "Yes, same mother, same father." This specificity is important among Somalis, because of the prevalence of half-sibling and step-sibling relationships. The half-siblings and step-siblings may have different mothers and live in different homes, but they are apt to spend time together and treat each other well, without the awkwardness that one might imagine could affect children of a man's first wife when relating to the children of a man's subsequent wives. At the same time, "same mother, same father," is a closer form of kinship.

The varieties of relationships and living arrangements are endless. We must be open to hearing about each person's reality. Our paperwork should allow us to record informal adoptive families, extended families that live together, gay and lesbian partners, step- and half-siblings, foster families, friends who are central to a family's life, and so on.

Among Latin Americans, Spaniards, Portuguese, and Italians, godparents are often considered family, although there is usually no blood relationship. When a parent names a person his child's godfather or godmother, the parent and godparent enters into a codified relationship with each other, and they are called in Spanish *compadres* or *comadres* and in Italian *compari* and *comari* (literally, cofathers or comothers). Godparents may be central to families on a daily basis or step in only in times of crisis or transition. When asking people from these groups about family, it is a good idea to inquire about godparents to see if they have an important influence and should therefore be included in interviews and interventions.

In many cultures a marriage does not merely join two individuals but also two extended families (illustrated vividly with Greek, Asian Indian, and Chinese families in the movies *My Big Fat Greek Wedding, Monsoon Wedding,* and *The Wedding Banquet,* respectively). In some cultures, the relationships among the sets of in-laws are dignified with a name—in Spanish, the in-laws become *consuegros* (literally "co-inlaws") and in Yiddish, *machatainisteh*, while the two extended families become *mishpucheh*. Many American Indian cultures make no distinction between birth relatives and relatives by marriage. A son-in-law is a son; a sister-in-law is a sister (Sutton & Broken Nose, 2005).

Dates of Birth

When working with immigrants, professionals sometimes notice that birth-dates seem to keep shifting or are hard to pin down. Every time I interpret for a Portuguese relative at a doctor's office and I ask her birthdate as we fill out forms, she says, "Which one?" She was born in a small village in Portugal where there was a law mandating that parents register their children within a couple of months of the child's birth. Because her parents were poor and lived far from the registry office, and because they did not want to attract "the evil eye" by taking her survival for granted before passing those crucial first months of life, her parents waited several months before registering her. To conform to the law, they had to say she was just 2 months old. Hence, she has two birthdays—an official one that is on all her documents and the real date of birth which the family celebrates. This kind of situation is not uncommon with immigrant families.

People who work with refugees sometimes notice an unusual number of people who say they were born on January 1 or July 1. When a family without documents applies for entrance to the United States in a refugee camp, often the officials will assign everyone January 1 or July 1 birthdates. The children often appear younger than their chronological age because of malnutrition, and so they are assigned birthdates that suggest they are younger than they truly are. (In some cases the parents will purposely say the children are younger than their true age because younger children receive priority access to food and shelter). Once these errors have been entered into official documents they are extremely difficult to change.

At times it is important to determine a child's true age. Uba (1994) recounts the case of a 17-year-old Laotian child whose documents said he was 11 years old. He was feeling the stirrings of puberty and eager to date and felt extremely uncomfortable in a class with other children who were 11. His parents did not want his true age revealed, however, because they would be cut off from welfare benefits once he was no longer officially a minor, and he would also be forced to leave high school prematurely and lose his opportunity to gain an education.

When a Bangladeshi friend immigrated to the United States, his father falsified his and his brother's documents to make them look a year younger. He thought it would be to his son's advantage to be considered precocious for his age. The son bemoans this decision, however, because it has delayed his ability to get a driver's license, drink alcohol legally, and sign legal documents. Making children appear younger is not uncommon. Nor is the reverse uncommon, where a family says their children are a year or more older than their actual age, so the children can enter public school one year earlier, enabling both parents to work outside the home.

Sometimes parents change a child's birthdate because the child has been born on a day or during a year considered to bring bad luck, such as the Day of the Dead for Mexican families, or the Year of the Rooster for Chinese families, or at an inauspicious time for Hindus. Other families create new stories including new dates to hide incidents that they consider shameful—such as a pregnancy resulting from rape or an affair, children born out of wedlock, and even previous marriages or liaisons.

People who come from rural societies or whose lives have been disrupted by war may simply have no idea of their "true" birthday on a Western calendar. People from other traditional agricultural societies often do not keep track of birthdates or celebrate birthdays. Children's maturity may be measured by how grown up they look and what they are able to do, rather than by a chronological date. The chronological age assigned by officials may not mean much to the parents, and they may not remember their children's official ages. Chinese families often celebrate the day a person was conceived as the birthday, rather than the day the person was born. There may also be confusion when translating dates from the Chinese to the Western calendar. In Europe the day is usually written before the month, so that the birthday of someone born on July 12, 1986, would be written 12/7/86 rather than 7/12/86, as would be true in the United States. (Canada uses both formats, in French and in English). European and U.S. dates are often transposed in this way on official documents.

TRUTH, LIES, AND IMMIGRATION

When working with people of uncertain immigration status or people who you know are undocumented, it is helpful to be able to say, "Our agency has a policy—we do not release information to immigration authorities." If your agency does not have such a policy, it should develop one—and this should be posted in several languages in the waiting room and in written materials. In some jurisdictions, however, law enforcement and child protective services may be required to report certain classes of crimes committed by undocumented people to the authorities. You should become aware of your responsibilities, and you may decline to ask certain questions to avoid risking damage to your agency's relationship with immigrant communities.

Fleeing war or persecution, displaced persons are often faced with situations in which they have to find "the right" story so they can obtain safety. They may believe they need to present themselves in one way to obtain entrance into refugee camps, present another story to gain entrance into their new country, and frame their situation in a third way to be granted citizenship. Rumors abound in refugee camps about what is an "acceptable" story to the authorities, and families with legitimate claims to refugee status sometimes distort their histories in response to these rumors. If their lies are discovered, the family is likely to face deportation, regardless of the true dangers they might face if deported.

As illustrated in the following example, getting basic demographic information from a refugee family or a family of recent immigrants may be especially difficult:

A Liberian father, Tamba, was tortured and threatened with death when civil war broke out in his country. He fled to the United States Embassy and was granted permission to travel to the United States with his family. Tamba brought his wife and their two children, and also his sister and their two children, claiming the sister as the wife's mother, and the two children as their own. He needed to lie to save his extended family. In the chaos of the war, they were able to obtain new documents and arrived safely in the United States as refugees.

However, these are big secrets to keep. The children entered school, knowing they had a "grandma" who was really an aunt, sisters who were really cousins, and so on. Their birthdays also had been falsified to make it all work out. This family was called into the principal's office because the 8-year-old daughter, Bindu, was caught lying about her homework to her teacher. The family punished the girl for lying by placing a hot pepper on her tongue—they thought they were responding appropriately to what they interpreted as the school's request that they punish her. The child told a teacher about the punishment, and the teacher called in child protective services. The investigator working with the family had a hard time figuring out who was who and what really happened. The family lied about basic demographic facts like birthdays and relationships. The lies looked suspicious, and the family appeared fearful, but not because they were trying to hide child abuse. Rather:

- They feared deportation for having lied upon entry.
- They feared losing their lease because they had so many people living in one apartment.
- They were afraid the niece and nephew—who they had said were

their son and daughter—would lose health benefits because they would no longer qualify under the father's medical plan.

- They feared their children would be held back at school if their true ages were revealed.
- They were afraid of authorities because they had been severely mistreated by authorities in Liberia.

This was a loving, close-knit family, who needed education about child rearing norms in their new country, not punitive intervention.

Children from families of all kinds are raised to tell lies—to hide immigration status or an illegal activity, to keep secret a birthday surprise, or to get the kid's-price meal at a restaurant. While lying about the details of ages and relationships may concern us and complicate our job as interviewers, it should not be seen as an indication that the family is generally untrustworthy.

How should we handle concerns about truthfulness? It is important to gain the individual or family's trust, clarify our professional role, and let the family know who will have access to the information they provide. We should acknowledge that in the process of immigration many families have had to tell new stories about their life. We should ask for the truth about things that matter but avoid punishing or embarrassing family members who lie about unimportant or unrelated matters. So, for instance, an interviewer could say to a family:

"I'm having trouble understanding certain issues here. There may be things you are afraid to tell me, or don't want to talk about in front of the children. I don't need to know everything today. But I would like to meet alone with the parents now to help me understand those points that are important for me to gather today."

By speaking with the parents alone, without children present, we allow the parents to save face.

In English we say, "The truth will make you free." In Spanish there is a saying, *La verdad no mata, pero incomoda* (truth doesn't kill, but it makes us uncomfortable). In fact, truth can kill people living under repressive governments. Telling stories that are not entirely truthful may have enabled certain immigrants and refugees to survive—a reality that is alien to most people growing up in more secure environments. Lying for self-protection is a hard habit to break. To do our jobs we may need to seek the truth, but we should try to do this sensitively after establishing trust, and without humiliating the interviewees.

PROMPTNESS AND ALTERNATIVES

The more delayed you are, the better you arrive.
—KASHMIRI SAYING

In many cultures, people have a much more fluid sense of time than in the United States, Canada, and Northern Europe, where time is seen as something to save, avoid wasting, and use wisely. We divide time into millennia, centuries, decades, years, months, weeks, days, hours, minutes, and seconds. This has been described as a linear sense of time. People who live with a linear sense of time are apt to follow schedules, plan to do only one thing at a time, and will subordinate their interpersonal relationships to their schedule. This linear sense of time is so deeply embedded into interview situations that we barely notice it. Most of us schedule a given amount of time for an interview and call the interview to a close regardless of what is happening in that moment, to meet the dictates of our schedules.

In many parts of the world, however, and among many people from ethnic minority groups in Western industrialized nations, people see time as dynamic, circular, and flowing from the ancestors' past into the descendents' future. "Time never moves forward in a straight line; it lives in cycles and what begins must end" (Koul, 2002, p. 32).

People with a more fluid sense of time or people who are less familiar with the Western calendar may have difficulty answering concrete questions about dates of family events, the onset of problems or illnesses, and special events such as medication schedules or appointments. If you need precision in terms of dates or times it may be helpful to check documents, if they are available, or try to ask questions that establish the sequence in relation to events that you can date precisely. For instance, "Did you feel ill over the weekend, when the kids were home from school?" or "Did you have those fears before you moved to Greenfield?" or "Did he come to your door before or after dinner?" If you are including estimated dates or times in official records, you should probably note that these are estimates, so people will not be penalized if the approximate dates are given differently at a later interview.

If your clients come from a non-Western culture, you may discover that they arrive early or late for engagements, regardless of the appointed time. Waiting time varies across cultures. Usually, high-status people make lower-status people wait longer. People who are accustomed to waiting a long time for appointments may arrive late habitually because they assume that a "3 o'clock appointment" is apt to begin at 4:30. They mean no insult by arriving late and are not apt to apologize because they think this is what is expected of them. Some Latin Americans I have worked with were as apt to arrive early as late for appointments. For instance, if I said, "I'll see you at 6 next Wednesday," they might reply, "Great! I'll be over right after work," and might show up at 5:30. This points out the difference between my conception of time as something fixed and precisely measurable, to be noted exactly in an appointment book, as compared to their sense of time as something that flows through a series of events from past to future. They were apt to have remembered to come to the appointment "after work" rather than at a specific time and are unlikely to have noted the time in an appointment book. However, if it is important for an interviewee to arrive at an exact time, first you should make sure that the time works with his or her schedule and then explain why promptness is important.

When I was teaching a graduate seminar some years ago, a Nigerian student would arrive at class each week consistently 15 or 20 minutes after it had begun. After a number of sessions I finally asked him, privately, if something specific was interfering with his arriving at class on time. He replied, "Oh, would you like me to be here from the beginning? Does class really start at 4 o'clock?" He was never late again. Clear communication about expectations is crucial.

Different cultures measure time in different ways, as well. In Somalia, when the sun rises is considered 1 o'clock. So for Somalis, 2 in the morning might be the equivalent of 8 in the morning in many Western industrialized nations. This could create confusion in an interview.

It is crucial that we not overrely on cultural explanations of tardiness, however. Sometimes people are late for very practical reasons, for instance because they cannot afford the transportation or child care that would enable them to attend appointments punctually. Sometimes they are delayed by their work schedules or the responsibilities of caring for family members, neighbors, or farm animals. It is easy to grow frustrated with people who arrive at scheduled meetings late—sometimes hours late. It is important to explore this issue with the interviewees rather than simply threatening them with, "If you're late for your next appointment, I will have to tell your social worker (or probation officer) that you are not cooperating." We must work with interviewees to resolve these very real problems. Perhaps we can meet the person in a more convenient location or at a more convenient time. Perhaps we can supply them with transportation or travel vouchers. Maybe we can offer them child care during the interview, or offer a stipend for someone to care for the child at home.

ASKING PEOPLE DIRECTLY ABOUT
THEIR BACKGROUNDS

It can be tricky to ask directly about people's race, ethnicity, religion, sexual orientation, or other membership groups. In some contexts, indeed, such as certain employment contexts, these kinds of questions may be illegal. In other contexts the answers to these questions may be optional, while in still others, people may have to fit certain criteria in order to obtain benefits, and so the answers to these questions are crucial. Try to determine which of these categories your interviews fit into when you consider inquiring about identity group memberships.

In some cases, a general question, such as "Tell me a little about your background," will yield the desired answer. In others, you will want to read a list of options and say, "Please tell me which of the following groups describes you best." Of course, many people feel that the standard categories of race, ethnicity, religion, sexual orientation, and even gender are inadequate to describe who they "really" are (see the section on notational bias in Chapter 10).

When deciding how to ask these kinds of questions, it can be helpful to think, first, about why the questions need to be asked. For instance, if you are asking about a person's ethnicity simply because it is a federal requirement to keep track of who falls into which categories, then it may make sense to read a list of options. If you were to ask a general question and people were to respond with a term that does not easily fall into a standard federal category, then you might be stumped as to how to record the answer. For instance, you could ask a woman how she defines her ethnicity and she might respond "I am a Caribbean tiger and I will do anything for my children." While that is certainly a revealing response, it might not help you decide which box to check on a federal form. On the other hand, if you are asking because you want to make sure you work with the person in a culturally competent way, then a question posed in a more general way, such as, "Please tell me what I need to know about you and your culture to work with you well," might be perfectly adequate.

Similarly, in medical interviews that include queries about sexuality, the pertinent question is not usually regarding people's sexual orientation per se (do they regard themselves as gay, straight, bisexual, etc.) as it is do they have sex with men, women, both, or neither? And perhaps you'll need to inquire about particular sex acts, avoiding assumptions. Many people who identify as straight have sexual liaisons with people of the same sex (see Chapter 10 on writing reports for more information on this area).

WHEN YOUR COMPETENCE OR APPROPRIATENESS IS QUESTIONED

Sometimes interviewees may reject us. At the first meeting they may look us up and down and simply say, "Uh hum. I'm not talking to you." Or they may fold their arms across their chest, sit back, and let us know through nonverbal behavior that they don't like or trust us and aren't afraid to make that clear. It can hurt our feelings to be viewed in this way, and it can be tempting to respond with hostility and defensiveness.

When an interviewee questions or rejects an interviewer because of his or her real or perceived gender, race, age, marital status, sexual orientation, family situation, ethnicity, religion, national origin, or other factors, the interviewer should try to remain calm and nondefensive. Accept, listen, and try to understand the nature of the objections. Your caring and careful attention alone may allay some of their concerns.

In some cases, perhaps a different interviewer should be summoned. This will depend partly on your agency policy, the circumstances of the interview, and the nature of the interviewee's objections. In other situations, after addressing specific concerns, the interviewee may be much relieved and able to proceed more comfortably. A non-Latino therapist who speaks fluent Spanish and works a lot with Puerto Ricans told me that she is frequently challenged by clients at the beginning of their work together. They express their disappointment at not having been assigned a Latino professional. She acknowledges their objections and tells them that this is a common concern for many of her Puerto Rican clients in the beginning. She suggests that they continue with the first session to test the waters and if after one half hour they still believe they'd be better off with a different kind of person, she would be happy to refer them to a Latino colleague. She says that this first session is usually sufficient to convince her clients that she cares for them, understands them, and is the right therapist for them. The fact that she is fluent in Spanish and intimately familiar with Puerto Rican culture improves her credibility. In the rare instances when they continue to state a preference for a Latino therapist, she facilitates this referral.

People from many countries will suspect that young-looking women have low status and assume that older men have more status. If they are being interviewed by a young woman, they may see this as signaling that their situation is of little importance. The interviewer whose status or abilities are being questioned should nondefensively describe her qualifications, her training, her licenses or certifications if she has them, and her experience. Sometimes a sense of humor can help, as in saying, "I've been told I look too young to be a doctor, but I'm working on the gray hair!"

To use another example, if a client asks you outright if you have children and you answer that you don't, they may assume that you are therefore incapable of assisting them with problems related to their children. It can be helpful to address this issue head on. "You asked me if I have children. Are you afraid I won't be able to understand your situation if I don't?" And then, perhaps, "While I'm not a mother/father [yet], I have worked with dozens of children your daughter's age, and so I have a sense of what children are like at that age, what some of the common issues are, and how to handle them."

Sometimes interviewees who have been through traumas or who are in the throes of an addiction ask potential helpers, "Have you ever . . . " questions, such as, "Have you ever had your best buddy blown up right next to you?" or "Have you ever been starving?" or "Have you ever been raped by your father?" While these questions may have a note of challenge in them, they are also an expression of hopelessness and skepticism about being helped. The interviewee may be trying to keep you at arm's length, hide shame with a patina of bravado, or convey the profound depths of the suffering and isolation caused by the trauma. A psychiatrist whose patients have included Holocaust survivors says he responds to patients who have lived through trauma with a comment such as, "Please tell me what happened, how you reacted to it then and how it lives in you now" (Walter Reich, cited in Satel, 2007). Through the invitation to make the traumatic experience clear and complete for the therapist, the patient steps out of his or her private world and is able to integrate the traumatic experience rather than being overwhelmed by it.

There are times when interviewers may need to ask interviewees numerous and precise questions to understand their experience. At other times, interviewers would do well to seek the help of someone who is experienced with a particular culture or problem. For instance, an interviewer who is unfamiliar with refugee camps in a particular country may need information about them to understand an interviewee's experience. The same can be said for an interviewer who is unfamiliar with heroin addiction, international adoption, torture, or other issues. Okawa (2008) provides the example of a Cameroonian asylum seeker who says he was taken out of his jail cell for his "morning coffee" each day. Only people familiar with torture in this country would understand that this refers to a brutal morning beating. When there are significant gaps between your experiences and those of the interviewee, it is incumbent upon you to read about the interviewee's culture, consult with cultural experts or the interpreter, where appropriate, seek trainings, and ask experienced colleagues and the interviewee for guidance.

Sometimes interviewers from more privileged groups are told, essentially, that they cannot understand what it's like to be on the receiving end of a raw deal in society. If this happens to you, it can be helpful to admit that your position gives you a different perspective, that you are committed to understanding the interviewee's viewpoint, and that you recognize his or her distress. For instance, "You are right. I don't know what it's like to raise a Black boy in this country. That must be so difficult. I empathize one hundred percent with your situation and am determined to help you in any way I can. I will be listening carefully so I can learn from you." Importantly, in this segment the interviewer did not minimize or try to explain away the interviewee's concerns but, rather, acknowledged them and their importance, at the same time trying to build a strong working alliance.

It can also be helpful to emphasize that you are part of a team, and that although you might not possess one of the characteristics the interviewee would value (because you are not male, Latino, gay, a parent, or whatever), you have colleagues who are and with whom you discuss cases confidentially on a regular basis. If you are currently in training and don't possess the degree or title that would grant you credibility in the interviewee's eyes, it may be helpful to emphasize that you work closely with your supervisor who does have the desired credential, and perhaps even introduce your supervisor to the interviewee. In some situations it may be best just to help the interviewee work with a different professional, who better fits his or her desired profile. It may be that, at this particular moment in the client's life, the client would be better served by someone who shares his or her own ethnic or cultural background, or another desired characteristic.

I remember interviewing potential candidates for a psychotherapy group that a colleague and I were going to be facilitating for adult survivors of child sexual abuse. Many asked us if we ourselves had been victimized, as a way of establishing our credibility. We replied with a statement on the order of: "I have not been through the same incident you went through, but I have been through experiences that have helped me understand your situation." This felt like the right amount of self-disclosure to use in that setting. (See the section of Chapter 3 on self-disclosure.)

You may want to reflect on why the interviewee chose to question your competence at this particular point. Did his or her expression of lack of confidence follow a particular line of questioning or something you did or said? Have you unintentionally conveyed disrespect or bias in some way? Acknowledging our errors is a powerful way to avoid repeating them. And it's a good way to improve rapport.

CROSSING THE CLASS DIVIDE

Most social scientists agree that the concept "social class" refers to opportunities, social capital, and material wealth. But they disagree as to how to measure social class, precisely how its influence is felt, and which variables might mediate its impact. In most studies social class is determined through questions about income, education, or occupational status. These questions are asked in a variety of ways in different studies and may not be measuring the same constructs (Bradley & Corwyn, 2002).

In its various definitions, social class is correlated with numerous social conditions including health, educational achievement, and occupational aspirations (Liu, Soleck, Hopps, Dunston, & Pickett, 2004). However, people from the same social class background are far from homogeneous, and their worldviews often differ widely, depending on their national or regional background, religion, occupation, and ownership of property, among other factors.

Social class can affect the worldview, skills, attitude, knowledge, values, roles, experiences, opportunities and assumptions of both the interviewer and the interviewee. Many of us respond to subtle indicators of social class on a regular basis. We may believe we're able to distinguish between a person who is newly rich and a person who comes from old money, even if the two are dressed identically, for instance. We may have beliefs that people should behave in a way that conforms to their social class: People who are considered in some way "untrue" to their class might be denigrated and viewed as spending "beyond their means" or as "poseurs," "gold-diggers," "oikers," or "trust-fund hippies."

Social class differences between interviewers and interviewees can create enormous gaps in understanding and connection, particularly if the interviewers are unaware that they harbor feelings of social class prejudice (classism). Such social class prejudices could influence the way in which we conduct an interview, the empathy we exhibit, the amount of time we devote to the interview, the outcome we recommend, and the final report we write.

When indulged to extremes, social class prejudice can be manifested toward people of a lower social class through derogatory remarks or attitudes about "trailer trash," "hillbillies," "rednecks," "yokels," "low-lifes," or "homies." Less frequently, people feel prejudice toward those of a higher social class and refer to them or think of them as "boojies," "rich bastards," "preppies," "Cosby kids," "spoiled brats," or "daddy's little girl." These social class prejudices are often combined with racial prejudices and stereotypes, resulting in terms such as "White trash," "cracker," "wetback," "Jewish American Princess," and "porch monkey."

As professionals, we usually conduct interviews in a downward direction on the societal power hierarchy with people who are poorer, less educated, more discriminated against, and in a variety of ways less socially powerful than ourselves. Our questions often reveal class-based assumptions about education, access to therapy, medical treatment, transportation, housing conditions, afterschool care and activities, and leisure time. To build rapport, interviewers often ask children about their bedroom, movies, toys, or holiday activities, without considering that low-income children may not have or even share a bedroom, may not have ready access to movies and toys, and—in some cases—may not celebrate the holidays. I remember speaking with a little girl who had eaten Thanksgiving dinner in a church basement—an experience that shamed her deeply, and which she did not want to discuss. I had asked about her Thanksgiving holiday with the idea that this would be an easy conversation starter, but she reacted with painful distress.

We must examine ourselves to identify and root out our prejudices against people of different social classes, whatever they may be. (Regardless of our own personal background, if we are professionals we have risen into the middle class.) Many professionals hold prejudices about the motivations, preferred outcomes, or favored interventions for people from different social classes, and they maintain these prejudices despite research that contradicts them. For instance, many psychotherapists believe low-income people respond poorly to insight-oriented therapy and better to group or behavioral therapies. Research does not support this notion, and it may be that middle- and upper-middle-class psychotherapists are simply less comfortable with their lower-income clients and less able to connect with them in session, and therefore recommend these less intimate approaches (Smith, 2005).

Smith (2005) reminds us that while "poor people" need adequate shelter, medical care, personal safety, and access to income, they also benefit from the usual benefits offered by psychotherapists, such as an empathic ear and opportunities to reflect on their life. Smith described some of the feelings she faced when beginning to work in a low-income community. She felt underappreciated, as clients did not sign up readily for her services. She felt impotent when her conscientious interventions did not return her stressed-out clients to pleasant lives. And she felt saddened on a regular basis by the cruel poverty she witnessed. She suggests that many psychologists (and I believe people from other professions as well) turn away from low-income clients to avoid these feelings. It is worth considering whether these issues are relevant to each of us when we work with lower-income people. We need to understand how these concerns show up in our work and how we can overcome class prejudice in order to meet interviewees' needs.

When the interviewer and interviewee are from the same minority ethnic group, issues of social class may supersede ethnic issues. That is, a middle-class African American professional who has been trained in the values of the dominant culture may not be perceived by a Black client as being "one of us" at all. An African American professor of psycholinguistics and sociolinguistics, who originally came from a low-income family, writes of his early mistrust of African American professionals: "I developed an intense mistrust and dislike for professionals, especially 'boozje' [bourgeois] Blacks. . . . Because Black professionals were always 'talking proper' and seemingly 'puttin' on airs,' they appeared superficial, insincere, and phony" (Smith, 2002, p. 19). Thus, while an interviewer or an interviewer's supervisor may expect that there will be easy rapport between two people of the same race, minority ethnic group, or national origin, the interviewee may feel a great distance from the interviewer because of social class differences.

Sometimes, of course, interviewers will meet with people who are of a higher social class than they are. Prejudices against people of a higher social class can include the (mis)perception of snobbism and elitism, the derogation of people who do office work as "pencil pushers" (Liu et al., 2004), and the assumption that people of a higher social class are all debutantes, airheads, corrupt, undeserving, lazy, insensitive, or debauched.

Great wealth brings on its own forms of stress, including fears of intrusive paparazzi and kidnappings and reluctance to trust others because people frequently befriend the wealthy to obtain their influence. Women who have married into wealth based at least partially on their beauty may feel their status is tenuous, experiencing great pressure to maintain their youthful appearance and approaching this task as a full-time job. Interviewees from wealthier social classes may question the interviewer's political perspective and press for information about his or her credentials. They may assume they will be accorded total confidentiality, and they may become angry if they are told confidentiality cannot be assured. They may be quick to threaten to sue. Interviewers should not allow these tactics to interfere with performing their jobs conscientiously.

THE MULTIPLE MEANINGS OF "YES"

When people from the dominant cultures in the United States, Canada, and Northern Europe say "yes," they usually mean they have understood and agreed with, approved, or accepted the topic that is being discussed. "Yes" means "yes" in direct, low-context cultures. However, "yes" can have a variety of meanings for people who have a different native language, who are from cultures that favor indirect, high-context communication, and for people who are from cultures where saying "no" to an interviewer would be considered rude. These people may say "yes" in response to queries but mean something different from the usual meaning of "yes." Asians and Pacific Islanders can mean the following when they say "yes":

It can mean (1) "Yes, I heard what you said (but I may or may not agree with you)"; (2) "Yes, I understand what you said (but I may or may not do what I understand)"; (3) "Yes, I can see this is important for you (but I many not agree with you on this)" or (4) "Yes, I agree (and will do what you said)." (Shusta et al., 2005, p. 148)

When people respond to a suggestion or query with, "yes," we need to make sure that they understood what we were asking and that their assent is genuine, not simply a show of politeness. The more familiar we are with a cultural group the more easily we can understand the kind of subtle communication behind a "yes" that means "yes" and a "yes" that means something else.

With some Asian interviewees you may receive a response to a question or suggestion that feels evasive or noncommittal. Because you are in a position of authority, they may resist saying "no" or responding truthfully to a question where they feel the answer would offend or embarrass you. They may decline to correct your mistakes or dispute incorrect assumptions. This communication style can be challenging to professionals who are accustomed to more direct and frank ways of speaking and the "efficient" use of words. Because people raised in Asian cultures tend to be more sensitive to context and nonverbal communication, they often are able to interpret and follow up on more subtle signs of disagreement. Be sure not to respond with impatience to what you may sense are evasive answers by Asian interviewees. You may need to give them opportunities to express themselves in a more comfortable way.

MAGICAL THINKING

"Magical thinking" is a term used by social scientists to describe the nonlogical ways people try to make sense of, and influence, their environment (Carey, 2007). Examples from Western industrialized nations include looking for signs in the environment that can predict or influence the future (such as finding a penny and picking it up for good luck); engaging in rituals to ward off bad luck (e.g., knocking on wood); avoiding certain practices to avoid bad luck (such as not opening an umbrella indoors); avoiding speaking of certain things ("speak of the devil and he'll appear") or believing that one's unrelated actions can influence the future (e.g., not changing one's clothing while one's favorite sports team is on a winning streak).

The custom of "knocking on wood" or "touching wood" is widespread around the world, but its origins are uncertain. Jews will say, *Keynehore* (no evil eye) when they say something positive, to let the Almighty know they are not taking it for granted. Muslims and Jews agree that an ornament of a hand with a colored eye shields its wearers from the powers of the evil eye. Much magical thinking also surrounds the care of newborns. For example, traditional Somali mothers wear earrings made from string placed through a clove of garlic, and the newborn wears a bracelet made from string and an herb to ward off the evil eye.

Most people engage in some form of magical thinking, and although they may recognize it as illogical, they have an attitude of "better safe than sorry." To many people, their own forms of magical thinking feel intuitively right. But other people's less familiar forms seem peculiar, illogical, or superstitious. For instance, even though I know it is "just a superstition," I knock on wood when saying something good about my children. I might also add the Portuguese expression *Que o diabo seja ceigo, sordo e mudo* (Let the devil be deaf, blind, and dumb), or *Keynehore*. I engage in these illogical acts because I don't want to take any chances on a misfortune befalling my children. However, fears of black cats and the number 13, avoiding walking under ladders or on cracks in the sidewalk, and purposely throwing salt over the left shoulder to avoid bad luck feel like illogical superstitions to me.

In many cultures, people are hesitant to discuss good news or offer praise, for fear that it will tempt fate or attract the evil eye. Koul (2002) describes how these beliefs work in the Kashmir:

> We never announce good news because we are obsessed with the evil eye.
> . . . Whenever anyone asks us how we are doing we look as though we are
> recovering from something, no one wants to look prosperous or well. We
> are not comfortable with prosperity and well-being, having seen it at close
> quarters only for a short while. . . . Our history has been under the joint
> custody of oppressive rulers and an earthly trinity of earthquakes, famine,
> and floods. These are etched into our genes and we never forget, even at the
> best of times. (p. 18)

In many countries babies are considered particularly vulnerable to forces of evil, probably harkening back to a time when infant mortality rates were high enough so that infants were, indeed, vulnerable in their early months. Among Latinos from some countries, one must touch a baby when praising the baby—failing to touch the child in this way might attract the evil eye. In many countries babies are either not named or are given what is considered a false name until they reach a certain age. Lee (2005) describes how a Korean family failed to give a child "a milk-name, like Dog Shit, which would have hidden from the gods how very precious he was to them" (pp. 46–47).

There are an endless variety of other beliefs around the world that would fall under the category of "magical thinking." When interviewing someone who mentions beliefs that seem like illogical or superstitious magical thinking to you, it is important to maintain a respectful attitude and listen carefully for the significance of the event from that person's viewpoint. You may need to ask questions of a cultural informant so you can determine whether the belief is, indeed, cultural, or whether it is a product of a person's idiosyncratic or delusional thinking. Remember, one person's religion is another person's magical thinking. Substantial portions of the world's population believe that wine in certain circumstances is the blood of the son of God and wafers are his body (Catholics), or that one should not speak God's true name (Jews), or that kissing or touching the Black Stone during the pilgrimage to Mecca (the Haj) will wash away one's sins (Islam).

THE MEANING OF DREAMS

Cultures also commonly differ in their beliefs about the meaning and importance of dreams. This can lead to confusion or misdiagnosis during interviews. Some cultures believe dreams are messages from deceased ancestors; some believe they contain prophecies or advice that is relevant to the future; some Westerners believe they are expressions of internal psychological conflict. Westermeyer (1987, cited in Ridley, 2005) describes the ethnic Chinese refugee who was diagnosed by a U.S. clinician as suffering from psychotic depression because of the client's belief that her dead mother had traveled from the place of the dead to accompany her to the next world. Westermeyer reports that he and his colleagues reinterpreted this symptom "as a culturally consistent belief in a depressed woman who had recently begun to see her deceased mother in her dreams (a common harbinger of death in the dreams of some Asian patients)" (p. 58) rather than as a symptom of psychosis.

Okawa (2008) reports that African refugees and asylum seekers interpret dreams of a deceased relative as either a sign that the deceased person is trying to communicate with them or a portent of what lies ahead for the dreamer. If the person you are interviewing describes dreams to you, be sure to ask what dreams mean in general, and what this particular dream means, before offering your own interpretation or explanation.

CONCLUDING OBSERVATIONS

We should avoid making assumptions about people from a different cultural background because of preconceived notions or even ideas suggested in this book. With awareness and sensitivity, we need to ask people about their current and past experiences both here and—where relevant—in their original country. It is important to understand the interviewees' traditions and essential to learn about their experiences *from them*.

We are bound to make mistakes and our interviews will occasionally suffer from misunderstandings. As with so many skills, our cultural competence will improve with time, as long as we are sincerely dedicated to it.

Questions to Think about and Discuss

1. Discuss three reasons why people from non-Western industrialized nations may be late to interviews and how you can handle this.
2. Imagine you are at your workplace and you discover that an interviewee has provided you with a birthdate that doesn't match his or her records. What might this mean? How would you handle this situation?
3. Discuss a cultural misunderstanding that you faced in an interview. What happened and what would you do differently if faced with the same situation today?

RECOMMENDED ADDITIONAL READING

McGoldrick, M., Giordano, J., & Garcia-Preto, N. (2005). *Ethnicity and family therapy* (3rd ed.). New York: Guilford Press.

Shweder, R. A., Minow, M., & Markus, H. R. (Eds.). *Engaging cultural difference: The multicultural challenge in liberal democracies* (pp. 432–452). New York: Russell Sage.

Afterword
Your Self as a Resource

One of the most difficult tasks we face as
human beings is communicating meaning
across our individual differences, a task
confounded immeasurably when we attempt
to communicate across social lines, racial lines,
cultural lines, or lines of unequal power.
　　　　　　　　　　　　　—Lisa Delpit

I would like to offer my applause to you, the reader, for engaging in this important effort to improve the cultural competence of your interviews. Needless to say, no single book, training, or continuing education course can turn an interviewer into an immediate expert at working with diverse people. We've covered a lot of territory in this book. You might wonder how you can juggle all these guidelines while also trying to listen to the person you're interviewing.

Focus on improving one or two areas at a time. For instance, start by making sure that you ask open-ended questions and allow enough time for people to give full answers. Once you feel confident using those skills, you can focus on practicing others.

Cross-Cultural Interviewing Practices

Skilled cross-cultural interviewers:

- Recognize that it is counterproductive to treat all people exactly alike.
- Acknowledge with interviewees, where appropriate, that there is a difference of cultures.
- Encourage interviewees to express their worldview and define their own experience, thus avoiding stereotypes.
- Become knowledgeable, sensitive, and aware of clients in their cultural setting.
- Use only those assessment instruments that are culturally appropriate and valid.
- Assure that the interview situation minimizes the stress experienced by culturally diverse interviewees, thus improving their comfort, their performance, and the likelihood of their full cooperation.
- Design recommendations and treatment plans that help interviewees take full advantage of the services available.
- Consider cultural explanations of behavior as well as individual, familial, economic, and other situational explanations.
- Recognize that diversity exists not only among groups but also within all groups.
- Act as change agents within their own organizations to improve practices with clients from cultural minority groups.
- Take into account issues of language and bilingualism. Avoid disadvantaging interviewees by obligating them to use a language in which they are not fluent.
- Understand and acknowledge differences in social power, and avoid confusing these differences with culture, personality, or pathology.
- Convey humility.
- Recognize the limitations of their own expertise and enlist the help of culturally similar interviewers or guides, as appropriate.
- Engage in continual self-examination to avoid imposing their own values, perspectives, or prejudices on others.
- Avoid overly simplistic notions of dysfunction by understanding the interviewees' worldview and experiences.

(Some items adapted from De Souza, 1996).

Rest assured that most people will appreciate your efforts to make them feel comfortable during interviews, even if they don't seem to show gratitude. Above all, remember that the most vital element is you: your *self* as a human being and your focus, presence, and dedication. Interviewees sense a general attitude of openness, friendliness, and support. So if you bungle a greeting or confuse an issue, don't despair. You can recover. Just retain your humility and sense of humor. Be willing to admit mistakes, ask pardon, and invite your interviewees to teach you. Be patient with yourself and know that your cultural competence will improve with time, as long as you remain firm in your commitment.

THE LIMITS OF OUR KNOWLEDGE

Despite all the research that has been done on interviews, particularly forensic interviews, there is still a great deal we don't know for sure. For example:

- How do professionals who've been trained in cultural competence differ in their interviews from professionals who have not received such training?
- What are the outcomes in a variety of fields when the interviewers and interviewees come from different cultures, as compared with the outcome when they have been matched for culture?
- Are the standard questions we ask regarding suicidality, and the factors we consider predictive of risk, the right questions for people from a variety of cultural groups?
- How does the setting of an interview affect its content and its resulting report? For instance, will a woman who has been battered appear very different if she is interviewed in her home, at a courthouse where she is fighting for custody of her children, at her lawyer's office, at a mandated evaluation, or in a shelter where she is interviewed by an advocate? How does the setting in each of these cases affect the impression she gives, and even her performance on instruments that purport to measure stable attributes such as intelligence, mental health, or ability to parent?
- Which people in which circumstances are best interviewed in person, and which people are best interviewed using a remote technology such as a telephone, video, or computer?
- How do interviews with bilingual people differ when they are conducted through an interpreter, by a bilingual interviewer, or in the person's second language without assistance?

The answers to these questions, and many others regarding cross-cultural interviewing, remain uncertain.

CULTURAL COMPETENCE AND SOCIAL JUSTICE

Cultural competence can help us engage and communicate more effectively with culturally diverse clients. It can help us conduct more accurate assessments and produce more helpful recommendations. However, cultural competence alone is not a panacea for all the problems our interviewees face. It cannot improve the conditions in which many immigrant, poor, and ethnic minority families live, increase their access to employment and education, or correct for bias in official systems.

Indeed, a little cultural awareness can be dangerous if it is used to exoticize the values, practices, and beliefs of members of ethnic minority groups, while the interviewer fails to examine the values, practices, and beliefs of the mainstream culture. We must add to our commitment to cultural competence an equal commitment to social justice—to providing all people, regardless of their identity groups, with equal access to opportunities. We must also practice cultural humility, striving for habits of self-reflection and self-critique that safeguard us from imposing our values on others. We must establish respectful partnerships with leaders of various cultures. And we must remember that the responsibility for bridging cultural differences does not reside in the client but rather in the provider, who must make a special effort to develop attitudes, services, and policies that are appropriate for clients from a range of backgrounds.

STEPPING FORWARD TOWARD CULTURAL COMPETENCE

The road toward cultural competence has a beginning and middle, but does not end. As I become more culturally competent, I realize how much I still have left to learn.

I hope this book has helped you move further ahead on your own journey toward cultural competence, avoiding interviews that degenerate into resentments, misunderstandings, and inaccuracies. I hope it will help you produce interviews that are not only fair, accurate, and efficient but that are also a satisfying experience of human connection.

References

Ahluwalia, M. K. (2008). Multicultural issues in computer based assessment. In L. Suzuki & J. Ponterotto (Eds.), *Handbook of multicultural assessment: Clinical, psychological, and educational applications* (3rd ed., pp. 92–105). New York: Jossey-Bass.

Altarriba, J., & Morier, R. G. (2004). Bilingualism: Language, emotion and mental health. In T. Bhatia & W. C. Ritchie (Eds.), *The bilingual handbook* (pp. 250–280). Malden, MA: Blackwell Publishing.

Alvarez, J. (2004). *The woman I kept to myself.* Chapel Hill, NC: Algonquin Books.

American Professional Society on the Abuse of Children. (1995). *Guidelines for the use of anatomical dolls.* Available from *www.APSAC.org*

American Professional Society on the Abuse of Children. (2002). *Guidelines on investigative interviewing in cases of alleged child abuse.* Available from *www.APSAC.org*

American Psychiatric Association. (2000). *Diagnostic and statistical manual* (4th ed., text rev.). Washington, DC: Author.

American Psychological Association. (2001). *Publication manual of the American Psychological Association* (5th ed.). Washington, DC: Author.

Anthony, T., Cooper, C., & Mullen, B. (1992). Cross-racial facial identification: A social cognitive integration. *Personality and Social Psychology Bulletin, 18,* 296–301.

Axtell, R. E. (1998). *Gestures: The do's and taboos of body language around the world* (rev. and exp. ed.). New York: Wiley.

Azar, S. (2006, November 17). *A social information processing perspective on the role of race and ethnicity in making judgments about parenting in child maltreatment cases.* Conference on Race, Class, Culture and Crisis, St. Johns University Law School, Queens, New York.

Baetens-Beardsmore, H. (1986). *Bilingualism: Basic principles* (2nd ed.). San Diego, CA: College-Hill Press.

Baker, N. G. (1981). Social work through an interpreter. *Social Work, 26,* 391–397.

Ballenger, C. (1998). *Teaching other people's children.* New York: Teachers College Press.

Bartholomew, R. E. (1995). Culture-bound syndromes as fakery. *Skeptical Inquirer, 19*(6), 36–41.

Bauer, M. (1996). The narrative interview. *Papers in social research methods, 1.* London: London School of Economics.

Bereiter, J. (2007, May 1). Psychiatric evaluation of children and adolescents: It takes time. *Psychiatric Times, 24*(6).

Bhatia, T., & Ritchie, W. C. (Eds.). (2004). *The bilingual handbook.* Malden, MA: Blackwell.

Biggs, M. (2007). *Just the facts: Investigative report writing* (3rd ed.). Upper Saddle River, NJ: Pearson/Prentice Hall.

Bird, H., Canino, G., Rubio-Stipec, M., Gould, M., Ribera, J., Sessman, M., et al. (1988). Estimates of the prevalence of childhood maladjustment in a community survey in Puerto Rico. *Archives of General Psychiatry, 45,* 1120–1126.

Bowekaty, M. B., & Davis, D. S. (2003). Cultural issues in genetic research with American Indian and Alaskan native people. *Ethics and Human Research, 25,* 12–15.

Boyd-Franklin, N. (2003). *Black families in therapy: Understanding the African American experience.* (2nd ed.). New York: Guilford Press.

Boykin, A. W. (2001). The challenges of cultural socialization in the schooling of African American elementary school children: Exposing the hidden curriculum. In W. Watkins, J. Lewis, & V. Chou (Eds.), *Race and education: The roles of history and society in educating African American students* (pp. 190–199). Needham, MA: Allyn & Bacon.

Bradford, D. T., & Muñoz, A. (1993). Translation in bilingual psychotherapy. *Professional Psychology: Research and Practice, 24,* 52–61.

Bradley, R. H., & Corwyn, R. F. (2002). Socioeconomic status and child development. *Annual Review of Psychology, 53,* 371–399.

Bryant-Davis, T., & Ocampo, C. (2005). The trauma of racism: Implications for counseling, research, and education. *Counseling Psychologist, 33,* 574–578.

Burnard, P. (2004). Some problems in using ethnographic methods in nursing research: Commentary and examples from a Thai nursing study. *Diversity in Health and Social Care, 1*(7), 45–51.

Burgoon, J. K., Buller, D. B., & Woodall, W. G. (1995). *Nonverbal communications: The unspoken dialogue* (2nd ed.). New York: McGraw Hill.

Canino, I. A., & Spurlock, J. (2000). *Culturally diverse children and adolescents: Assessment, diagnosis, and treatment* (2nd ed.). New York: Guilford Press.

Caplan, P. J. (2004). Confusing terms and false dichotomies in learning disabilities. In P. J. Caplan & L. Cosgrove (Eds.), *Bias in psychiatric diagnosis* (pp. 109–113). New York: Jason Aronson.

Carey, B. (2006, November 11). What's wrong with a child? Psychiatrists often disagree. *New York Times.* Available at *www.nytimes.com/2006/11/11/health/psychology/11kids.html*

Carey, B. (2007, January 23). Do you believe in magic? *New York Times,* pp. F1, 6.

Centers for Disease Control and Prevention and Agency for Toxic Substance and Disease Registry. (1999). Employee scientific ethics training program (Not available to the public).

Chan, C. S. (1999). Culture, sexuality and shame: A Korean American woman's experience. In Y. M. Jenkins (Ed.), *Diversity in college settings: Directives for helping professionals* (pp. 77–85). New York: Routledge.

Chan, S., & Lee, E. (2004). Families with Asian roots. In E. W. Lynch & M. J. Hanson (Eds.), *Developing cross-cultural competence* (3rd ed., pp. 219–298). Baltimore: Brookes.

Charney, R. (2001). *Teaching children to care: Classroom management for ethical and academic growth, K–8*. Turners Falls, MA: Northeast Foundation for Children.

Chen, W. L., O'Connor, J. J., & Radin, E. L. (2003). A comparison of the gaits of Chinese and Caucasian women with particular reference to their heelstrike transients. *Clinical Biomechanics, 18,* 207–13.

Crago, M. B. (1992). Communicative interaction and second language acquisition: An Inuit example. *TESOL Quarterly, 26,* 487–505.

Davidson, B. (2000). The interpreter as institutional gatekeeper: The social–linguistic role of interpreters in Spanish–English medical discourse. *Journal of Sociolinguistics, 4*(3), 379–405.

Davis, S. L., & Bottoms, B. L. (2002). Effects of social support on children's eyewitness reports: A test of the underlying mechanism. *Law and Human Behavior, 26,* 185–215.

DelBello, M. P. (2002, March 1). Effects of ethnicity on psychiatric diagnosis: A developmental perspective. *Psychiatric Times, 19*(3).

Delgado, M., Jones, K., & Rohani, M. (2005). *Social work practice with refugee and immigrant youth in the United States.* New York: Pearson.

Delpit, L. (1995). *Other people's children: Cultural conflict in the classroom.* New York: New Press.

Delpit, L. (2002). No kinda sense. In L. Delpit & J. K. Dowdy (Eds.), *The skin that we speak* (pp. 31–48). New York: New Press.

Delpit, L., & Dowdy, J. K. (Eds.). (2002). *The skin that we speak.* New York: New Press.

De Souza, R. (1996, October). *Transcultural care in mental health.* Paper presented at the annual Australian and New Zealand Conference of Mental Health Nurses, Auckland, Aotearoa, New Zealand.

Dowdy, J. K. (2002). Ovuh dyuh. In L. Delpit & J.K. Dowdy (Eds.), *The skin that we speak* (pp. 3–13). New York: New Press.

Dunham, K., & Senn, C. Y. (2000). Minimizing negative experiences: Women's disclosure of partner abuse. *Journal of Interpersonal Violence, 15,* 251–261.

Dunkerly, G. K., & Dalenberg, C. J. (1999). Secret-keeping behaviors in black and white children as a function of interviewer race, racial identity, and risk for abuse. *Journal of Aggression, Maltreatment and Trauma, 2,* 13–35.

Dyregrov, A., Gupta, L., Gjestad, R., & Mokanoheli, E. (2000). Traumatic exposure and psychological reactions to genocide among Rwandan children. *Journal of Traumatic Stress, 13,* 3–21.

Ellsworth, P. C. (1994). Sense, culture and sensibility. In S. Kitayama & H. R. Markus

(Eds.), *Emotion and culture* (pp. 23–50). Washington, DC: American Psychological Association.

Ensler, E. (2001). *The vagina monologues.* New York: Virago Press.

Erickson, B. M. (2005). Scandinavian families: Plain and simple. In M. McGoldrick, J. Giordano, & N. Garcia-Preto (Eds.), *Ethnicity and family therapy* (3rd ed., pp. 641–653). New York: Guilford Press.

Erzinger, S. (1999). Communication between Spanish-speaking patients and their doctors in medical encounters. In G. X. Ma & G. Henderson (Eds.), *Rethinking ethnicity and health care: A sociocultural perspective* (pp. 122–140). Springfield, IL: Charles C. Thomas.

Faller, K. (Ed.). (2007). *Interviewing children about sexual abuse: Controversies and best practice.* New York: Oxford University Press.

Family Planning Advocates of New York State. (2006). *Promoting cultural competency among family planning providers: Lessons from the field.* New York: Planned Parenthood Federation of America.

Folman, R. D. (1998). "I was tooken": How children experience removal from their parents preliminary to placement into foster care. *Adoption Quarterly, 2,* 7–35.

Fontes, L. A. (1992, December). Considering culture and oppression in child sex abuse: Puerto Ricans in the United States. *Dissertation Abstracts International, 53*(6-A), 1797.

Fontes, L. A. (1995). *Sexual abuse in nine North American cultures: Treatment and prevention.* Newbury Park, CA: Sage.

Fontes, L. A. (1997). Conducting ethical cross cultural research on family violence. In G. K. Kantor & J. L. Jasinski (Eds.), *Out of the darkness: Contemporary perspectives on family violence* (pp. 296–312). Thousand Oaks, CA: Sage.

Fontes, L. A. (1998). Ethics in family violence research: Cross-cultural issues. *Family Relations, 47,* 53–61.

Fontes, L. A. (2002). Child discipline and physical abuse in immigrant Latino families: Reducing violence and misunderstanding. *Journal of Counseling and Development, 80,* 31–40.

Fontes, L. A. (2004). Ethics in violence against women research: The sensitive, the dangerous, and the overlooked. *Ethics and Behavior, 14,* 141–174.

Fontes, L. A. (2005a). *Child abuse and culture: Working with diverse families.* New York: Guilford Press.

Fontes, L. A. (2005b). Physical discipline and abuse. In *Child abuse and culture: Working with diverse families* (pp. 108–134). New York: Guilford Press.

Fontes, L. A. (2007). *Sin vergüenza:* Addressing shame with Latino victims of child sexual abuse and their families. *Journal of Child Sexual Abuse, 16,* 61–82.

Fontes, L. A., Cruz, M., & Tabachnick, J. (2001). Views of child sexual abuse in two cultural communities: An exploratory study with Latinos and African Americans. *Child Maltreatment, 6,* 103–117.

Franco, E. M. (2006). Intrafamilial childhood sexual abuse and a culture of silence: Experiences of adult Mexican survivors with disclosure. Unpublished master's thesis, Smith College School of Social Work, Northampton, Massachusetts.

Genzberger, C. A. (1994). *Japan business.* Petaluma, CA: World Trade Press.

Gilbert, J., & Langrod, J. (2001). Polish identity and substance abuse. In S. L. A. Straussner (Ed.), *Ethnocultural factors in substance abuse treatment* (pp. 234–249). New York: Guilford Press.

Giles, H., & Niedzielski, N. (1998). Italian is beautiful, German is ugly. In L. Bauer & P. Trudgill (Eds.), *Language myths* (pp. 85–93). New York: St. Martins Press.

Givens, D. (2005). *Love signals.* New York: St. Martins Press.

Givens, D. (2006). *The nonverbal dictionary of gestures, signs, and body language cues.* Available at *members.aol.com/nonverbal2/diction1.htm*

Goldin-Meadow, S. (2003). *Hearing gestures: How our hands help us think.* Cambridge, MA: Harvard University Press.

Gopaul-McNicol, S., & Thomas-Presswood, T. (1998). *Working with linguistically and culturally different children.* New York: Allyn & Bacon.

Greenfield, P. M. (1997). You can't take it with you: Why abilities assessments don't cross cultures. *American Psychologist, 52*(10), 1115–1124.

Greenwald, R. (2005). *Children and trauma.* Binghamton, NY: Haworth.

Grieger, I. (2008). A cultural assessment framework and interview protocol. In L. Suzuki & J. Ponterotto (Eds.), *Handbook of multicultural assessment: Clinical, psychological, and educational applications* (3rd ed., pp. 132–162). New York: Jossey-Bass.

Grossman, H. (1995). *Teaching in a diverse society.* Needham Heights, MA: Allyn & Bacon.

Gunaratnam, Y. (2003a). More than words: Dialogue across difference. In M. Sidell, L. Jones, J. Katz, A. Peberdy, & J. Douglas (Eds.), *Debates and dilemmas in promoting health: A reader* (2nd ed., pp. 112–121). Basingstoke, UK: Palgrave.

Gunaratnam, Y. (2003b). *Researching "race" and ethnicity.* Thousand Oaks, CA: Sage.

Hall, E. T. (1973). *The silent language.* New York: Anchor Books.

Harris-Hastick, E. F. (2001). Substance abuse issues among English-speaking Caribbean people of African ancestry. In S. L. A. Straussner (Ed.), *Ethnocultural factors in substance abuse treatment* (pp. 52–74). New York: Guilford Press.

Hashwani, S. S. (2005). Pakistanis. In J. G. Lipson & S. L. Dibble (Eds.), *Culture and clinical care* (pp. 360–374). San Francisco: UCSF Nursing Press.

Heredia, R. R., & Brown, J. M. (2004). Bilingual memory. In T. Bhatia & W. C. Ritchie (Eds.), *The bilingual handbook* (pp. 225–248). Malden, MA: Blackwell.

Heslin, R. (1974). *Steps toward a taxonomy of touching.* Paper presented at the meeting of the Midwestern Psychological Association, Chicago.

Hockenberry, M. J., Wilson, D., & Winkelstein, M. L. (2005). *Wong's essentials of pediatric nursing* (7th ed.). St. Louis, MO: Mosby.

Hoffman, E. (1989). *Lost in translation.* New York: Dutton.

Ide, K. (1995). Not telling stories: A Japanese way. *Family Journal, 3,* 259–264.

Im, E. (2005). Koreans. In J. G. Lipson & S. L. Dibble (Eds.), *Culture and clinical care* (pp. 317–329). San Francisco: UCSF Nursing Press.

Javed, N. S. (1995). Salience of loss and marginality: Life themes of "immigrant women of color" in Canada. In J. Adelman & G. Enguídanos (Eds.), *Racism in the lives of women* (pp. 13–22). New York: Harrington Park Press.

Javier, R. A. (1995). Vicissitudes of autobiographical memories in a bilingual analysis. *Psychoanalytic Psychology, 12,* 429–38.

Joe, J. R., & Malach, R. S. (2004). Families with American Indian roots. In E. W. Lynch & M. J. Hanson (Eds.), *Developing cross cultural competence* (pp. 109–134). Baltimore: Brookes.

Juarbe, T. C. (2005). Puerto Ricans. In J. G. Lipson & S. L. Dibble (Eds.), *Culture and clinical care* (pp. 389–403). San Francisco: UCSF Nursing Press.

Kim, B-L. C., & Ryu, E. (2005). Korean families. In M. McGoldrick, J. Giordano, & N. Garcia-Preto (Eds.), *Ethnicity and family therapy* (pp. 349–362). New York: Guilford Press.

Kim, H. S., & Markus, H. R. (2002). Freedom of speech and freedom of silence: An analysis of talking as cultural practice. In R. A. Shweder, M. Minow, & H. R. Markus (Eds.), *Engaging cultural difference: The multicultural challenge in liberal democracies* (pp. 432–452). New York: Russell Sage.

King, N. M., & Churchill, L. R. (2000). Ethical principles guiding research on child and adolescent subjects. *Journal of Interpersonal Violence, 15*, 710–720.

Kitayama, S., & Markus, H. R. (Eds.). (1994). *Emotion and culture.* Washington, DC: American Psychological Association.

Knapp, M. L., & Hall, J. A. (2005). *Nonverbal communication in human interaction* (6th ed.). Belmont, CA: Wadsworth.

Kolata, G. (2007, June 26). Study says chatty doctors forget patients. *New York Times.* Available at *www.nytimes.com/2007/06/26/health/26doctors.html*

Koul, S. (2002). *The tiger ladies: A memoir of Kashmir.* Boston: Beacon Press.

LaFromboise, T., Coleman, H. L. K., & Gerton, J. (1993). Psychological impact of biculturalism: Evidence and theory. *Psychological Bulletin, 114*, 395–412.

Lane, W. G., Rubin, D. M., Monteith, R., & Christian, C. W. (2002). Racial differences in the evaluation of pediatric fractures for physical abuse *Journal of the American Medical Association, 288*, 1603–1609.

Lee, E. (1997). *Working with Asian Americans: A guide for clinicians.* New York: Guilford Press.

Lee, M. M. (2005). *Somebody's daughter.* Boston: Beacon Press.

Lipson, J. G., & Askaryar, R. (2005). Afghans. In J. G. Lipson & S. L. Dibble (Eds.), *Culture and clinical care* (pp. 1–13). San Francisco: UCSF Nursing Press.

Lipson, J. G. (1994). Ethical issues in ethnography. In J. M. Morse (Ed.), *Critical issues in qualitative research methods* (pp. 333–345). Newbury Park, CA: Sage.

Lipson, J. G., & Dibble, S. L. (2005). *Culture and clinical care.* San Francisco: UCSF Nursing Press.

Liu, W. M., Soleck, G., Hopps, J., Dunston, K., & Pickett, T. (2004). A new framework to understand social class in counseling: The social class worldview model and modern classism theory. *Journal of Multicultural Counseling and Development, 32*, 95–122.

Lombardi, F. (2000, June 24). Most Hispanics fear cops: Poll finds concern about NYPD brutality and bigotry. *New York Daily News,* p. 8.

Lynch, E. W., & Hanson, M. J. (Eds.). (2004). *Developing cross-cultural competence* (3rd ed.). Baltimore: Brookes.

Maiter, S., & George, U. (2003). Understanding context and culture in the parenting approaches of immigrant South Asian mothers. *Affilia, 18*, 411–428.

McGoldrick, M., Giordano, J., & Garcia-Preto, N. (Eds.). (2005). *Ethnicity and family therapy* (3rd ed.). New York: Guilford Press.

Meleis, A. I. (2005). Arabs. In J. G. Lipson & S. L. Dibble (Eds.), *Culture and clinical care* (pp. 42–57). San Francisco: UCSF Nursing Press.

Miller, J. G. (1984). Culture and the development of everyday social explanation. *Journal of Personality and Social Psychology, 46*, 961–978.

Mirsky, L. (2007). Restorative Justice Practices of Native American, First Nation and Other Indigenous People of North America: Part Two. Accessed online on July 8, 2007 at *www.realjustice.org/library/natjust2.html*

Morris, D. (1994). *The human animal*. New York: Crown.

Morrison, J., & Anders, T. F. (1999). *Interviewing children and adolescents: Skills and strategies for effective DSM-IV diagnosis*. New York: Guilford Press.

Nieto, S., & Bode, P. (2007). *Affirming diversity: The sociopolitical context of multicultural education* (5th ed.). New York: Allyn & Bacon.

Novak, T. T. (2005). Vietnamese. In J. G. Lipson & S. L. Dibble (Eds.), *Culture and clinical care* (pp. 446–460). San Francisco: UCSF Nursing Press.

O'Dwyer, P. (2001). The Irish and substance abuse. In S. L. A. Straussner (Ed.), *Ethnocultural factors in substance abuse treatment* (pp. 199–215). New York: Guilford Press.

Ogbu, M. A. (2005). Nigerians. In J. G. Lipson & S. L. Dibble (Eds.), *Culture and clinical care* (pp. 343–359). San Francisco: UCSF Nursing Press.

Okawa, J. (2008). Considerations for the cross-cultural evaluation of refugees and asylum seekers. In L. A. Suzuki & J. G. Ponterotto (Eds.), *Handbook of multicultural assessment: Clinical, psychological, and educational applications* (3rd ed., pp. 165–194). New York: Jossey-Bass.

Orbach, Y., & Lamb, M. E. (2000). Enhancing children's narratives in investigative interviews. *Child Abuse and Neglect, 24*, 1631–1648.

Orfield, G., & Lee, C. (2006). *Racial transformation and the changing nature of segregation*. Cambridge, MA: Civil Rights Project at Harvard University.

Parron, D. L. (1997). The fusion of cultural horizons: Cultural influences on the assessment of psychopathology in children. *Applied Developmental Science, 1*, 156–159.

Perez Foster, R. (1999). *The Power of language in the clinical process: Assessing and treating the bilingual person*. New York: Jason Aronson.

Pezdek, K., & Taylor, J. (2002). Memory for traumatic events in children and adults. In M. Eisen, J. Quas, & G. Goodman (Eds.), *Memory and suggestibility in the forensic interview* (pp. 165–184). Mahwah, NJ: Erlbaum.

Piller, I., & Pavlenko, A. (2004). Bilingualism and gender. In T. K. Bhatia & W. C. Ritchie (Eds.), *The handbook of bilingualism* (pp. 489–511). Malden, MA: Blackwell.

Pitchforth, E., & van Teijlingen, E. (2005). International public health research involving interpreters: A case study from Bangladesh. *BMC Public Health, 25*. Available online.

Ponterotto, J. G., Casas, J. M., Suzuki, L. A., & Alexander, C. M. (Eds.). (2001). *Handbook of multicultural counseling*. Thousand Oaks, CA: Sage.

Portes, A., & Rombaut, R. G. (2001). *Legacies: The story of the immigrant second generation*. Los Angeles: University of California Press.

Potter, C. (2002). Improving prospects. *Pittsburgh City Paper*. Accessed on line (n.d.).

Presser, H. B. (1980). Puerto Rico: Recent trends in fertility and sterilization. *Family Planning Perspective, 12*(2), 102–106.

Purcell-Gates, V. (2002). ". . . . As soon as she opened her mouth!": Issues on language, literacy, and power. In L. Delpit & J. K. Dowdy (Eds.), *The skin that we speak* (pp. 121–141). New York: New Press.

Pynoos, R. S., Steinberg, A. M., & Goenjian, A. (1996). Traumatic stress in childhood and adolescence: Recent developments and current controversies. In B. A. van der Kolk, A. C. McFarlane, & L. Weisaeth (Eds.), *Traumatic stress* (pp. 331–358). New York: Guilford Press.

Richie, B. (1996). *Compelled to crime: The gender entrapment of battered black women.* New York: Routledge.

Ridley, C. R. (2005). *Overcoming unintentional racism in counseling and therapy* (2nd ed.). Thousand Oaks, CA: Sage.

Ritchie, W. C., & Bhatia, T. (2004). Social and psychological factors in language mixing. In T. Bhatia & W. C. Ritchie (Eds.), *The bilingual handbook* (p. 336–352). Malden, MA: Blackwell.

Roach, P. (1998). Some languages are spoken more quickly than others. In L. Baeur & P. Trudgill (Eds.), *Language myths* (pp. 150–158). New York: St. Martins Press.

Roberts, D. (2002). *Shattered bonds: The color of child welfare.* New York: Basic Books.

Rogoff, B. (2003). *The cultural nature of human development.* New York: Oxford University Press.

Samuels, S., Gonzalez, J., & Lockett, P. (2006). Do you have to speak English to raise your own child? Paper presented at the meeting of the American Professional Society on the Abuse of Children, Nashville, TN.

Santiago-Rivera, A. L., & Altarriba, J. (2002). The role of language in therapy with the Spanish-English bilingual client. *Professional Psychology: Research and Practice, 33,* 30–38.

Santos, R. M., & Chan, S. (2004). Families with Pilipino roots. In E. W. Lynch & M. J. Hanson (Eds.), *Developing cross-cultural competence* (3rd ed., pp. 299–344). Baltimore: Brookes.

Sapphire. (1996). *Push.* New York: Random House.

Satel, S. (2007, June 12). "Been there?" Sometimes that isn't the point. *New York Times.* Available at *www.nytimes.com/2007/06/12/health/psychology/12essa.html*

Sattler, J. M. (1998). *Clinical and forensic interviewing in children and families.* San Diego: Author.

Saywitz, K. J., Goodman, G. S., & Lyon, T. D. (2002). Interviewing children in and out of court: Current research and practice implications. In J.E. B. Myers, L. Berliner, J. Briere, C. T. Hendrix, C. Jenny, & T. A. Reid (Eds.), *The APSAC handbook* (pp. 349–377). Newbury Park, CA: Sage.

Schrauf, R. W. (2003, September 3). A protocol analysis of retrieval in bilingual autobiographic memory. *International Journal of Bilingualism, 7,* 235–256.

Sharifzadeh, V. S. (2004). Families with Middle Eastern roots. In E. W. Lynch & M. J. Hanson (Eds.), *Developing cross-cultural competence* (3rd ed., pp. 473–414). Baltimore: Brookes.

Shibusawa, T. (2005). Japanese families. In M. McGoldrick, J. Giordano, & N. Garcia-Preto (Eds.), *Ethnicity & family therapy* (3rd ed., pp. 339–348). New York: Guilford Press.

Shusta, R. M., Levine, D. R., Wong, H. Z., & Harris, P. R. (2005). *Multicultural law enforcement* (3rd ed.). Upper Saddle River, NJ: Pearson/Prentice Hall.

Smith, E. (2002). Ebonics: A case history. In L. Delpit & J. K. Dowdy (Eds.), *The skin that we speak* (pp. 15–30). New York: New Press.

Smith, L. (2005). Psychotherapy, classism and the poor: Conspicuous by their absence. *American Psychologist, 60*, 687–696.

Sommers-Flanagan, R. (2007). Ethical considerations in crisis and humanitarian interventions. *Ethics and Behavior, 17*, 187–202.

Sommers-Flanagan, J., & Sommers-Flanagan, R. (2003). *Clinical interviewing* (3rd ed.). New York: Wiley.

Springman, R. E., & Wherry, J. N. (2006). The effects of interviewer race and child race on sexual abuse disclosures in forensic interviews. *Journal of Child Sexual Abuse, 15*, 99–116.

Steele, L. C. (2007, January 23). *Native American children and the forensic interview.* Workshop delivered at the 21st annual conference on Child Maltreatment, Chadwick Center, San Diego, CA.

Stern, P., & Meyers, J. E. B. (2002). Expert testimony. In J. E. B. Myers, L. Berliner, J. Briere, C. T. Hendrix, C. Jenny, & T. A. Reid (Eds.), *The APSAC handbook* (2nd ed., pp. 379–402). Newbury Park, CA: Sage.

St. Hill, P. F. (2005). West Indians/Caribbeans. In J. G. Lipson & S. L. Dibble (Eds.), *Culture and clinical care* (pp. 461–473). San Francisco: UCSF Nursing Press.

Sternberg, R. J., & Grigorenko, E. L. (2008). Ability testing across cultures. In L. Suzuki & J. Ponterotto (Eds.), *Handbook of multicultural assessment: Clinical, psychological, and educational applications* (3rd ed., pp. 449–469). New York: Jossey-Bass.

Stokes, E. (1992). Maori research and development. In M. K. Hohepa & G. H. Smith (Eds.), *The issue of research and Maori* (Monograph No. 9). Auckland, New Zealand: University of Auckland Research Unit for Maori Education.

Straussner, S. L. A. (Ed.). (2001). *Ethnocultural factors in substance abuse treatment.* New York: Guilford Press.

Sue, S., & Sue, D. (2007). *Counseling the culturally diverse* (5th ed.). New York: Wiley.

Sue, S., Fujino, D. C., Hu, L., Takeuchi, D. J., & Zane, N. W. S. (1991). Community mental health services for ethnic minority groups: A test of cultural responsiveness hypothesis. *Journal of Consulting and Clinical Psychology, 59*(4), 533–540.

Suleiman, L. P. (2003). Beyond cultural competence: Language access and Latino civil rights. *Child Welfare, 84*, 185–200.

Sutherland, A. H. (2005). Roma (Gypsies). In J. G. Lipson & S. L. Dibble (Eds.), *Culture and clinical care* (pp. 404–414). San Francisco: UCSF Nursing Press.

Sutton, C. T., & Broken Nose, M. A. (2005). American Indian families: An overview. In M. McGoldrick, J. Giordano, & N. Garcia-Preto (Eds.), *Ethnicity & family therapy* (3rd ed., pp. 43–54). New York: Guilford Press.

Suzuki, L. A., & Ponterotto, J. G. (Eds.). (2008). *Handbook of multicultural assessment: Clinical, psychological, and educational applications* (3rd ed.). New York: Jossey-Bass.

Thomas, K. W., & Kilmann, R. H. (1974). *Thomas-Kilmann conflict mode instrument.* Tuxedo, NY: Xicom.

Tomm, K. (1988). Interventive interviewing: Part III. Intending to ask lineal, circular, strategic, or reflexive questions? *Family Process, 27*, 1–15.

Uba, L. (1994). *Asian Americans: Personality patterns, identity, and mental health.* New York: Guilford Press.

U.S. Department of Health and Human Services, Office of Minority Health. (2001,

March). *National standards for culturally and linguistically appropriate services in health care* [Final report]. Washington, DC: Author.

U.S. Department of Justice, Civil Rights Division. (2004, September 21). *Executive order 13166: Limited English Proficiency Resource Document: Tips and Tools from the field.* Washington, DC: Author.

Volpp, L. (2005). Feminism versus multiculturalism. In N. Sokoloff (Ed.), *Domestic violence at the margins* (pp. 39–49). NJ: Rutgers University Press.

Webb, N. B. (2001). *Culturally diverse parent–child and family relationships.* New York: Columbia University Press.

Webb, N. B. (Ed.). (2004). *Mass trauma and violence: Helping families and children cope.* New York: Guilford Press.

Wex, M. (2005). *Born to kvetch.* New York: St. Martin's Press.

Wierzbicka, A. (1994). Emotion, language and cultural scripts. In S. Kitayama & H. R. Markus (Eds.), *Emotion and culture* (pp. 133–196). Washington, DC: American Psychological Association.

Wilson, E. G. (2008). *Against happiness.* New York: Farrar, Straus and Giroux.

Wilson, L. C., & Williams, D. R. (1998). Issues in the quality of data on minority groups. In V. C. McLoyd & L. Steinberg (Eds.), *Studying minority adolescents* (pp. 237–250). Mahwah, NJ: Erlbaum.

Yoshihama, M. (2001). Immigrants-in-context framework: Understanding the interactive influence of socio-cultural contexts. *Evaluation and Program Planning, 24,* 307–318.

Yoshino, K. (2006). *Covering: The hidden assault on our civil rights.* New York: Random House.

Zachariah, R. (2005). East Indians. In J. G. Lipson & S. L. Dibble (Eds.), *Culture and clinical care* (pp. 146–162). San Francisco: UCSF Nursing Press.

Zuniga, M. E. (2004). Families with Latino roots. In E. W. Lynch & M. J. Hanson (Eds.), *Developing cross-cultural competence* (3rd ed., pp. 179–218). Baltimore: Brookes.

Index